ARISTOTLE

DE SENSU AND DE MEMORIA

ARISTOTLE

DE SENSU AND DE MEMORIA

TEXT AND TRANSLATION
WITH INTRODUCTION AND COMMENTARY

BY

G. R. T. ROSS, D.Phil. (Edin.)

CAMBRIDGE :
at the University Press
1906

CAMBRIDGE
UNIVERSITY PRESS

University Printing House, Cambridge CB2 8BS, United Kingdom

Published in the United States of America by Cambridge University Press, New York

Cambridge University Press is part of the University of Cambridge.

It furthers the University's mission by disseminating knowledge in the pursuit of education, learning and research at the highest international levels of excellence.

www.cambridge.org
Information on this title: www.cambridge.org/9781107418646

© Cambridge University Press 1906

First published 1906
First paperback edition 2014

A catalogue record for this publication is available from the British Library

ISBN 978-1-107-41864-6 Paperback

PREFACE.

IN the following pages I have attempted to give an adequate translation of the first two tractates belonging to the Parva Naturalia and I have appended a commentary which, I hope, will elucidate the many difficulties occurring in the interpretation of the text.

As regards the text I have been fortunate in having to my hand the admirable edition prepared for the Teubner series by the late W. Biehl. Before its appearance many of the difficulties seemed absolutely hopeless, but now there are but few passages where emendation seems to be desirable or, at least, where any alteration that can come nearer to the *ipsissima verba* of Aristotle may be successfully devised.

As my interest in preparing this edition was not mainly textual, I have refrained from discussing variant readings at great length unless they were of importance in determining the actual doctrine of the treatise. My purpose was to give a rendering of the Greek which should be accurate and should meet the needs of students of philosophy who, not being expressly classical scholars, have hitherto had no adequate means of becoming acquainted with these two important works. I have not prepared an apparatus criticus, but simply reproduce Biehl's text, indicating at the foot of the page little else than the alterations I have made. For full information as to the MS. sources of our text I refer to Biehl's introduction. Suffice it to say that the MSS. fall into two main classes, L S U and E M Y; the former, though often agreeing with the excerpts found in Alexander's commentary and drawn from a source of high antiquity, yet seem to be specimens of an 'improved' version in which the crabbedness of the original text has been smoothed down, though often with a loss of the significance which a more thorough-going interpretation might have found in the concise and often awkward phrasing of the authentic statements. The E M Y group (of which Paris E—10th century—is the most important), though full of misspellings and inaccuracies, seem to have suffered less from editorial tampering, and thus apparently give us hints as to the genuine reading; they are often supported by the ancient Latin translation of William de Moerbeka used by Thomas Aquinas. Unfortunately the commentators generally have followed the MSS. of the former group, especially Vatican L (14th century), and often expend great pains on explaining passages where their version is hopeless.

In my commentary I have tried not only to give such explanations of ordinary words and expressions as a student not yet versed in the Aristotelian philosophy will find useful, but to contribute an adequate elucidation of the undoubted difficulties which continually arise. In dealing with these I have derived much assistance from M. Rodier's monumental edition of the *De Anima*. Many of the ἀπορίαι in the *De Sensu* arise also in connection with the larger psychological treatise and, as a result of M. Rodier's labours, the path is now much clearer than formerly. Mr Beare's work on *Greek Theories of Elementary Cognition* came to hand just after I had finished the correction of the proofs of the present volume. Though I notice some points in which we are not in agreement, I see many more in which I should have been able to profit by his great learning if the result of his researches had been accessible at an earlier date.

It should be stated that the present work originally formed a thesis, for which the University of Edinburgh awarded me, in April, 1904, the degree of Doctor of Philosophy. Since that date it has been revised and slightly enlarged.

It remains for me to thank the Syndics of the Cambridge University Press for undertaking the publication of this volume, and to express my gratitude also to the Press Reader and Staff for their valuable assistance. I am much indebted also to Mr J. A. Smith, of Balliol College, Oxford, for many important criticisms and suggestions. Above all my thanks are due to Mr W. D. Ross, of Oriel College, Oxford, who has read the whole work both in proof and in manuscript and whose counsels and criticisms have guided me at every turn.

G. R. T. ROSS.

May, 1906.

NOTE. I should like to point out to readers that though I have used Bekker's paging for purposes of reference, it has been found necessary to take a larger number of lines than he requires for the printing of each of his columns. Hence there is a tendency towards a discrepancy (which increases as we approach the foot of the Bekker page) between the number of the line in which a word or passage stands in this edition and its line-number in Bekker's text.

G. R. T. R.

TABLE OF CONTENTS.

		PAGES
I.	INTRODUCTION	1—40
II.	TEXT AND TRANSLATION OF THE *DE SENSU* . .	41—99
III.	TEXT AND TRANSLATION OF THE *DE MEMORIA* .	100—119
IV.	COMMENTARY ON THE *DE SENSU*	121—243
V.	COMMENTARY ON THE *DE MEMORIA* . . .	244—286
VI.	APPENDICES	287—292
VII.	INDICES	293—303

INTRODUCTION

SECTION I. THE PARVA NATURALIA.

THE two treatises styled briefly the *De Sensu* and the *De Memoria* form the initial members of that collection of tractates on separate psychological topics known to the Latin commentators as the *Parva Naturalia*. The full list of these 'opuscules' is not found in *De Sensu*, ch. 1, but practically the whole of the topics to be discussed are there set forth. They are essays on psychological subjects of very various classes, and there is so much detail in the treatment that, if incorporated in the *De Anima*, they would have detracted considerably from the unity of the plan of that work. Consequent on the separateness of the subjects in the *Parva Naturalia*, the method of treatment is much more inductive than in the *De Anima*. There, on the whole, the author is working outwards from the general definition of soul to the various types and determinations of psychic existence, while here, not being hampered by a general plan which compels him to move continually from the universal to the particular, he takes up the different types of animate activity with an independence and objectivity which was impossible in his central work.

Some plan, of course, there must be in any coherent scientific exposition, and Aristotle seems to proceed from a discussion of those activities which are ἴδιαι to animals, *i.e.* belong to animals *quâ* animate, to those which are κοιναί, viz. affections which, though found in animals, are not

uniquely a feature of animate existence; to the former
category belong sensation and memory etc., to the latter
evidently such phenomena as νεότης καὶ γῆρας, ζωὴ καὶ
θάνατος. I have selected the first two treatises of the
former class, on Sense and on Memory, for translation and
comment. They have perhaps more importance for general
psychological doctrine than any of the others, and in them
certain metaphysical problems of unusual interest are raised.

Section II. The De Sensu.

The περὶ αἰσθήσεως καὶ αἰσθητῶν—Sense and its Objects,
is not merely a treatise on the subjects referred to in the title
but takes in also an account of the organs of sensation, not
an account of each organ in detail but of the general character
and ultimate constituents of the sensitive members. This
occurs in chapter 2, and thereafter the objects of the special
senses are discussed not merely as relative to sense but in
their own proper nature as modifications of external reality.
It is this which distinguishes the account of sense given here
from that in the *De Anima*; there the objective physical
nature of that which stimulates the sense organ is only
glanced at. The treatment of taste and odour is particularly
minute, and here we get involved in the details of the
Aristotelian physics which now-a-days seems so crude and
remote from our habits of thought. In fact, in the whole
of this treatise we seem to be immersed in detail, and there
is less of the wide generalisation and speculative insight
which characterise Aristotle's chief psychological work.

In the treatment of the special sense objects there are
notable omissions. Not a word is said about touch, while
the physical process involved in hearing has little more than
a reference made to it[1].

In chapters 6 and 7 Aristotle goes on to discuss
certain problems which have arisen in the course of the

---

[1] In ch. 6, 445 b 3 sqq.

discussion, problems lying at the root of all perceptive process. First, do the objects of perception have any part too minute to be perceived? Are there any imperceptible magnitudes? The answer is no; but this is not stated without an important reservation. Considered separately the minute parts of an object are only potentially perceptible, though taken in conjunction with the other parts that go to make up the total object, they do make an impression on the sense and hence are actually perceptible. The simple converse of this proposition is proved at the end of chapter 7. Every sensible object has magnitude; whatever has magnitude has parts and there is no atomic object of sensation. If you suppose an object to be so far removed as, while yet remaining visible, to be perfectly indivisible to the eye, it must occupy a mere point in space; any further removal from us would render it invisible, while any nearer approach would give it magnitude. It then occupies a point where the distance at which it is invisible and that at which it is visible meet; but, since a point is an absolute numerical identity and is without parts, the object occupying this point must be simultaneously visible and invisible—an absurd conclusion.

In the second part of chapter 6[1] Aristotle raises points about the process involved in the stimulation of sense by a distant object, deciding that in the case of sight it is instantaneous. In chapter 7, he inquires about the principle of coordination in sense perception. He decides that, except in the case of sensations which fuse, we cannot account for the simultaneous perception of two objects unless we assume that there is some unitary principle over and above the special senses which, though numerically a unit like a point, yet has a double aspect, like the point, which may be regarded as the terminus of each of the two lines which it separates; or again the unity of the central sensitive principle may be regarded on the analogy of that of the self-identical object which yet may have diverse attributes. This central sense is λόγῳ or

[1] 446 a 22 sqq.

τῷ εἶναι plural, though it is ἐν ἀριθμῷ. Its organ is localised in the heart, and to it other functions as well as those of coordination are ascribed[1].

Section III. The De Memoria.

The full title of this treatise is περὶ μνήμης καὶ ἀναμνήσεως (Memory and Recollection), and the two subjects occupy respectively the first and second of the two chapters which the book contains.

Memory (μνήμη) depends upon the retention of a sense stimulation after the object producing it has ceased to affect us. The stimulus appears to persist in the heart and is then known as an image (φάντασμα). Memory consists in regarding this φάντασμα as the image of the absent object and not merely as an object of consciousness that does not refer to a reality other than itself. The condition to be fulfilled, if the image of an object is to be regarded as objective, is the union with it of the image representing the time which has elapsed since the experience took place[2].

Memory may occur either through the persistence of the original sense stimulation or through its reinstatement by another process which has been originally experienced in connection with it. This latter process of reinstatement it is which Aristotle distinguishes by the term ἀνάμνησις. In its most typical meaning it is the purposive revival of a previous experience by a process of active search among the contents of mind, but apparently involuntary recollection is also grouped along with the voluntary[3]. In describing the process Aristotle formulates definitely for the first time the three well-known laws of the Association of Ideas, the laws of Similarity, Contiguity, and Contrast. With some subsidiary discussions, *e.g.* that which shows the dependence of

---

[1] *De Mem.* and Section IX. below.

[2] *De Mem.* ch. 2, 452 b 26 sqq.

[3] Cf. *De Mem.* ch. 2, 451 b 26.

memory and recollection on bodily processes, the treatise on memory closes. On the whole this treatise is on a higher level and contains more suggestive thoughts than the previous one.

SECTION IV. ARISTOTLE'S PHYSIOLOGY.

In order to understand the relation in Aristotle of the Physiology to the Psychology of sense and memory we must go back to the *De Anima* and seek the sources of our discussion there. The common terms for the phenomena belonging to both faculties alike are πάθος—modification, and κίνησις—change or process. But the question is, of what are they the changes or modifications? They are πάθη of the soul, but all the πάθη (with the exception of νοῦς[1]) are common to soul and body alike (*De An.* I. ch. I) and are as much affections of the body as of the soul. The true φυσικός—scientist—who studies the phenomena of life must not leave out of account the material embodiment of the psychic processes. Sight is, as it were, the soul of the eye but it cannot be studied apart from the eye; and this holds good of all psychical phenomena generally. At the same time Aristotle does not lose sight of the superiority of the mental aspect of the facts. The soul generally is an ἐνέργεια or ἐντελέχεια; that is to say, in manifesting soul the body realises its proper end and fulfils its proper function. ἐντελέχεια means perfection and properly (like ἐνέργεια) refers to something mental. Aristotle illustrates the relation of soul to body, by that existing between a manufactured article (an axe) and the idea realised in it. Here once more the ἐνέργεια or εἶδος is something mental (though of course the cases are different, as the εἶδος of an axe is not an immanent motive principle regulating the existence of the thing through a series of changes, as the soul of a man maintains his bodily life). Similarly an act of perception which is a πάθος—a passive affection, in so far as it involves

[1] *De An.* II. ch. I, 413 a 7.

a bodily affection, is, as an act of mind, an ἐνέργεια and not a mere πάθος or κίνησις[1]. Just as in the act of perception or knowledge the passive bodily determination serves as the instrument for the realisation of a mental act; so in the passive alteration which must be experienced in building up a state of knowledge there is involved a transition which is not ἀλλοίωσις—qualitative change, in the usual acceptation, but is the realisation of a determinate state of mind the existence of which alone makes the processes of transition intelligible. We may generalise then and say that only in so far as they are bodily affections are mental phenomena processes or passive modifications; mind as such is ἀπαθής; in thinking we are not passively affected[2].

This is especially true of the highest faculty of consciousness, νοῦς or νόησις, the apprehension of concepts, but the question need not be raised here whether in the human soul this impassivity or pure spontaneity of thought is anything that has a separate existence. Aristotle's answer in his special discussion of the subject in *De An.* III. ch. 5, leaves no room for doubt that in his view it is not so. The human νοῦς is παθητικός, *i.e.* it is merely the cognitive aspect of a process ultimately material.

Thus Aristotle's theory of the relation of mind and body may in a way be designated as a doctrine of psychophysical parallelism. But this should not blind us to the fact that with him the mental aspect of the process is no epiphenomenon. Mind occupies the higher place in the scale. It is the important member of the pair of correlatives, is the end for which the bodily changes exist and has all the dignity implied in the epithets ἐνέργεια, εἶδος and ἐντελέχεια. Having made this reservation we may be quite untroubled at finding in his account of sensation and memory what looks like the crudest materialism. Objects exist in the physical world external to and in relation with an organism; they, whether when in contact with it, or at a distance, act upon this

---

[1] *De An.* II. ch. 5 *passim.*
[2] Cf. *De An.* II. ch. 5, 417 b 8; cf. also I. ch. 3, 407 a 32.

organism and produce changes, whether mechanical (mere φορά), or qualitative (ἀλλοίωσις), in certain of its members. The reception of these changes in the sense organ *is* perception. But why should the mere production of a process in a bodily part be an apprehension of the object which causes it? We must remember what Aristotle says about sense being δεκτικὴ τοῦ εἴδους, and what he affirms about the sense holds equally of the sense organ. In fact, he frequently talks of a sense and its organ without discrimination of the two[1]. Evidently then what gets inside the organ must be the εἶδος of the external object. If we think of the εἶδος or knowable character of the object as existing independently in the external world, then the εἶδος which is present in the sensorium cannot be numerically the same; it will be only specifically identical with it or analogous to it. With regard to the subjective processes persistent in the central sensorium and representative of absent objects this seems to be the view held[2]. Again with sense a similar position seems at times to be taken up. The eye is transparent and receives the light which exists in the external medium[3], and similarly the movement of the air which sound is, is something ἀλλότριος[4], and merely sets in activity a corresponding movement in the air of the internal ear. But from another point of view it seems erroneous to talk of the εἶδος in the object and that in the organ as being numerically different. You may not talk of the same concept when realised in two distinct individuals as being numerically different; it is rather the individuals that are numerically distinct, while in concept, *i.e.* specifically, they are one. Thus it is in εἶδος that the object and the organ are one. The εἶδος of the object is its ἐνέργεια. Hence the ἐνέργεια of the object and that of the sense organ are one; it is only in respect of particular existence (τῷ εἶναι) that they can be regarded as distinct[5].

---

[1] *De Sens.* ch. 2, 438 a 13 note ; cf. *De An.* III. ch. 2.
[2] *De Mem.* ch. 2, 452 b 16 note.
[3] *De Sens.* ch. 2, 438 b 11.
[4] *De An.* II. ch. 8, 420 a 17.
[5] Cf. *De An.* III. ch. 2, 426 a 15 and 425 b 27.

A grave difficulty[1] arises here; the object as it is for knowledge will, on this showing, only exist in the act of perception; it will have merely potential existence before this. Such is the view taken in *De An.* III. ch. 2, and *Metaph.* IV. ch. 5, 1010 b 30 sqq.; but there Aristotle is quite sure that though the sense object as such only exists in perception yet its ὑποκείμενον (substrate) exists independently. There is, however, no way of characterising this substrate if all the qualities given in sensation are abstracted from it, and yet it is clear that, when Aristotle talks of the ὑποκείμενα of sense objects, he cannot mean the mere undifferentiated πρώτη ὕλη. He cannot, on the other hand, mean by them objects with geometrical and kinetic qualities only, the subterfuge by which atomistic physics avoids the difficulty of the independence of the external object; Aristotle did not believe in atoms. Accordingly we continually find expressions which imply that the ἐνέργεια or ἐντελέχεια already exists as realised in some way in the external object[2]. In truth, the fact that the external object is the agent in perception and transmits its character to the sense, shows that it must already possess that character[3]. It is from this point of view that Aristotle discusses the physiology of the sense organs.

It is obvious that, if the sensoria are to be capable of receiving the same εἶδος as that existing in the external object, they must consist of the same ὕλη; if, on the other hand, the subjective affection were merely an ἀνάλογον of the external as is suggested in *De Mem.* ch. 2, 452 b 17 it would hardly be necessary for the ὕλη to be identical. The latter, of course, is the modern conception. Molecular disturbances in the brain correspond one by one to different transferences of energy in the external world; every event in the universe can have an appropriate and more or less adequate symbolisation in the human brain. But one would

---

[1] Cf. below, Sec. X. of Introduction, for a further discussion of the objectivity of objects of sense.

[2] *e.g. De An.* II. ch. 5, 418 a 3.

[3] This is implied in *De An. loc. cit.* 417 a 6 sqq.

hardly say that the formula of the neural process (if it could be found) was the same as that which expressed the production of a red light or the flight of a projectile, nor would the oscillation of particles in the brain be in the least *like* those external phenomena. Aristotle, on the other hand, tried to think of the subjective κίνησις as occurring *in pari materia* with the external event, and probably where he refers to the subjective εἶδος as an ἀνάλογον of the external he does so because he is thinking of the processes in the central organ involved in memory; the heart, probably to be identified as the organ of memory, is not of the same character as the external transparent medium; but the eye, the organ of the special sense of sight, is[1].

Section V. Physiology of the Special Senses.

The qualitative identity of the organ with the vehicle or medium in which the objective sensuous quality is generated is most conspicuous in the case of sight and hearing. The συμφυὴς ἀήρ of the ear[2] and the transparent pupil accept, in the one case the impulsive movement set up in the external air, in the second the light which is the basal principle of all specific modifications of colour. The primary constituent of the visible εἶδος of things is light. Light is the activity of a transparent element which penetrates all bodies in differing degrees and, at the extremity of solid bodies, shows as colour. This colour is either positive or negative, black or white, and all other colours are mixtures of those two elements in different proportions[3]. The visible form of a thing is therefore the determinate mixture of these two constituents and, when we see, this (by a propagative process said to be not a transition in time[4]) gets, as it were, stamped upon the sense-organ[5]. We hear that it is the

[1] *De Sens.* ch. 2, 438 b 7 sqq.
[2] *De Sens.* ch. 2, 438 b 21; *De An.* II. ch. 8, 420 a 3.
[3] *De Sens.* ch. 3, 439 b 19 sqq. [4] Cf. *De Sens.* ch. 6, 446 b 31.
[5] *De An.* III. ch. 12, *sub fin.*, and *De Mem.* ch. 1, 450 a 33; also *De An.* II. ch. 12, 424 a 19.

colour which stimulates the medium[1] and consequently the
sense, and one would thus suspect that the colour was
something different from the process which it produces.
But that can hardly be so; the colour or modification of
light must be the visible form of the object, and it is that or
something qualitatively identical with it which enters the eye.
The process of transition in the medium which results in the
establishment of vision, or indeed of any of the mediated acts
of sense perception, seems to be conceived as consisting in a
pushing forward of this sensuous character until it actually
gets embedded in the percipient organ. In the case of
hearing this process is mere φορά—change in place, whereas
in smell it is a continuous qualitative change—ἀλλοίωσις, and
in sight something still higher, something not a transition
at all in the sense of occupying time[2]. There must be,
however, some object which originates the process, which
itself does not move. This is, we must suppose, the ὑποκείμενον of the sensuous character. It is, however, Aristotle's
practice to allude both to the object which causes sensation
and to its sensuous character, the sound or colour, by the single
word τὸ αἰσθητόν.

It had been the ambition of the earlier psychologists to
identify each sense organ with one of the four elements. On
the theory that like is perceived by like each organ will
perceive the qualities of that element with which its nature
is identical. Aristotle shows that, prior to perception, the
organ must be *unlike* the quality perceived. The sense organs
are not all composed of a single element. As we have seen
two are (the eye and the ear); but the organ of smell consists of both air and water, or perhaps one element in some
animals, the other in others, while πῦρ, if present anywhere,
enters into all and γῆ into that of touch[3]. But we do not by
any organ perceive the qualities actually possessed by the
substance composing it. The qualities possessed by any of
the elements are tactual, while those apprehended by the

---

[1] *De An.* II. ch. 7, 418 a 31.

[2] Cf. *De Sens.* ch. 6, 446 b 30 and also *De An.* III. ch. 12, 434 b 30 sqq.

[3] Here I follow the account in *De An.* III. ch. 1, 425 a 3 sqq.

senses of sight, hearing, and smell are not tactual. The organ fulfils its function in being the vehicle or neutral receptacle of qualities existing in a vehicle of the same nature outside it. In being neutral in this way the organ will be capable of receiving the opposite determinations which characterise the contents of each sense. In the case of the qualities apprehended by touch, the organs, being composed of the various elements, must show a μεσότης of the various tactual qualities; this must mean a combination in equal proportions of those qualities in order that something neutral and capable of registering the variations on this side and that of the mean point may be formed. This organ would naturally be the flesh, which is a composite formed from all the elements, and we should expect that its λόγος τῆς μίξεως was the μεσότης in question, but though at times this is his doctrine, in the *De Anima* Aristotle apparently will not have it so, probably, however, meaning only that the external surface of the body is not the sensorium but rather the medium which communicates tactual impressions, the real organ or ἔσχατον αἰσθητήριον being the heart. This, however, is after all a fleshly organ, and in fact, on the analogy of the senses of sight and hearing, the medium must be of the same nature as the receptive organ, for it has to be capable of transmitting the stimulus which ultimately reaches the organ and so causes perception[1]. Evidently he conceives of the exterior flesh of the body transmitting the tactual properties of things, heat, cold, hardness, softness, etc., by a progressive qualitative alteration like the propagation of odour in the air, or, in a way, of light in the transparent medium. Since in this case the organ and the medium alike are bodily members and they receive and transmit the differentiae of other elements than earth, they cannot consist of one element alone; they cannot be the hard

---

[1] For confirmation of this view cf. *De Part. Animal.* II. ch. 8, 653 b 24. Talking of the flesh he says: ταύτης (ἁφῆς) δ' αἰσθητήριον τὸ τοιοῦτον μόριόν ἐστιν, ἤτοι τὸ πρῶτον ὥσπερ ἡ κόρη τῆς ὄψεως, ἢ τὸ δι' οὗ συνειλημμένον, ὥσπερ ἂν εἴ τις προσλάβοι τῇ κόρῃ τὸ διαφανὲς πᾶν. The flesh functions both as organ and as medium, cf. Bäumker, *Des Aristoteles Lehre von den Aussern und Innern Sinnesvermögen*, pp. 55, 56.

parts of the body, *e.g.* bone, etc., which must be referred to earth[1], and hence there is nothing left for them to be but the flesh.

The eye consists of water; though air would have served, being also transparent, yet water is more easily retained in position[2]. The material out of which it is constructed is derived from the brain, which Aristotle describes as an organ with an excess of moisture[3]. The material of the organ of hearing is simply a συμφυὴς ἀήρ. The ultimate organ of touch seems, as we have seen, to be the heart, and consists of flesh, a compound of all the elements. Yet, though not consisting of γῆ alone, the flesh, as something σωματῶδες, *i.e.* solid, seems to contain a preponderance of γῆ, that element which is most characteristically a σῶμα[4]. This fact may lend some countenance to a statement made at the end of the second chapter of the *De Sensu*[5], according to which the organ of touch consists of earth. This assertion as it stands without qualification is in flat contradiction with the teaching in the *De Anima*, and it is noteworthy that it occurs in a passage where Aristotle is not stating his own final opinions, but is discussing in a tentative way some possible working interpretation of the theory which assigns a special element to each organ[6]. Aristotle there tries to combine with it his own theory that the organ is, before perception, only potentially of the nature of the determination which it perceives. But this will conflict with the doctrine that the organ of touch actually consists of γῆ; for, in order to perceive the qualities of γῆ, it will need to be only potentially of that nature, and is, in fact, Aristotle says, warm, being connected with the heart, the seat of the animal heat, and *quâ* hot it must have the character opposite to γῆ (which is cold).

---

[1] Cf. *De An.* III. ch. 13, 435 a 20 and *De Part. Animal.* II. ch. 1, 647 a 14.

[2] *De Sens.* ch. 2, 438 a 15.

[3] *De Sens.* ch. 2, 438 b 30, and *De Gener. Animal.* II. ch. 6, 744 a 5 sqq.

[4] Cf. *De Part. Animal.* II. ch. 1, 647 a 19 sqq. and ch. 8, 653 b 29, and cf. also notes to *De Sens.* ch. 5, 445 a 20 sqq.

[5] 438 b 32.

[6] Cf. *De Sens.* ch. 2, notes to 438 b 17 sqq., and Bäumker *op. cit.* pp. 47, 48.

Similarly the organ of smell will be only potentially warm, if the nature of odour lies in heat. This will accord with a derivation of the sensorium of smell, like that of vision, from the watery substance of the brain. But, though heat is required for the diffusion of the odorous principle, it is not that principle, and consequently the theory breaks down once more. His own doctrine, as we have seen, is that the organ consists both of air and of water or of either one or the other.

The organ of taste is the tongue, though, as in the sense of touch, there is a reference back to a still more primary organ—the heart[1]. Aristotle regards taste as a subvariety of touch, evidently on the ground both that contact with the object is necessary in each alike and that taste discriminates in an indirect way the tactual properties of things which go to make up their nature as the possible constituents of nutriment[2]. A certain independence, however, is allowed to the tongue, and, since tastes only exist in humid matter, the tongue must have a neutral humidity[3],—once more the doctrine that the sense organ shows a μεσότης of opposite determinations. In this case, however, the parallel to the other senses cannot be consistently worked out. The opposite determinations in taste are not excess and deficiency of ὑγρότης but rather τὸ γλυκύ and its negative τὸ πικρόν, which are ultimately reduced to τὸ κοῦφον and τὸ βαρύ respectively. Again, in the passage from *De An.* II. ch. 10 referred to above, Aristotle confuses two distinct conceptions; if the tongue is only potentially humid, as he says, it cannot be described as of a neutral humidity.

The above inconsistencies only show the enormous difficulty in giving any coherent account of the process of sense stimulation in terms of the ancient physics. They in no way detract from the value of the central principle involved—that the organ is of a nature capable of manifesting in itself the contrary determinations which characterise the objective qualities falling under any one specific sense; that apart

---

[1] Cf. *De Part. Animal.* II. ch. 10, 656 a 29 and *De Sens.* ch. 2, *loc. cit.*
[2] *De Sens.* ch. 4 *passim.*   [3] *De An.* II. ch. 10, 422 a 34 sqq.

from stimulation by an object the organ is perfectly neutral as regards these determinations, and hence may in certain cases (touch[1] at any rate) be regarded as a μεσότης, for the mean is neutral as regards opposite determinations and hence is κριτικόν.

Section VI.   The Physiology of the so-called Common Sense.

In addition to the special senses there is an unifying or central function of sense by means of which we perceive the κοινὰ αἰσθητά, *i.e.* the determinations of number, unity, figure, magnitude, and change involved in the apprehension of the special sensations of colour, sound, hardness, etc. Figure and magnitude are perceived at least by two senses, viz. sight and touch[2], and unity seems to be an idea involved in the functioning of each single sense alike[3]. Again, the comparison and discrimination of qualities belonging to different senses require a unifying principle in some way over and above the particular sense organs[4]. Indeed, the simultaneous discrimination of qualities given by the same sense seems to require the existence of such a principle[5]. Lastly, to this also is to be ascribed the self-consciousness that accompanies all perception, *e.g.* the perception that we see, hear, and feel, etc.[6]

This central function of sense[7] is localised in an internal

---

[1] The explicit references are only to touch (*De An.* II. ch. 11, 424 a 4, III. ch. 13, 435 a 21, *Meteor.* IV. ch. 4, 382 a 19) and the discrimination of pleasure and pain (*De An.* III. ch. 7, 431 a 11).

[2] Cf. *De Sens.* ch. 4, 442 b 8.

[3] Cf. *De An.* III. ch. 1, 425 a 20 and *De Sens.* ch. 7, 447 b 27. It is specific unity which is perceived by the functioning of a single sense.

[4] *De An.* III. ch. 2, 426 b 12 sqq.

[5] Cf. *De An. loc. cit. infra* and III. ch. 7, 431 a 17 sqq. ; also *De Sens.* ch. 7, 449 a 1 sqq. and notes.

[6] Cf. *De Somno,* ch. 2, 455 a 15 sqq. ; *De An.* III. ch. 2, 425 b 12 sqq.

[7] It is well to note that the mere fact of talking about ' *the* common sense' or ' *the* central sense' may give a wrong impression of the way in which Aristotle conceived this faculty to exist. Aristotle, in fact, does not talk except in one instance (*De Mem.* ch. 1, 450 a 12) of κοινὴ αἴσθησις but usually of τὰ κοινὰ

organ, and that is universally admitted to be the heart[1]. But great difficulties arise when we attempt to determine whether it is the heart as a whole which is the organ, or only some part of or constituent in it. Great uncertainty also surrounds the question as to how the central and the peripheral organs are connected, and similarly what is the exact relation between the inner faculty and the special senses. As to the physiology of the central organ there is but little said in the two treatises which we are discussing (the passages, *De Mem.* ch. 1, 450 b, and ch. 2, 453 a 16, do not help us much), while as to the connection between central and end organ there is not a word. Accordingly a full discussion of this subject belongs rather to a treatise dealing with the *De Somno, De Insomniis,* and *De Juvent., De Resp.,* etc. At present it will be sufficient to examine the main contentions of Neuhäuser[2] as to the subject in question in so far as they derive confirmation or the reverse from passages in our text.

Neuhäuser maintains (1) that, though many passages[3] would lead us to believe that the perception of the special sense qualities is localised in the end organs, this is not really so. The stimulation communicated from the external objects or the medium to the end organ is continued right up to the heart. Perception does not result unless the heart is in a

αἰσθητὰ and τὸ κοινὸν αἰσθητήριον. It is not a sense functioning in independence of the special senses, as any one of these may function in independence of the others ; as such it would require to have a special organ independent of the other sense-organs — a doctrine against which he argues in *De An.* III. ch. 1, 425 a 13–21. The common sense is, in fact, that common function which all the special senses possess, namely that of discrimination, which, as common to all, is contrasted with the special receptivity which each has for the separate kinds of objective quality, *e.g.* sound, colour, etc. It is this function of discrimination which requires the coordination of the stimuli received by the special sense organs in a central or common sensorium. Perhaps then, in strictness, we should talk not about a common sense but about the common discriminative function of sense. Cf. section X. below and Neuhäuser, *Aristoteles Lehre von den sinnlichen Erkennt-nissvermögen,* pp. 30 sqq.

[1] Cf. *De Juvent.* ch. 3, 469 a 10, ch. 4, 469 b 3. *De Gener. Animal.* II. ch. 6, 743 b 25, *De Part. Animal.* II. ch. 10, 656 b 24 etc.

[2] *Aristoteles Lehre von den sinnlichen Erkenntissvermögen und seinen Organen,* pp. 30–132.

[3] Cf. Bäumker, pp. 79, 80.

condition in which it can function[1], hence it is the presence of the κινήσεις in the central organ that constitutes perception. Secondly (2), the medium of communication between the peripheral and central organs consists of πόροι—canals (in the case of the three senses of sight, hearing, and smell), which are filled with a substance identical with that which composes the end organs themselves[2]. This he extracts from statements[3] (*a*) that these organs are in connection with the heart, (*b*) that πόροι from them extend into the veins of the brain, (*c*) that the organs of hearing and smell are themselves really πόροι full of air[4] (σύμφυτον πνεῦμα), and (*d*) that in the case of the eye its substance has issued through the πόροι from the brain[5]; finally (*e*), it is neither the blood nor any bloodless part which is the organ of sensation, but a structure created out of the blood. Thirdly (3), the central organ of sensation is not the heart itself, but a substance found in its middle chamber and designated by Aristotle[6] τὸ καλούμενον θερμόν and also πνεῦμα. We hear as well that this substance is analogous to the element found in the stars (ἀνάλογον οὖσα τῷ τῶν ἄστρων στοιχείῳ), yet it is not πῦρ, though we generally identify τὸ ἄνω σῶμα—the aether, with fire, and we hear elsewhere[7] that the ψυχή is ὥσπερ ἐμπεπυρευμένη—suffused with fire. The point is that this substance is different from the elements of the sublunary world and seems to serve as a basis or substratum for terrestrial conscious life, just as the upper aether serves as the substratum for the psychical existence of the heavenly bodies. It is frequently named τὸ φυσικὸν θερμόν, τὸ σύμφυτον θερμόν, and is to be identified with τὸ σύμφυτον πνεῦμα, of which we hear so much in the περὶ ζῴων κινήσεως[8].

    Neuhäuser seems to show pretty conclusively[9] that the

---

[1] *De Somno*, ch. 2, 455 a 33 and b 11.

[2] Neuhäuser, *op. cit.* pp. 123 sqq.

[3] Cf. *De Part. Animal.* II. ch. 10, 656 a 27 sqq., 656 b 16; *De Gen. Animal.* II. ch. 6, 743 b 32 sqq.

[4] Cf. *De Sens.* ch. 2, 438 b 21.   [5] *De Sens.* ch. 2, 438 b 29.

[6] In *De Gen. Animal.* II. ch. 3, 736 b 30 sqq.

[7] *De Juventut.* ch. 4, 469 b 6–17; *De Resp.* ch. 8, 474 b 12, ch. 16, 478 a 29.

[8] Cf. Neuhäuser, *op. cit.* pp. 94, 95.

[9] pp. 104, 105 and p. 85.

heart is properly characterised as the place in which the central organ or faculty of perception is situated, not as the organ itself (except surely in the case of the sense of touch[1]); again, if the organ of consciousness is not the heart as a whole but only some constituent in it, the seat of this organ is probably the middle chamber[2] of the heart.

Now these contentions may all be just, but the question arises whether this element· or anything of the nature of a substance will serve as a counterpart of that principle of unity which, according to Aristotle, the common sense must be. This σύμφυτον θερμὸν or σύμφυτον πνεῦμα must be a substance and hence quantitative. Aristotle tells us that the primary organ of sensation or that which perceives must be a magnitude[3]. It is the sense or its concept which is non-quantitative. Now in the *De Anima*, III. ch. 2, 427 a 1 sqq., he likens the principle of unity to something for which the only analogue is a point, the point which, while remaining indivisibly one, has yet a double reference as the end of the two segments respectively of a line which it divides. This is also the doctrine to be extracted from *De An.* III. ch. 7, 431 a 19 sqq. and *De Sens.* ch. 7, 448 b 19—449 a 22[4]. In the latter passage he takes up the supposition that different qualities could be simultaneously discriminated by an organ which, while not atomic, was yet atomic in the sense of being completely continuous. Such a description would fit, if not the heart, that supposed internal substance of celestial affinities which it contains[5]. The hypothesis is negated, and Aristotle passes on to the conclusion of the *De Anima*—that that which accounts for the holding of different sensations in unity must be actually a perfect unity, though in aspect diverse. It is true that he also compares the unity of this psychic principle

---

[1] In the passage in *De Part. Animal.* II. ch. 1, 647 a 28, where he talks of a μόριον (evidently the heart) being capable of receiving all sense-qualities he is probably referring to tactual αἰσθητά.

[2] Neuhäuser, *op. cit.* p. 86.

[3] *De An.* II. ch. 12, 424 a 17 sqq.

[4] Cf. notes ch. 7, below *loc. cit.*

[5] The heat in the heart is καθαρωτάτη; *De Gen. Animal.* II. ch. 6, 744 a 29.

to the unity of an object with diverse qualities[1]. But, as we shall see, this involves no difference of theory; the ascription of two attributes to one spatial thing involves a reference to an identity which is itself not spatial.

Hence we come to the conclusion that Aristotle in accounting for 'apperception' has to make reference to a unity that cannot be described as a material organ. It is true that in consonance with his general psycho-physical parallelism he should be forced to try to think of it as an organ, but it has that characteristic which nothing corporeal can possess; it is ἄτομόν τι[2]. Hence we cannot conceive both the soul and its immediate substrate (numerically the same as the central organ of sensation) as unity[3].

It is naturally just here that the parallelism of mind and body, αἴσθησις and αἰσθητήριον, should break down. It is just in coordinating and distinguishing the contributions of the senses that the ἐνέργεια of a typical act of mind comes in. It is as referred to a unity that sensations are anything for mind. Now *quâ* ἐνέργεια, *i.e. quâ* mental, a psychical phenomenon is nothing passive and nothing to be ascribed to body. Mind in its proper nature is ἀπαθής, and hence, if we were to ascribe the function of apperception of sensations to anything, it would need to be assigned to the νοῦς, which is ἀπαθής, and "comes in from outside[4]." The essence of my contention is, that it is impossible to ascribe to an organ that which, not being an instance of πάσχειν—passive alteration, it is the function of nothing corporeal to account for. Unless Aristotle were to maintain that the substrate of the soul, the σύμφυτον θερμόν or πνεῦμα, were not extended (which would be the same as making it immaterial) he could not attribute to it the unification of consciousness. As facts are, he says or implies in *De An.* II. ch. 12 *ad init.* that the organ is a μέγεθος.

At the same time this psychical substance may very well

---

[1] Both here and in *De An.*

[2] I note that Neuhäuser, p. 110, agrees with me in thinking that τῷ ἀτόμῳ καὶ ἐσχάτῳ, *De Mem.* ch. 2, 451 a 28, refers to the organ of sensation.

[3] Neuhäuser, p. 104.

[4] *De Gen. Animal.* II. ch. 3, 736 b 28 τὸν νοῦν μόνον θύραθεν ἐπεισιέναι.

be the organ which accounts for the *plurality* of impressions which are united in one act by the mind. It may be this which is the delicate structure capable of receiving and retaining the multitude of impressions which function in memory. In our treatise (the *De Memoria*) there is nothing which bears this out. We hear about processes in τὸ αἰσθη-τικόν being interfered with by the too great pressure of the parts above them[1], and of defects of memory being due to excessive fluidity or hardness of the receptive structure[2]. This last description would surely suit the heart as a whole better than the mysterious πνεῦμα which it contains. It really does not matter which was Aristotle's theory; anything extended will suffice, so far as space goes, for the reception of a plurality.

On the subject of the connection between central and end organ there are, in our treatises, no materials to enable us to come to a decision. We hear[3] of affections going on καὶ ἐν βάθει καὶ ἐπιπολῆς, i.e. both in the central and the end organ, and we hear that it is the κίνησις going on *in the eyes* which causes us to have light sensations still when we turn aside out of the sun into the dark. Of course it may still be the case that perception does not occur until the κίνησις reach the heart, but it is not necessary to believe that the medium of communication was, according to Aristotle, qualitatively the same as that of the end organ, and that the process transmitted to the heart was hence qualitatively the same as that realised in the end organ[4]. An impression in the central organ is known as a φάντασμα[5]; the question is whether an αἴσθημα is, as Neuhäuser maintains, numerically the same as and only in aspect different from a φάντασμα. Without committing ourselves to an answer it might be profitable to point out that a possible solution is that,

---

[1] *De Mem.* ch. 2, 453 b 1.   [2] Ch. 1, 450 b 1 sqq.
[3] *De Insom.* ch. 2, 459 b 7.
[4] Neuhäuser thinks that in maintaining this doctrine Aristotle anticipated the discovery of the nerves (due to Herophilus) or at least invented an analogue to them.
[5] Cf. *De Mem.* ch. 1, 450 a 11.

though consciousness cannot arise unless the central organ be stimulated, the stimulation reaching it might be only analogous[1] to and not identical with the modification of the peripheral organs.

SECTION VII. THE OBJECTS OF SPECIAL SENSATION.

(*a*) Colour. The ground-work of all colour phenomena is τὸ διαφανές, which is a κοινὴ φύσις, a common characteristic, of two of the four elements, namely air and water. We translate τὸ διαφανές as the transparent *medium*, but though it functions as a medium between the coloured object and the eye, it is not merely as a medium that Aristotle considers it. It is most frequently referred to simply as τὸ διαφανές without the further qualification that it is a medium. It is properly a vehicle or ground-work for the manifestation of colour. It penetrates all bodies to a greater or less degree[2] (doubtless Aristotle means all composite bodies, which contain air and water in some proportion), and it is in so far as they are thus permeated by it that they are capable of showing colour. The colour of a solid body is the limit, *i.e.* the surface, not of the body itself but of the διαφανές in it[3]. That is the colour seen, but the same nature extends right through the body. Similarly bodies that are not opaque but consist of a diaphanous substance altogether (αὐτῶν τῶν διαφανῶν)[4] show colour[5]. But that colour is light. This brings us to the consideration that it is not merely the existence of the transparent vehicle that causes colour or light phenomena to arise. In itself it is a mere δύναμις; it must be raised to the state of ἐνέργεια by the presence of fire in it[6]. Hence light is the 'colour' of the diaphanous quality in bodies and is due to some other determining cause (κατὰ συμβεβηκός); it is not anything self-existent. It is equally defined as the ἐνέργεια or ἐντελέχεια τοῦ διαφανοῦς.

---

[1] Cf. note to *De Mem.* ch. 2, 452 b 16, 17.
[2] *De Sens.* ch. 3, 439 b 9. [3] 439 a 34 sqq.
[4] 439 b 13. [5] 439 b 1. [6] 439 a 20 sqq.

The presence of fire causes the existence of actual light, the positive determination of the transparent medium, its absence that of darkness, the privation of light. These are the contrasted determinations for substances typically transparent: in definitely bounded (opaque) bodies, in which, it is implied, τὸ διαφανές does not exist in the same degree or purity, the contrasted determinations are black and white[1]. Thus far there is no particular difficulty in the Aristotelian conception; light and colour are determinations ultimately identical, of the type ἐνέργεια, affecting a material or vehicle which, apart from these determinations, is neutral to them. Light is to be perceived as an all-pervasive character of transparent substances equally and instantaneously present in every part. But when we come to consider the action of a coloured object upon the eye, and remember that it is said to affect the vision by means of a κίνησις through the medium[2], it seems natural to consider this κίνησις to be light. When, in *De Sensu,* chapter 6[3], Aristotle talks of light proceeding from the sun through the medium to the eye, it is evidently thought of as the stimulation which causes sight. Similarly, when in the latter part of the same chapter[4] he affirms that all parts of the medium are affected at the same time[5], *e.g.* that light travels instantaneously (and hence is not really a κίνησις), he seems to be still thinking of it as an activity exerted by the object on the eye (τὸ γὰρ φῶς ποιεῖ τὸ ὁρᾶν). Yet in other passages it seems to be rather the indispensable condition of the operation of a coloured object on the eye. The colour stimulates the transparent medium which already is in a condition of actuality, *i.e.* is illuminated; objects are seen ἐν φωτί[6]. Again, in *De Sensu,* ch. 2, 438 b 4, light is referred to as possibly itself the medium. It is the κίνησις through the medium, whether that be light or air (in a state of illumination), that causes vision. Hence from this point of view light is not the activity exerted by the object on the sense organ but merely the condition of the exertion of this

[1] *De Sens.* ch. 3, 439 b 17.   [2] Ch. 2, 438 b 5.
[3] Ch. 6, 446 a 30 sqq.   [4] 446 b 30 sqq.
[5] 447 a 10.   [6] *De An.* II. ch. 7, 419 a 7 sqq.

activity. When in chapter 6 Aristotle denies that light is a κίνησις (equally whether that κίνησις be of the type φορά— spatial transference, or ἀλλοίωσις—qualitative alteration[1]) he is still thinking of it as an activity, and the substance of his contention is, that that ἐνέργεια, which was elsewhere treated as the indispensable condition of that activity, is *itself* the activity which accounts for vision. It is very difficult to ·get the two conceptions to blend. The transference of the εἶδος of the object to the sense organ can only be thought of as a κίνησις, *i.e.* a process involving time. The activity as such is caused by the coloured object, whereas the ἐνέργεια is caused by the presence of the illuminating fire. Yet Aristotle, misled by the apparent instantaneousness of light, wished to conceive as not a κίνησις that which could only be a κίνησις and to raise it to the rank of an ἐνέργεια, *i.e.* something not physical at all.

The fundamental colour-tones are black and white, and Aristotle thinks to account for all other tints by the mixture of these two. He apparently wishes to make out that a mixture or rather chemical union of the substances which are black and white will give the chromatic tints[2]. One might have thought that common observation would have refuted this, and it is true that he does not say exactly this but merely "when substances unite so do their colours." True union of any two substances is one in which the original character of the component substances is lost and a third distinct qualitative character emerges as characterising every minutest part of the compound. To our modern chemical theory this holds true only if we stop our subdivision of the composite at the molecule. Any further analysis is supposed to give us parts which are not qualitatively identical, *i.e.* the molecule is supposed to split into atoms which have the qualities of the diverse component substances. But to Aristotle this was not so; the minutest conceivable sub- division of a true compound would still yield parts which were qualitatively identical with the whole. The compound

---

[1] Cf. notes ch. 6 *ad loc.*   [2] Cf. *De Sens.* ch. 3, 440 b 15 sqq.

was ὁμοιομερές[1]. Of such a sort was the mixture of black and white resulting in the chromatic tones supposed to be. Mere juxtaposition of the minute parts of differently coloured substances resulted only in the production of an indeterminate neutral tint which varied with the acuteness of our perception and our remoteness from the object. It is noteworthy that, if one were to define black and white[2] in the modern way as the capacity of a surface to reflect none or all of the light cast upon it, one could still describe the chromatic tints as intermediate between these, as diverse aptitudes for reflecting one portion and absorbing the rest of the total light. But of course nothing like this is to be found in Aristotle. What is suggestive in his theory is his contention that the difference of the composite tones depends upon the different proportions of the ingredients entering into them. This is an attempt to assimilate the theory of colours to that of harmonies; the pleasantest colours are those in which the proportions are simplest. This idea, if erroneous, is interesting as showing his readiness to recognise that mathematical relations enter into the constitution of reality. These relations are arithmetical; from mere geometrical characteristics you cannot derive any new quality, but, given a pair of opposed fundamental sensuous attributes, you can by a proportionate combination of the two account for the intermediate qualities. The same theory is worked out also in connection with flavour.

---

[1] Cf. notes to ch. 3, 440 a 34 sqq.

[2] In *Metaph.* x. ch. 7, 1057 b 8 sqq. white and black are distinguished as τὸ διακριτικὸν χρῶμα and τὸ συγκριτικὸν χρῶμα, and one might suspect that this implied some theory that white was the active and black the passive element in colour mixture in conformity with the principle in *Meteorol.* IV. ch. 1, 378 b 22 τὸ γὰρ συγκριτικὸν ὥσπερ ποιητικόν τι ἐστίν. But from various passages in the *Topics, e.g.* III. ch. 5, 119 a 30, IV. ch. 2, 123 a 2, we find that it is white which is τὸ διακριτικὸν χρῶμα. It is also said to be διακριτικὸν ὄψεως. I suppose the fact alluded to by this term is that it dissipates and exhausts the energy of the sense organ. If indeed the term is properly Aristotelian and not simply taken by way of illustration from some current popular theory, it is to be connected with the doctrine referred to in *De An.* III. ch. 13, 435 b 13 and elsewhere, that excessive stimulation destroys the sense organ, and white being the purest and most characteristic colour will tend to this extreme.

(*b*) Sound is not treated at length in the *De Sensu*, and
the theory of taste and smell involves to a still greater degree
than that of light the crudities of the Aristotelian psychics.
Not that we should speak with entire disrespect of the generalisation which assigned the constituents of all things to but
four ultimate elements. The grouping of substances together
according as they were dry, fluid, gaseous, or manifested
warmth, implied something more than a mere universal of
sense in each case. The distinctions reappear in modern
science not as the designations of different primitive substances but as marking distinct states in which all matter
can exist. At least τὸ ξηρόν or γῆ, τὸ ὑγρόν or ὕδωρ, and ὁ
ἀήρ correspond to the solid, the liquid, and the gaseous states,
and in the celestial fire—τὸ ἄνω σῶμα—which though not
identical with is yet analogous to πῦρ, Aristotle in a way
shadows forth the conception of the ether.

(*c*) Flavour is, according to the *De Sensu*, a qualitative[1]
affection of liquid by dry substance. This modification is
effected by the agency of heat (heat is the cooperating cause
—συναίτιον), and the process by which it is produced is a sort
of solution of the dry in the liquid (πλύσις, ἐναποπλύνειν[2]).
Knowing Aristotle's theory of the qualitative modification of
one substance by another[3], we shall, however, refuse to regard
this as a diffusion of the particles of the solid in the liquid.
It is no mechanical diffusion, but what we should call a
chemical union of the dry with the moist; it is, in fact, a
union more intimate than our chemical union is supposed to
be. If it were not so, then really the particles of the solid
would stimulate the sensation, and there would be some
ground for the Democritean theory that it was the different
shapes of these particles that produced the different flavours.
This Aristotle entirely rejects[4]; though taste is a tactual
sense, that does not mean that it is acted upon by the spatial
and mechanical properties of the minute parts of bodies,

---

[1] ποιόν τι τὸ ὑγρὸν παρασκευάζει, ch. 4, 441 b 21.
[2] *De Sens.* 441 b 17, cf. also ch. 5, 445 a 15.
[3] Cf. above in connection with colour mixture.
[4] Ch. 4, 442 a 31 sqq.

analogous to those properties discerned by touch when the bodies have an appreciable mass. It is not the particle impinging on the tongue that causes the taste, but the qualitative modification of the liquid medium which is identified as the flavour. If we lived amidst this vehicle[1], surrounded by it as we are by the air, then it would act as a medium just exactly as the air does in odour or sound, and the sense of taste would be a mediated one. In assigning the sense of taste as a subvariety of touch[2], Aristotle no doubt has in mind the fact that, as things are, it is only effected by contact with a portion of the substance in which the qualitative modification known as flavour subsists; he also, of course, has in view his theory that the fundamental qualities of flavour, sweetness and bitterness, are really indices of the tactual properties of food which go to determine its value as nutriment. The sweet—τὸ γλυκύ—is identified with the light— τὸ κοῦφον, *i.e.* with that light substance which can be raised up by the supposed vital heat operative in digestion and so get incorporated in the organism. The bitter—τὸ πικρόν— being heavy, sinks down and passes away as excrement[3]. Those actual properties, be it noted, are not spatial or dynamical according to Aristotle, but qualities given by the special sensations of touch, and it is upon such tactual attributes of objects that their value or hurtfulness for our organisms depends[4].

All other tastes than sweet and bitter are composites of those two qualities in different proportions, exactly as the chromatic tones are compounds of black and white[5].

(*d*) For odour to exist we require the prior production of flavour; we must already have τὸ ἔγχυμον ὑγρόν, *i.e.* liquid modified by flavour, or, what is the same thing[6], τὸ ἔγχυμον ξηρόν, dry substance which has produced a qualitative modification on liquid. The further solution of this flavoured substance in either air or water is, it seems, that which

---

[1] *De Sens.* ch. 6, 447 a 8.
[2] Ch. 4, 441 a 3.
[3] 441 b 26 sqq.
[4] *De An.* III., ch. 13, 435 b 4 sqq.
[5] Cf. above (*a*) on colour.
[6] Cf. notes to ch. 5, 442 b 31.

produces odour[1]. The diffusing agency is again heat[2], but it must be a *fresh* diffusion of the sapid substance which produces odour; if not, odour to creatures living in water would be identical with taste, whereas Aristotle distinctly assigns the sense of smell as such to them[3]. Similarly odour to animals that respire is not simply the presence in air of exactly the same thing that in liquid causes taste; it is a 'diffusion' in the air of the flavour itself, not of the cause of the flavour. But, since flavour is the basis of odour, differences in the latter correspond to the varieties of the former[4], and the scents derive their names from those distinguishing the tastes to which they correspond, owing to the similarity of the actual sensations[5].

Animals that respire perceive odour by means of the air in which it is 'diffused' entering the nostrils. The characteristic which modifies the air seems to be thus transferred to the organ, which Aristotle probably thought was composed of air alone in respiring animals[6]. The air in entering the organ displaces a membrane[7] and so effects communication. But in animals which dwell in water, the organ (probably consisting of water) is uncovered, just as the eyes also of fishes have no protecting covering; though the manner of perception is different the sense is still the same, for it is the same objective quality which affects them as in us causes smell[8].

Thus far odours are strictly parallel to flavours, and serve as an index to the character of the food from which they proceed. But we can classify them in a different way and not according to the taste to which they correspond; or rather, as Aristotle says, there are two different varieties or groups of odour. As we saw, heat is required in the propagation of all[9], *i.e.* the δύναμις or φύσις of odour contains the heat. Now in man[10] this heat entering the nostrils tempers the cold

---

[1] *De Sens.* ch. 5, 443 b 7.   [2] 443 b 17.   [3] 443 a 4, 444 b 21.
[4] 443 b 9.   [5] Cf. *De An.* II. ch. 9, 421 b 1.
[6] Cf. *De An.* III. ch. 1, 425 a 5 (θατέρου τούτων sc. ἀέρος καὶ ὕδατος) and cf. section v. above.
[7] *De Sens.* ch. 5, 444 b 24.   [8] Cf. notes to 444 b 21.
[9] Cf. 444 a 27.   [10] Ch. 5, 444 a 19 sqq.

which is supposed to prevail in the brain and its neighbourhood. Odours then appear to have a direct effect upon health and to be regarded as pleasant or the reverse in proportion as their action is beneficial or not. It is thus that Aristotle accounts for the appreciation felt by man for the scents of flowers and perfumes which have no association with edible things, an appreciation not felt by the lower animals. In the latter the brain, not being nearly so large in proportion to their size, does not apparently need this tonic influence. Thus Aristotle assigns to what we should call an aesthetic satisfaction a purely physiological and naturalistic explanation.

SECTION VIII.   PERCEPTION AS QUANTITATIVE.

In chapters 6 and 7 of the *De Sensu* Aristotle raises the question (1) whether all perception is of a quantum[1] and (2) whether all quanta are perceptible[2]. Both are answered in the affirmative ; the reasons for maintaining the former principle we have already seen[3]. Spatial quantity is to be identified as the continuous (τὸ συνεχές), and the continuous is just that in which there is no least part, in which you never come to the indivisible; objects of perception may, however, appear to be indivisible and therefore non-quantitative[4]. What this admission amounts to we must now discuss. In raising the problem whether there are an infinite number of perceptible parts in any object (*e.g.* whether all quanta are perceptible), Aristotle points out that the different species of qualities belonging to any one sense must form a limited number[5]. They can all be arranged in a linear series with the simple qualities most opposed to each other forming the extreme points and the others arranged in proximity to the two poles in accordance with the preponderance of the one or the other element respectively in them. But though thus arranged in linear fashion, they do not form a continuum, *i.e.* in analysing the whole of which they are constituent parts, you come

---

[1] *De Sens*. ch. 7, 449 a 12 sqq.
[2] Ch. 6, 445 b 3 sqq. ; cf. also ch. 7, 448 a 21 sqq.
[3] Sec. II. above.   [4] Ch. 7, 448 b 17.   [5] Ch. 6, 445 b 24.

ultimately to units which cannot be subdivided, *i.e.* you come to the indivisible. Hence there must be a finite number of parts or steps between the ends of the scale. This is a general proposition that holds good equally of a series of cognate qualities and of the number of middle terms to be interposed between subject and predicate in the proof of any proposition[1]. It is true equally of any finite magnitude. There must be a finite number of assignable parts (equal, ἴσα, cf. ch. 6, note *ad loc.*) between point A and point B, or else Achilles can never overtake the tortoise[2]. What then becomes of the assertion that all quantities are perceptible, *i.e.* that no matter how far you analyse the object the parts obtained are still something for sense ? Aristotle solves the difficulty by pointing out that it is one thing for a part to be perceived by itself and another as in the whole. We come to a limit at which a part ceases to be *per se* actually (ἐνεργείᾳ) an object of perception. The very minute parts of bodies are in their individuality only potentially (δυνάμει) perceptible. As taken along with the others and going to compose the whole they are, no doubt, actually perceptible. They do produce an effect upon the sense, but taken in their individuality they do not ; in fact, if a very minute part of any substance is actually isolated from the whole it is altered qualitatively and reduced to the nature of the new medium in which it is placed[3]. The conclusion of the whole doctrine is, that the sum of distinct objects of consciousness into which any total can be divided is limited, and that, for explicit consciousness, such units are indivisible. All specific existences are as such indivisible, and the mind can grasp absolute unity. This must be the truth underlying the statements that sense objects can appear indivisible ; as objects of mind they may be indivisible, though, as existences in the physical world and hence continuous, they cannot really be so[4].

---

[1] Cf. notes, *De Sens.* ch. 6, 445 b 24.   [2] Cf. *Physics*, VI. ch. 9, 239 b 14 sqq.

[3] *De Sens.* ch. 6, 446 a 8 sqq.

[4] Cf. *Metaph.* x. ch. 3, 1054 a 27 where it is pointed out that τὸ πλῆθος and τὸ διαιρετόν is μᾶλλον αἰσθητόν, and unity and the indivisible only known by opposition to these.

Aristotle's distinction between the actual and the potential perceptibility of a sense object may throw some light upon the conception of the subconscious existence of ideas which is so much in evidence in modern psychology. To many writers it seems to be the case that ideas or sensations may go on diminishing in intensity until they reach a zero point—the threshold of consciousness, after which they pass over into the subconscious region and go on existing as 'petites perceptions' with a separate individuality just as good as that which they had before. They are not 'unconscious mental modifications,' *i.e.* they are still in some way present to consciousness, for, it appears, they may go on diminishing still further in intensity until they reach a zero of total oblivion. Now such a conception of an intermediate subconscious zone interposed between the conscious and the unconscious is quite self-contradictory[1]. A sensation in its individuality is either an object of consciousness or it is not; if it is not you may call it subconscious if you like, meaning by that that in conjunction with others it produces an effect upon the mind, but in its individuality it is not an object of consciousness of any grade whatsoever. The subconscious 'region' should then be defined, not as a *region*, but as that state of an object in which, as a separate thing, it cannot be distinguished, but still in conjunction with others helps to produce a total psychical disposition. Whether the object can ever become a distinct element in consciousness *per se* depends upon circumstances. Sometimes by straining the attention or banishing other stimuli we can detect separate sensations hitherto unnoticed; sometimes sensations which, we know, must to a more acute sense appear distinct, are known to us only in the total volume which they produce. So too with ideas and memories, some can be aroused in their individuality by recollection, while others are real only in so far as by their former existence they modify our total present mood.

Aristotle's doctrine of the infinite divisibility of sensation

---

[1] This is what Lewes (Aristotle, p. 253) seems to have in mind in criticising Hamilton's theory of 'latent' knowledge. He by no means, however, makes his point clear.

(as above explained) fits in well with his general polemic against the atomic theory. With his expressly physical objections to atoms we are not here concerned. What his teaching amounts to is, that, though the characters of the minute parts called atoms are supposed to explain the sensational quality of the total substance which they compose, they themselves as occupying space will have parts and hence will want explaining by the nature of their minute parts and so on *ad infinitum*. Merely mathematical or mechanical qualities will not explain the special differentiae perceived by sense, and the atoms themselves, if corporeal, cannot be thought of as having merely mathematical and mechanical properties. To think of them we must invest them with the attributes known to us by sense. Hence instead of assuming that the sense-quality of an appreciable object is due to the configuration alone of its parts, it is as well to suppose that those parts have qualitative affections which, if not identical with those of the whole, are yet like them sensuous and contribute in some way to the resultant nature of the total object.

SECTION IX. APPERCEPTION.

Apperception is, of course, a term not corresponding to any expression in Aristotle, but by it we may designate that function of sense in which it judges (κρίνει) and by so doing coordinates in the same indivisible act different objects. The physiology of the matter we have already dealt with ; Aristotle localises the function in a central organ and hence it may be held to correspond to what is known to modern science as the action of the higher centres as opposed to the stimulation of end organ and lower ganglia merely. The latter affection does not result in perception of the typically human kind, which requires that higher coordination which has often been referred to by the current psychological term 'apperception.' The term αἰσθάνεσθαι with Aristotle includes discrimination (κρίνειν), and though in the discussion in the *De Sensu* he almost invariably employs the former term, whereas in the *De Anima* the latter emerges more conspicuously, he does not mean to distinguish two different functions by the different expressions. Αἰσθάνεσθαι implies both receptivity and discrimination, and would not be αἴσθησις without discrimination. Accordingly, when Aristotle asks how perception of two objects at the same time is possible, he is not asking how two impressions may be *received* at the same time; the sense organ, being a μέγεθος and having an indefinite plurality of parts within it, can easily account for that—the different parts may be differently modified. What he wants to find out is how the different determinations can be simultaneously discriminated, for that requires simultaneous existence in the same individual entity, not merely in different parts of it. Discrimination and coordination go together; as he shows in the *De Anima*[1], the consciousness which discriminates must be single. The objects perceived must not be present in separate moments[2] or to a divided consciousness.

In chapter 7 of the *De Sensu*, Aristotle without first hinting at his theory of how an indivisible unit of consciousness is possible, and thus leaving the field free for any other theory, asks whether discrimination of different sense elements in an indivisible moment can be effected. He distinguishes the cases of (1) perception of opposite qualities belonging to the same sense, *e.g.* black and white, and (2) determinations due to different senses—sweet and white. If, he says, such discrimination were likely to occur, it would be most natural to expect it in the case of the ἐναντία[3]— contrary determinations of one single sense,—μᾶλλον γὰρ ἅμα ἡ κίνησις τῆς μίας—[4] for the modifications due to black and white colour being localised in the same organ are more 'together' than those caused by sweetness and white-ness (which exist in different organs), and hence they have more chance of being coordinated. But, as it turns out, when

[1] III. ch. 2, 426 b 17 sqq.   [2] *De Sens.* ch. 7, 448 a 21 sqq.
[3] 447 b 23.   [4] 447 b 9.

two modifications occur together one either drives out the other or modifies it in some way, and, in the latter case, it is so modified in return that a third and new modification arises in which the individuality of the component elements is lost. Two equal and contrary determinations might completely annul each other [1], but when we get qualities belonging to the same sense simultaneously presented, what does occur is μίξις, a fusion of the two elements, as in the case of harmony ; they form one thing, a compound, and though they are, as forming such a thing, present to consciousness, their individuality is lost and hence they cannot be discriminated.   In an obscure passage [2] which Biehl has had to reconstruct almost entirely, Aristotle rejects the theory that this discrimination can be effected by the determination in different ways of the different parts of an organ which are yet continuous with each other This leads up to his own theory that, if either contrary or diverse qualities are to be simultaneously perceived there must be an absolutely indivisible psychical unity which can yet be viewed in two different ways at the same time.   Its nearest analogue is, as has been said [3], the mathematical point, or the unity of an object which possesses diverse attributes.   It has been debated whether those two solutions of the difficulty are the same, or whether the latter, if satisfactory for the case of qualities like white and sweet, belonging to different senses, will not be insufficient to account for the *harder* [4] case of contrary modifications like black and white.   A passage in the *De Anima* [5] might make us think so, but, as Rodier in his elucidation of *De An.* III. ch. 7 [6] points out, there is no real discrepancy between the two theories. Opposed qualities—ἐναντία—though existing in different parts of the same total object must (if between them they cover the whole extent of the ground) meet in a common indivisible point if they are still to be ascribed to the same object, and diverse characters (ἕτερα) like white and sweet, which do not exist in different *parts* of the substance, must be deemed (as

---

[1] *De Sens.* ch. 7, 447 a 27.   [2] 448 b 19 sqq.
[3] Section VI.   [4] Cf. notes to 449 a 4 sqq.
[5] III. ch. 2, 426 b 28 sqq.   [6] *Traité de l'Âme*, Vol. II. p. 501.

long as the substance has those qualities) to belong equally to its minutest parts, *i.e.* to be held together in a unity which, like the point, is absolutely indivisible. Of such a nature, then, is the psychic faculty involved in discrimination. It would be natural, if we followed out the parallelism between mind and body mechanically, to imagine that there was some corporeal organ which had the same properties, and there is a passage in the *De Memoria*[1], where, having evidently the organ of consciousness in mind, Aristotle refers to it as atomic; hence there is some countenance for Neuhäuser's theory that this organ is the mysterious vital heat of heavenly or transcendent origin. But as we have seen, nothing corporeal can fulfil the functions of an absolute indivisible unity; the unity of apperception is generally styled ἔν τι τῆς ψυχῆς[2], and perhaps the emphasis is on the latter word. We might have expected that it would have been in some way affiliated with the operation of νοῦς, which is non-spatial and has a really transcendent origin. The account of the activity of νόησις in *De An.* III. ch. 6, is almost entirely parallel to his description of the higher function of sense. However, the tendency of Aristotle to treat νοῦς simply as the highest of the intellectual faculties—that of pure conceptual thought—prevents us from making this identification; but, on the other hand, his refusal to see in discrimination of any kind mere passivity or determination by what is foreign to one's own being, leads us to surmise that the faculties of Sense and of Reason must be in essence one. This no doubt is his real belief but, as usual, it is veiled by his cautious manner of presenting the subject.

SECTION X. MEMORY AND RECOLLECTION.

The text of the treatise on Memory and Recollection presents some difficulties in interpretation which are perhaps still greater than those met with in the *De Sensu*. The worst

---

[1] Ch. 2, 451 a 28. Cf. above, Section VI.
[2] Cf. *De Sens.* ch. 7, 449 a 10, 448 b 23.

of these occur in passages where (*e.g.* 452 a 18 sqq., 452 b 16 sqq.)
symbols are employed, and in one case at least it is not
claimed that a perfectly satisfactory explanation has been
arrived at.

The main results of the treatise now claim our attention.

(1)   Memory (μνήμη) is used in a very restricted sense,
one much narrower than that assigned to it in modern
psychology.   It does not comprise retention: that rather is
an element present in the general faculty of Imagination, of
which Memory is a special determination.   A sense impression which persists as a psychic change resulting from an
actual perception[1] is an image (φάντασμα); it is the ascription of this image to some object existing in past time which
is memory in the proper sense.   In φαντασία generally
(though not apparently always[2]) the object which has
produced the originating sense-impression is not present,
but that fact does not constitute the mental state a memory.
The sense of time, either determinate or indeterminate, must
enter into the apprehension before we can be said to remember.   Thus Memory is relatively a high mental function,
and though it is not denied of several of the lower animals,
it is nothing which need emerge in that assimilation of
present to past which must be found in any consciousness
which profits by experience.

(2)   Aristotle thus thinks that a mental image may be
used and become an object of thought without the reference
to historical reality which memory implies.   It was quite
natural that he should do so.   As we have already seen,
the κίνησις in the body reproduces some κίνησις which has
existed in the external world, and the tendency of his
thought is to ascribe as nearly as possible identity of nature
to the two; at least his whole theory of sense-perception
implies this.   Hence, if a bodily κίνησις give knowledge of
external reality in sense perception, there is no reason why
it should not do so when the source of sense stimulation is
no longer present.   Certainly it is only when we remember

---

[1] *De An.* III. ch. 3, 429 a 1, 428 b 11 sqq.
[2] Cf. *De Mem.* ch. 1, note to 449 b 32.

in the strict sense, that the bodily κίνησις, which functions as νόημα or θεώρημα—an object of thought, gives us knowledge of the external object which caused the perception to which it is due; nevertheless it has an objective character, just as the animal in a picture has a definite nature as an object of consciousness independent of the reference to the actual living model from which it was copied or which suggested it[1]. From this account of the matter it might appear that Aristotle believed that the physiological modification in our bodies was the object of our thought when we imagined anything. So it is in a way, but it is only physiological *per accidens*; it is the same εἶδος whether existing in the external world or in the human body. To our minds the disparateness between the physiological and the merely physical seems extreme and we can think of the physiological process only as being some very remote symbolization of the external; not so was it to Aristotle, by whom the complexity of organic structures was very inadequately comprehended. It is noteworthy that the difference of the physiological and the physical seems to have been much more clearly realised by the time of Spinoza, who, when defining mind as 'idea corporis,' avoids the objection we have instanced above by explaining that our ideas involve the nature both of the external bodies and of the human organism[2]; he holds, however, that in perceiving the external we perceive also the nature of our own body. Nevertheless, the fact that no thought is the thought of the physiological process occasioning it, but is rather the consciousness of that which this process symbolizes, need not conflict with Aristotle's definition of memory or his account of the objective nature of a φάντασμα apart from memory. Just as the animal in a picture has an existence καθ' αὐτό—*quâ* animal, and not merely as a certain arrangement of paint devised to represent a living animal, so the φάντασμα may have an objective character without referring to the particular event or object to which it owes its origin.

---

[1] 450 b 23 sqq.   [2] *Ethics*, II. Prop. XVI. and Corollaries.

When it does so refer and is used as an εἰκών or μνημό-
νευμα¹, the representation of the object is coincident with a
representation (either definite or vague) of the time which has
elapsed since it was present to sense, and it is this coincidence²
alone which gives memory in the true sense.

To modern thought it may seem strange that Aristotle
should regard a φάντασμα, a mere alteration in the bodily
organs, as something objective. But one must remember
that this κίνησις was to him something of a definite pattern,
as definite as that of any object external to the human
organism, and that the knowledge of the one would not
differ from that of the other in point of 'objectivity.' The
stimulation of the sense organs by an external object might
originally cause the κίνησις. But this stimulation is nothing
else than the communication of the εἶδος of the external
object to the human organism. It is this εἶδος which forms
the content of thought, and whether existing in the external
physical object or in the sense organ it is equally objective.
The psychological problem as to how we perceive and remember and think is never for Aristotle the question of
how mind knows a real object. This latter, a metaphysical
difficulty, is quite distinct. That real objects existed and
could be known was the assumption from which he started.
Knowing was a fact which must be accepted, but how a
corporeal organism could manifest this function wanted explanation. The presence of the actual fact thought of in the
body of the thinking being and at the moment of thought
was the only solution he could offer. It is for modern
physiology to discover a better. But his was an attempt
in the right direction and a very natural answer also, for his
question was, not how *mind* thinks, but how *we*—embodied
creatures—think.

If it be asked : 'Is. Aristotle's a theory of representative
knowledge or perception?' we must answer no, at least it is
not so in the modern sense of such a theory. In a sense, no
doubt, there is representation ; between the individual and a

¹ *De Mem.* 451 a 3.   ² ch. 2, 452 b 26.

body external to his organism the κίνησις in the sense organs mediates, but between 'mind' and its object nothing interposes, and our apprehension of an external object is direct, —the immediate awareness of an objective, real character of things. Hence Aristotle could think of a φάντασμα which was not due to an object at the moment stimulating the senses, but was merely retained in the organs, as having objectivity apart from memory. This was so because the εἶδος or character it had was equally real whether in the body or out of it. Memory in fact adds nothing to the objectivity of the φαντάσματα involved in it. It is merely the union of the κίνησις caused by lapse of time and the φάντασμα originated by an external thing.

(3) The characteristic of involving continuous quantity, spatial or temporal, which cleaves to sense perception[1] infects also imagery, and hence memory. Thus memory must be assigned to the faculty of sense and its organ; it is not a function of pure thought[2]. The function of pure thought (νοῦς) is the apprehension of concepts apart (κεχωρισμένα) from this continuity which forms their ὕλη νοητή; the concept (νόημα) is to the image as the equation to a curve is to the curve in which it is realised. But memory, the apprehension of time, which is a continuum, can thus never belong to pure thought as such. Hence we may conclude (indeed, if my interpretation of ch. 1, 450a 20 be correct, we find it stated) that higher beings whose activity is purely intellectual do not share in memory.

(4) Differences in powers of memory Aristotle accounts for by the condition of the bodily organ (which is identical with the central organ of sensation). In language suggested largely by a passage in the *Theaetetus*[3] of Plato he describes the causes of variation between different individuals and the different ages of life. Generally speaking too great 'fluidity' of the receptive structure causes impermanence of the impression; too great 'density' occasions a difficulty in getting

---

[1] Cf. *De Sens.* ch. 6, 445 b 32.
[2] *De Mem.* ch. 1, 450 a 12 sqq. and notes.
[3] *Theaetetus*, 191 c sqq.

any experience ever impressed. Similarly in the process of recollection (which we shall next proceed to discuss) bodily conditions influence the recall of ideas either by impeding[1] the series of changes which occur in the central sensorium or by causing it to diffuse and so cause emotional disturbance[2].

(5) Recollection (ἀνάμνησις) is to be distinguished from memory, the ascription of an image to some event in the past, which may be due either to the persistence[3] of a sense-impression or to its reinstatement afresh; ἀνάμνησις is just that process of reinstatement and is so to be defined. It must, however, be carefully distinguished from the process involved in learning (which was identified with it by Plato). We may actually have reproduced in us by learning some knowledge previously possessed which might have been recalled but has totally passed into oblivion; under those circumstances the process is quite different from recollection; the latter process is self-conducted, while, for the former, we require instruction. Again, the basis from which we start is different in the two cases; much more than the meagre knowledge required in order to be capable of receiving instruction will be necessary, if we are to recall the previous idea unaided.

The objects to be recalled are twofold; they are either those which have a necessary connection with one another, like the concepts and judgments in mathematical science, or again they may be contingently related. The former are easily remembered, the latter not so, but in both cases the order of recall depends upon the experienced connection of the facts[4], and the connection is either that of like with like, or of things contiguous or opposed. The ease with which an idea may be recalled depends upon the frequency of the repetition of the particular series of connections by which it is reinstated. Frequent repetition due to custom produces a natural disposition[5] which tends to actualisation just like any other δύναμις or φύσις. Here,

---

[1] *De Mem.* ch. 2, 453 b 1. [2] 453 a 16 sqq. [3] 451 b 1 sqq.
[4] 451 b 32. [5] 452 a 29 sqq.

however, just because the disposition is due to custom, it is liable to be interfered with, just as any tendency in nature may be thwarted, only more so.

The laws of Association here formulated by Aristotle (Contiguity, Similarity, and Contrast) are obviously merely principles governing the reinstatement of ideas previously experienced. Hence their scope is much narrower than that assigned to them by modern psychology. Aristotle certainly held no 'Associationist Theory of Knowledge,' but for that the most recent theorists are hardly likely to blame him. There are, however, other psychical operations like 'complication,' his αἴσθησις κατὰ συμβεβηκός, which many writers would rank generally under 'association' but which he left unaffiliated to the process involved in recollection. This discreteness in his treatment of mental functions is no doubt due to his empirical way of approaching his data and his caution in all but the widest generalisations.

(6) Finally we hear that recollection is a higher activity than mere memory. It is peculiar to man[1]. Though it may operate involuntarily[2] it is typically a purposive operation[3] and is to be regarded as a kind of search, like the search for the middle term in demonstration or for the means to effect the fulfilment of an end in practical deliberation. Its purposiveness seems to argue to its higher nature; it is in this way illustrative of the ἀπάθεια which belongs to mind *per se*[4]. In recollecting the soul seems to be active, producing an activity which proceeds *towards*[5] the organs of sense. Apart from the aspect of activity we must, however, recognise that, in recollection, there is a process going on in the organs of sense or rather in the central sensorium. The various ideas which reinstate one another are all to be described as κινήσεις, and the end of a process of recollection seems to be attained when one particular κίνησις is produced which seems to constitute a terminus to the series—namely the

---

[1] *De Mem.* ch. 2, 453 a 11.   [2] 451 b 26.

[3] Cf. Prof. Laurie's *Institutes of Education*, p. 233 sqq.

[4] Cf. Section IV. above *ad init.*

[5] *De An.* I. ch. 4, 408 b 17.

κίνησις corresponding to the idea to be recalled. It is throughout implied that these κινήσεις, prior to the act of recollection, are dormant; that is to say they are not, until revived, κινήσεις. What then persists or what is the κίνησις when it is dormant? Aristotle talks of the impression on the organ being like an imprint—τύπος, and, no doubt, he must have thought of the impression left by an experience as being some kind of structural modification of the organ. He talks of the subjective affections involved in apprehending magnitudes as being σχήματα[1] like the objective magnitudes themselves. He does not work out his theory of the persistence of impression, but doubtless the dormant impression is merely something of the nature of a σχῆμα (at least in the case of the perception of magnitude), while the affection whether when first experienced or when revived is of the nature of a κίνησις, though a κίνησις which still has a spatial configuration and can be represented by a motion passing along a determinate path—as in the construction of a triangle. At any rate we find no hint in Aristotle of that modern theory which would make psychical dispositions consist in the faint functionings of the same parts as are brought into play when an idea is explicitly realised.

---

[1] Cf. *De Insom.* ch. 3, 461 a 8 sqq.

ΠΕΡΙ ΑΙΣΘΗΣΕΩΣ ΚΑΙ ΑΙΣΘΗΤΩΝ

ΠΕΡΙ ΑΙΣΘΗΣΕΩΣ ΚΑΙ ΑΙΣΘΗΤΩΝ

I

Ἐπεὶ δὲ περὶ ψυχῆς καθ' αὑτὴν διώρισται καὶ περὶ
τῶν δυνάμεων ἑκάστης κατὰ μόριον αὐτῆς, ἐχόμενόν ἐστι
ποιήσασθαι τὴν ἐπίσκεψιν περὶ τῶν ζῴων καὶ τῶν ζωὴν
ἐχόντων ἁπάντων, τίνες εἰσὶν ἴδιαι καὶ τίνες κοιναὶ
5 πράξεις αὐτῶν. τὰ μὲν οὖν εἰρημένα περὶ ψυχῆς ὑποκείσθω, περὶ δὲ τῶν λοιπῶν λέγωμεν, καὶ πρῶτον περὶ
τῶν πρώτων. φαίνεται δὲ τὰ μέγιστα, καὶ τὰ κοινὰ καὶ
τὰ ἴδια τῶν ζῴων, κοινὰ τῆς ψυχῆς ὄντα καὶ τοῦ σώματος,
οἷον αἴσθησις καὶ μνήμη καὶ θυμὸς καὶ ἐπιθυμία καὶ
10 ὅλως ὄρεξις, καὶ πρὸς τούτοις ἡδονή τε καὶ λύπη· καὶ
γὰρ ταῦτα σχεδὸν ὑπάρχει πᾶσι τοῖς ζῴοις. πρὸς δὲ
τούτοις τὰ μὲν πάντων ἐστὶ τῶν μετεχόντων ζωῆς κοινά,
τὰ δὲ τῶν ζῴων ἐνίοις. τυγχάνουσι δὲ τούτων τὰ μέγιστα τέτταρες συζυγίαι τὸν ἀριθμόν, οἷον ἐγρήγορσις
15 καὶ ὕπνος, καὶ νεότης καὶ γῆρας, καὶ ἀναπνοὴ καὶ
ἐκπνοή, καὶ ζωὴ καὶ θάνατος· περὶ ὧν θεωρητέον, τί
τε ἕκαστον αὐτῶν, καὶ διὰ τίνας αἰτίας συμβαίνει.
φυσικοῦ δὲ καὶ περὶ ὑγιείας καὶ νόσου τὰς πρώτας ἰδεῖν
ἀρχάς· οὔτε γὰρ ὑγίειαν οὔτε νόσον οἷόν τε γίγνεσθαι
20 τοῖς ἐστερημένοις ζωῆς. διὸ σχεδὸν τῶν περὶ φύσεως
οἱ πλεῖστοι καὶ τῶν ἰατρῶν οἱ φιλοσοφωτέρως τὴν τέχνην
436b μετιόντες, οἱ μὲν τελευτῶσιν εἰς τὰ περὶ ἰατρικῆς, οἱ δ'

I

Now that we have given a definite account of soul in its essential nature and of each of its faculties individually, the next thing to do is to consider animals and all things possessed of life and to discover which activities are specific and which they have in common.

Assuming as a basis our exposition about the soul, let us 5 discuss the remaining questions, beginning with those that are primary.

The most important of the characteristics of animals, both generic and specific, evidently belong to soul and body in common, *e.g.* sense-perception and memory, passion, desire and appetite generally, as well as pleasure and pain. These 10 are found practically in all animals.

But further, certain of the phenomena in question are common to all things which participate in life, while others are shared by particular kinds of animals. Of these the most important fall into four pairs of correlatives, to wit, waking and sleep, youth and age, the inhalation and expulsion of 15 breath, life and death. These phenomena call for discussion, and we must investigate both the nature of each and the reasons for its existence.

It falls within the province of the natural scientist to survey the first principles involved in the subject of health and disease, for to nothing lacking life can either health or sickness accrue. Hence pretty well the most of our in- 20 vestigators of nature do not stop until they have run on into medicine, and those of our medical men who employ their 436 b

ἐκ τῶν περὶ φύσεως ἄρχονται περὶ τῆς ἰατρικῆς. ὅτι
δὲ τὰ λεχθέντα κοινὰ τῆς τε ψυχῆς ἐστὶ καὶ τοῦ σώματος, οὐκ ἄδηλον. πάντα γὰρ τὰ μὲν μετ' αἰσθήσεως
5 συμβαίνει, τὰ δὲ δι' αἰσθήσεως· ἔνια δὲ τὰ μὲν πάθη
ταύτης ὄντα τυγχάνει, τὰ δ' ἕξεις, τὰ δὲ φυλακαὶ καὶ
σωτηρίαι, τὰ δὲ φθοραὶ καὶ στερήσεις. ἡ δ' αἴσθησις
ὅτι διὰ σώματος γίγνεται τῇ ψυχῇ, δῆλον καὶ διὰ τοῦ
λόγου καὶ τοῦ λόγου χωρίς. ἀλλὰ περὶ μὲν αἰσθήσεως
10 καὶ τοῦ αἰσθάνεσθαι, τί ἐστι καὶ διὰ τί συμβαίνει τοῖς
ζῴοις τοῦτο τὸ πάθος, εἴρηται πρότερον ἐν τοῖς περὶ
ψυχῆς. τοῖς δὲ ζῴοις, ᾗ μὲν ζῷον ἕκαστον, ἀνάγκη
ὑπάρχειν αἴσθησιν· τούτῳ γὰρ τὸ ζῷον εἶναι καὶ μὴ
ζῷον διορίζομεν. ἰδίᾳ δ' ἤδη καθ' ἕκαστον ἡ μὲν ἁφὴ
15 καὶ γεῦσις ἀκολουθεῖ πᾶσιν ἐξ ἀνάγκης, ἡ μὲν ἁφὴ διὰ
τὴν εἰρημένην αἰτίαν ἐν τοῖς περὶ ψυχῆς, ἡ δὲ γεῦσις
διὰ τὴν τροφήν· τὸ γὰρ ἡδὺ διακρίνει καὶ τὸ λυπηρὸν
αὐτῇ περὶ τὴν τροφήν, ὥστε τὸ μὲν φεύγειν τὸ δὲ διώκειν,
καὶ ὅλως ὁ χυμός ἐστι τοῦ θρεπτικοῦ πάθος. αἱ δὲ
20 διὰ τῶν ἔξωθεν αἰσθήσεις τοῖς πορευτικοῖς αὐτῶν, οἷον
ὄσφρησις καὶ ἀκοὴ καὶ ὄψις, πᾶσι μὲν τοῖς ἔχουσι
σωτηρίας ἕνεκεν ὑπάρχουσιν, ὅπως διώκωσί τε προαισθανόμενα τὴν τροφὴν καὶ τὰ φαῦλα καὶ τὰ φθαρτικὰ
437 a φεύγωσι, τοῖς δὲ καὶ φρονήσεως τυγχάνουσι τοῦ εὖ
ἕνεκα· πολλὰς γὰρ εἰσαγγέλλουσι διαφοράς, ἐξ ὧν ἥ
τε τῶν νοητῶν ἐγγίνεται φρόνησις καὶ ἡ τῶν πρακτῶν.
αὐτῶν δὲ τούτων πρὸς μὲν τὰ ἀναγκαῖα κρείττων ἡ ὄψις
5 καθ' αὐτήν, πρὸς δὲ νοῦν καὶ κατὰ συμβεβηκὸς ἡ ἀκοή.
διαφορὰς μὲν γὰρ πολλὰς καὶ παντοδαπὰς ἡ τῆς ὄψεως
ἀγγέλλει δύναμις διὰ τὸ πάντα τὰ σώματα μετέχειν
χρώματος, ὥστε καὶ τὰ κοινὰ διὰ ταύτης αἰσθάνεσθαι

---

436 b 19   γευστικοῦ L U Alex., θρεπτικοῦ etiam Bas. et Sylb. | post θρεπτικοῦ
addunt μορίου exceptis E M Y et scripti et impressi, atque addit etiam τῆς ψυχῆς P
vet. tr., θρεπτικοῦ sine ullo additamento probant etiam Hayduck et Biehl.

art in a more scientific fashion, use as the first principles of medicine truths belonging to the natural sciences.

There is no lack of evidence that the phenomena we have mentioned are shared by both soul and body in common, for they all either occur in concomitance with sensuous experience or are due to it. Some are modifications, some 5 permanent dispositions of sensuous experience, while some protect and preserve and others destroy and annul it.

That the psychical function of sensation depends upon the body is clear both *à priori* and apart from such evidence. However, the nature of sense and its function and the reason why this phenomenon is found in animals, have already been 10 explained in the Psychology. Animals *quâ* animal must possess sensation, for it is by means of this that we distinguish animate from inanimate.

To each animal in its own proper nature touch and taste must necessarily accrue, touch for the reason given in the 15 Psychology, taste owing to the fact that it takes nutriment; for by taste the pleasant and unpleasant are distinguished in food, so that as a consequence the one is pursued and the other shunned; to put it generally, flavour is a determination of that which is nutritive.

In animals with the power of locomotion, are found the senses which are mediated by something external, to wit, 20 smell, hearing, and sight. These exist uniformly for the purpose of the self-preservation of the animals possessing them, in order that they may become aware of their food at a distance and go in pursuit of it and that they may avoid what is bad and injurious. Where intelligence is found they 437 a are designed to subserve the ends of well-being; they communicate to our minds many distinctions out of which develops in us the intelligent apprehension alike of the objects of thought and of the things of the practical life. Of these three sight is *per se* more valuable so far as the needs of life are concerned, but from the point of view of thought and accidentally, hearing is the more important. 5 The characteristics are many and various which the faculty of sight reports, because all bodies are endowed with colour;

μάλιστα (λέγω δὲ κοινὰ σχῆμα καὶ μέγεθος, κίνησιν,
10 ἀριθμόν)· ἡ δ' ἀκοὴ τὰς τοῦ ψόφου διαφορὰς μόνον,
ὀλίγοις δὲ καὶ τὰς τῆς φωνῆς. κατὰ συμβεβηκὸς δὲ
πρὸς φρόνησιν ἡ ἀκοὴ πλεῖστον συμβάλλεται μέρος.
ὁ γὰρ λόγος αἴτιός ἐστι τῆς μαθήσεως ἀκουστὸς ὤν, οὐ
καθ' αὑτὸν ἀλλὰ κατὰ συμβεβηκός· ἐξ ὀνομάτων γὰρ
15 σύγκειται, τῶν δ' ὀνομάτων ἕκαστον σύμβολόν ἐστιν.
διόπερ φρονιμώτεροι τῶν ἐκ γενετῆς ἐστερημένων εἰσὶν
ἑκατέρας τῆς αἰσθήσεως οἱ τυφλοὶ τῶν ἐνεῶν καὶ
κωφῶν.

II

Περὶ μὲν οὖν τῆς δυνάμεως ἣν ἔχει τῶν αἰσθήσεων
20 ἑκάστη, πρότερον εἴρηται. τοῦ δὲ σώματος ἐν οἷς ἐγγίγνεσθαι πέφυκεν αἰσθητηρίοις, νῦν μὲν ζητοῦσι κατὰ
τὰ στοιχεῖα τῶν σωμάτων· οὐκ εὐποροῦντες δὲ πρὸς
τέτταρα πέντ' οὔσας συνάγειν, γλίχονται περὶ τῆς
πέμπτης. ποιοῦσι δὲ πάντες τὴν ὄψιν πυρὸς διὰ τὸ
25 πάθους τινὸς ἀγνοεῖν τὴν αἰτίαν· θλιβομένου γὰρ καὶ
κινουμένου τοῦ ὀφθαλμοῦ φαίνεται πῦρ ἐκλάμπειν· τοῦτο
δ' ἐν τῷ σκότει πέφυκε συμβαίνειν, ἢ τῶν βλεφάρων
ἐπικεκαλυμμένων· γίνεται γὰρ καὶ τότε σκότος. ἔχει
δ' ἀπορίαν τοῦτο καὶ ἑτέραν. εἰ γὰρ μὴ ἔστι λανθάνειν
30 αἰσθανόμενον καὶ ὁρῶντα ὁρώμενόν τι, ἀνάγκη ἄρ' αὐτὸν
ἑαυτὸν ὁρᾶν τὸν ὀφθαλμόν. διὰ τί οὖν ἠρεμοῦντι τοῦτ'
οὐ συμβαίνει; τὰ δ' αἴτια τούτου, καὶ τῆς ἀπορίας καὶ
τοῦ δοκεῖν πῦρ εἶναι τὴν ὄψιν, ἐντεῦθεν ληπτέον. τὰ γὰρ
λεῖα πέφυκεν ἐν τῷ σκότει λάμπειν, οὐ μέντοι φῶς γε
437 b ποιεῖ, τοῦ δ' ὀφθαλμοῦ τὸ καλούμενον μέλαν καὶ μέσον
λεῖον φαίνεται. φαίνεται δὲ τοῦτο κινουμένου τοῦ ὄμματος διὰ τὸ συμβαίνειν ὥσπερ δύο γίγνεσθαι τὸ ἕν.
τοῦτο δ' ἡ ταχυτὴς ποιεῖ τῆς κινήσεως, ὥστε δοκεῖν
5 ἕτερον εἶναι τὸ ὁρῶν καὶ τὸ ὁρώμενον. διὸ καὶ οὐ

thus by this sense especially are perceived the common sensibles (by these I mean figure, magnitude, motion, and number). 10

But hearing gives merely differences in sound and, in a few cases, in articulate utterance too. Hearing, however, has the greatest share in the development of intelligence, though this is an accidental function. Speech being audible is instrumental in causing us to learn; but this function it possesses not *per se* but accidentally, for speech is a complex 15 of words, every one of which is a conventional symbol. A consequence is that of those who from birth have been without one or other of those two senses, the blind are more intelligent than deaf-mutes.

II

We have already given an account of each of the sense faculties. But each develops, according to the course of 20 nature, in a bodily sense organ, and these we shall proceed to discuss.

Present-day investigators attempt to reduce them to the ultimate elements of all bodies; but, since the senses are five, they have a difficulty in reducing them to the four elements, and the fifth causes them anxious consideration.

Sight they all ascribe to fire owing to the misunderstanding of a certain phenomenon, viz. when the eye is 25 pressed and moved, fire appears to flash out from it; and it is the nature of this phenomenon to occur in the dark, or when the eyelids are closed, for then, too, there is darkness.

But this theory—that sight is of the nature of fire—raises a fresh difficulty; for, if it is impossible for that which is conscious of and sees some object to be unaware that it does 30 so, the eye will of necessity perceive itself. Why then is this not the case when the eye is at rest?

From the following considerations we shall discover the cause of this circumstance and of the apparent identity of fire and vision. It is the nature of smooth things to shine in the dark, but, nevertheless, they do not produce light; now what we call the "black" and "middle" of the eye has a 437 b smooth appearance and it shows on the eye moving, for the reason that this occurrence is a case of the reduplication of a single thing. The swiftness of the motion effects this, causing that which sees and that which is seen to appear to be distinct. Hence also if the motion is not swift and does not 5

γίγνεται, ἂν μὴ ταχέως καὶ ἐν σκότει τοῦτο συμβῇ·
τὸ γὰρ λεῖον ἐν τῷ σκότει πέφυκε λάμπειν, οἷον κεφαλαὶ
ἰχθύων τινῶν καὶ ὁ τῆς σηπίας θολός· καὶ βραδέως
μεταβάλλοντος τοῦ ὄμματος οὐ συμβαίνει, ὥστε δοκεῖν
10 ἅμα ἓν καὶ δύο εἶναι τό θ' ὁρῶν καὶ τὸ ὁρώμενον.
ἐκείνως δ' αὐτὸς αὑτὸν ὁρᾷ ὁ ὀφθαλμός, ὥσπερ καὶ ἐν
τῇ ἀνακλάσει, ἐπεὶ εἴ γε πῦρ ἦν, καθάπερ Ἐμπεδοκλῆς
φησὶ καὶ ἐν τῷ Τιμαίῳ γέγραπται, καὶ συνέβαινε τὸ
ὁρᾶν ἐξιόντος ὥσπερ ἐκ λαμπτῆρος τοῦ φωτός, διὰ τί
15 οὐ καὶ ἐν τῷ σκότει ἑώρα ἂν ἡ ὄψις; τὸ δ' ἀποσβέννυσθαι φάναι ἐν τῷ σκότει ἐξιοῦσαν, ὥσπερ ὁ Τίμαιος
λέγει, κενόν ἐστι παντελῶς· τίς γὰρ ἀπόσβεσις φωτός
ἐστιν; σβέννυται γὰρ ἢ ὑγρῷ ἢ ψυχρῷ τὸ θερμὸν καὶ
ξηρόν, οἷον δοκεῖ τό τ' ἐν τοῖς ἀνθρακώδεσιν εἶναι πῦρ
20 καὶ ἡ φλόξ, ὧν τῷ φωτὶ οὐδέτερον φαίνεται ὑπάρχον.
εἰ δ' ἄρα ὑπάρχει μὲν ἀλλὰ διὰ τὸ ἠρέμα λανθάνει ἡμᾶς,
ἔδει μεθ' ἡμέραν τε καὶ ἐν τῷ ὕδατι ἀποσβέννυσθαι τὸ
φῶς, καὶ ἐν τοῖς πάγοις μᾶλλον γίνεσθαι σκότον· ἡ γοῦν
φλὸξ καὶ τὰ πεπυρωμένα σώματα πάσχει τοῦτο· νῦν δ'
25 οὐδὲν συμβαίνει τοιοῦτον. Ἐμπεδοκλῆς δ' ἔοικε νομίζοντι ὁτὲ μὲν ἐξιόντος τοῦ φωτός, ὥσπερ εἴρηται πρότερον,
βλέπειν· λέγει γοῦν οὕτως·

ὡς δ' ὅτε τις πρόοδον νοέων ὡπλίσσατο λύχνον,
χειμερίην διὰ νύκτα πυρὸς σέλας αἰθομένοιο,
30 ἅψας παντοίων ἀνέμων λαμπτῆρας ἀμοργούς,
οἵτ' ἀνέμων μὲν πνεῦμα διασκιδνᾶσιν ἀέντων,
πῦρ δ' ἔξω διαθρῶσκον, ὅσον ταναώτερον ἦεν,
λάμπεσκεν κατὰ βηλὸν ἀτειρέσιν ἀκτίνεσσιν·
ὡς δὲ τό τ' ἐν μήνιγξιν ἐεργμένον ὠγύγιον πῦρ
438 a λεπτῇσιν ὀθόνῃσι λοχάζετο κύκλοπα κούρην·
αἱ δ' ὕδατος μὲν βένθος ἀπέστεγον ἀμφινάοντος,
πῦρ δ' ἔξω διαθρῶσκον, ὅσον ταναώτερον ἦεν.

ὁτὲ μὲν οὕτως ὁρᾶν φησίν, ὁτὲ δὲ ταῖς ἀπορροίαις ταῖς
5 ἀπὸ τῶν ὁρωμένων.

occur in the dark, the phenomenon does not take place. It is the nature of smooth things to shine in the dark, as *e.g.* the heads of certain fishes and the juice of the cuttle-fish. When the eye moves slowly, the effect—the apparent simultaneous identity and duality of that which sees and that which is seen—is not produced. But in the former case—that of 10 swift movement—the eye sees itself as it does too when reflected in a mirror; this is so, for, if it really consists of fire, as Empedocles alleges and we read in the *Timaeus*, and if vision is produced by the issuing forth of light from the eye as it were from a lantern, why does not sight function in the dark as well as by day?

The explanation in the *Timaeus*, that the sight issuing 15 from the eye is extinguished in the darkness, is quite without point, for what can the extinction of light mean? Heat and dryness are annulled by damp or cold, as we see in the case of the fire and flame in burning coals; but neither of these 20 is a characteristic of light. If they are and we do not detect their presence owing to the smallness of their amount, light would of necessity be extinguished in broad daylight too, when it was wet, and darkness would increase in frosty weather. This at any rate, viz. extinction, is what happens to flame and burning bodies, but nothing of the kind occurs in the phenomenon in question.

Empedocles evidently holds the view at times, that we 25 see upon the issuing of light from the eye, as we mentioned before. At any rate these are his words:

" As who a journey intendeth, himself with a candle equippeth
Thorough the blustering night with its fiery radiance gleaming,
And, to ward off every gust, in lantern-case fits it,   30
That this may part to this side and that the breath of the wild winds
While the fire pierces through, inasmuch as its nature is subtler,
And shines over the threshold with splendour that naught can conquer,
Thus too the world-old fire was confined in the delicate membranes
And lies hid 'neath the screens of the spherical-fashionëd pupil;   438 a
These keep in check the ocean of water that circles around it,
But the fire pierces through, inasmuch as its nature is subtler."

Sometimes he says this is the way in which we see, but at other times he explains it by a theory of effluxes issuing from the objects seen.   5

R.   4

5 Δημόκριτος δ' ὅτι μὲν ὕδωρ εἶναί φησι,
λέγει καλῶς, ὅτι δ' οἴεται τὸ ὁρᾶν εἶναι τὴν ἔμφασιν,
οὐ καλῶς· τοῦτο μὲν γὰρ συμβαίνει ὅτι τὸ ὄμμα λεῖον,
καὶ ἔστιν οὐκ ἐν ἐκείνῳ ἀλλ' ἐν τῷ ὁρῶντι· ἀνάκλασις
γὰρ τὸ πάθος. ἀλλὰ καθόλου περὶ τῶν ἐμφαινομένων
10 καὶ ἀνακλάσεως οὐδέ πω δῆλον ἦν, ὡς ἔοικεν. ἄτοπον
δὲ καὶ τὸ μὴ ἐπελθεῖν αὐτῷ ἀπορῆσαι διὰ τί ὁ ὀφθαλμὸς
ὁρᾷ μόνον, τῶν δ' ἄλλων οὐδὲν ἐν οἷς ἐμφαίνεται τὰ
εἴδωλα. τὸ μὲν οὖν τὴν ὄψιν εἶναι ὕδατος ἀληθὲς μέν,
οὐ μέντοι συμβαίνει τὸ ὁρᾶν ᾗ ὕδωρ ἀλλ' ᾗ διαφανές·
15 ὃ καὶ ἐπὶ τοῦ ἀέρος κοινόν ἐστιν. ἀλλ' εὐφυλακτότερον
καὶ εὐπιλητότερον τὸ ὕδωρ τοῦ ἀέρος· διόπερ ἡ κόρη
καὶ τὸ ὄμμα ὕδατός ἐστιν. τοῦτο δὲ καὶ ἐπ' αὐτῶν τῶν
ἔργων δῆλον· φαίνεται γὰρ ὕδωρ τὸ ἐκρέον διαφθειρο-
μένων, καὶ ἐν τοῖς πάμπαν ἐμβρύοις τῇ ψυχρότητι
20 ὑπερβάλλον καὶ τῇ λαμπρότητι. καὶ τὸ λευκὸν τοῦ
ὄμματος ἐν τοῖς ἔχουσιν αἷμα πῖον καὶ λιπαρόν· ὅπερ
διὰ τοῦτ' ἐστί, πρὸς τὸ διαμένειν τὸ ὑγρὸν ἄπηκτον.
καὶ διὰ τοῦτο τοῦ σώματος ἀρριγότατον ὁ ὀφθαλμός
ἐστιν· οὐδεὶς γάρ πω τὸ ἐντὸς τῶν βλεφάρων ἐρρίγωσεν.
25 τῶν δ' ἀναίμων σκληρόδερμοι οἱ ὀφθαλμοί εἰσι, καὶ
τοῦτο ποιεῖ τὴν σκέπην. ἄλογον δὲ ὅλως τὸ ἐξιόντι τινὶ
τὴν ὄψιν ὁρᾶν, καὶ ἀποτείνεσθαι μέχρι τῶν ἄστρων, ἢ
μέχρι τινὸς ἐξιοῦσαν συμφύεσθαι, καθάπερ λέγουσί
τινες. τούτου μὲν γὰρ βέλτιον τὸ ἐν ἀρχῇ συμφύεσθαι
30 τοῦ ὄμματος. ἀλλὰ καὶ τοῦτο εὔηθες· τό τε γὰρ συμφύεσθαι τί ἐστι φωτὶ πρὸς φῶς; ἢ πῶς οἷόν θ' ὑπάρχειν;
438 b οὐ γὰρ τῷ τυχόντι συμφύεται τὸ τυχόν. τό τ' ἐντὸς
τῷ ἐκτὸς πῶς; ἡ γὰρ μῆνιγξ μεταξύ ἐστιν. περὶ μὲν
οὖν τοῦ ἄνευ φωτὸς μὴ ὁρᾶν εἴρηται ἐν ἄλλοις· ἀλλ'
εἴτε φῶς εἴτ' ἀήρ ἐστι τὸ μεταξὺ τοῦ ὁρωμένου καὶ τοῦ
5 ὄμματος, ἡ διὰ τούτου κίνησίς ἐστιν ἡ ποιοῦσα τὸ ὁρᾶν.
καὶ εὐλόγως τὸ ἐντός ἐστιν ὕδατος. διαφανὲς γὰρ τὸ

Democritus is in the right in saying that the eye consists 5
of water, but his theory that sight is the mirroring of an
object is wrong. This phenomenon indeed—the visibility of
an object as in a mirror—occurs in the case of the eye
because it is smooth, and exists not in it (the reflecting eye)
but in the spectator; for the phenomenon is one of reflection.
But he seems to have attained to no clear general theory of
the mirroring and reflection of objects. It is ridiculous too 10
that it never entered his head to ask why the eye alone sees
and none of the other things in which images are mirrored.

Thus his theory is true that the sight-organ consists of
water; but the eye functions not *quâ* aqueous but *quâ*
transparent; this property it shares with air as well. But 15
water is more easily kept in, being denser than air; and hence
the pupil and the eye are composed of water.

The facts themselves make this clear; what issues from
the eyes when they are seriously hurt is evidently water, and
when they are quite in the embryonic stage it is excessively
cold and brilliant. Further, in sanguineous animals the white 20
of the eye is fat and oily; this is designed to keep the
moisture unfrozen. Hence the eye is less liable to be chilled
than any other part of the body; no one ever felt cold under
the eye-lids. In bloodless animals, however, the eyes have a
hard skin and this it is which protects them. 25

The theory is wholly absurd that sight is effected by
means of something which issues from the eye and that it
travels as far as the stars or, as some say, unites with
something else after proceeding a certain distance.

Than this latter a better theory would be, that the union
is effected in the eye—the starting point; but even this is
childish. What can the union of light with light mean? 30
How can it come about? The union is not that of any 438 b
chance light with any other chance light whatsoever. Again
how can the internal light unite with the external? The
membrane of the eye divides them.

We have elsewhere stated that vision without light is
impossible; but whether it is light or air that intervenes
between the object seen and the eye, it is the motion
propagated through this that produces sight. Thus, as our 5
theory would lead us to infer, the interior of the eye consists

ὕδωρ. ὁρᾶται δὲ ὥσπερ καὶ ἔξω οὐκ ἄνευ φωτός, οὕτως καὶ ἐντός· διαφανὲς ἄρα δεῖ εἶναι. καὶ ἀνάγκη ὕδωρ εἶναι, ἐπειδὴ οὐκ ἀήρ. οὐ γὰρ ἐπὶ τοῦ ἐσχάτου ὄμματος 10 ἡ ψυχὴ ἢ τῆς ψυχῆς τὸ αἰσθητικόν ἐστιν, ἀλλὰ δῆλον ὅτι ἐντός· διόπερ ἀνάγκη διαφανὲς εἶναι καὶ δεκτικὸν φωτὸς τὸ ἐντὸς τοῦ ὄμματος. καὶ τοῦτο καὶ ἐπὶ τῶν συμβαινόντων δῆλον· ἤδη γάρ τισι πληγεῖσιν ἐν πολέμῳ παρὰ τὸν κρόταφον οὕτως ὥστ᾽ ἐκτμηθῆναι τοὺς πόρους 15 τοῦ ὄμματος, ἔδοξε γενέσθαι σκότος ὥσπερ λύχνου ἀποσβεσθέντος, διὰ τὸ οἷον λαμπτῆρά τινα ἀποτμη-θῆναι τὸ διαφανές, τὴν καλουμένην κόρην. ὥστ᾽ εἴπερ τούτων τι συμβαίνει, καθάπερ λέγομεν, φανερὸν ὡς εἰ δεῖ τοῦτον τὸν τρόπον ἀποδιδόναι καὶ προσάπτειν ἕκα-20 στον τῶν αἰσθητηρίων ἑνὶ τῶν στοιχείων, τοῦ μὲν ὄμματος τὸ ὁρατικὸν ὕδατος ὑποληπτέον, ἀέρος δὲ τὸ τῶν ψόφων αἰσθητικόν, πυρὸς δὲ τὴν ὄσφρησιν. ὃ γὰρ ἐνεργείᾳ ἡ ὄσφρησις, τοῦτο δυνάμει τὸ ὀσφραντικόν· τὸ γὰρ αἰσθητὸν ἐνεργεῖν ποιεῖ τὴν αἴσθησιν, ὥσθ᾽ 25 ὑπάρχειν ἀναγκαῖον αὐτὴν ὃ δυνάμει πρότερον. ἡ δ᾽ ὀσμὴ καπνώδης ἀναθυμίασίς ἐστιν, ἡ δ᾽ ἀναθυμίασις ἡ καπνώδης ἐκ πυρός. διὸ καὶ τῷ περὶ τὸν ἐγκέφαλον τόπῳ τὸ τῆς ὀσφρήσεως αἰσθητήριόν ἐστιν ἴδιον· δυνά-μει γὰρ θερμὴ ἡ τοῦ ψυχροῦ ὕλη ἐστίν. καὶ ἡ τοῦ 30 ὄμματος γένεσις τὸν αὐτὸν ἔχει τρόπον· ἀπὸ τοῦ ἐγκεφάλου γὰρ συνέστηκεν· οὗτος γὰρ ὑγρότατος καὶ ψυχρότατος τῶν ἐν τῷ σώματι μορίων ἐστίν. τὸ δ᾽ 439 a ἁπτικὸν γῆς. τὸ δὲ γευστικὸν εἶδός τι ἀφῆς ἐστίν. καὶ διὰ τοῦτο πρὸς τῇ καρδίᾳ τὸ αἰσθητήριον αὐτῶν, τῆς τε γεύσεως καὶ τῆς ἁφῆς· ἀντίκειται γὰρ τῷ ἐγκεφάλῳ αὕτη, καὶ ἔστι θερμότατον τῶν μορίων. καὶ

---

438 b, 18 ὡς εἰ δεῖ (Biehl)] ὡς δεῖ E M Y et omnes edd., ὡς εἰ δεῖ reliqui codd. vet. tr. et sine dubio Alex., etiam Bäumker, Arist. Lehre von den Sinnesvermögen S. 47, ita scribi vult, cui assentitur Zeller, Gesch. der gr. Ph. II. 2, S. 538.

of water; for water is transparent. Just as we cannot see without the presence of light outside the eye, so without light inside the eye vision is impossible; this is the reason why the eye must be transparent, and since it is not air it must be water.

The reason for these contentions is that the consciousness, or the psychical faculty of sense perception, does not reside 10 on the surface of the eye but evidently within; this is why the interior of the eye must be transparent and receptive of light. The facts make this plain; for there have been cases of people wounded in war by a blow grazing the temple in such a way that the passages of the eye were severed, to whom darkness seemed to ensue just as when 15 a light is put out; this was because the transparency we call the pupil was severed like a lamp that has its wick cut.

Thus if our account is at all in accordance with fact and if, as in the fashion proposed, we should reduce the sensoria to the elements and correlate each of the former with one of the latter, it is clear we should ascribe the eye's power of 20 sight to water and the capacity of perceiving sounds to air and the sense of smell to fire.

This is because that which has the faculty of smell is potentially what smell is in actuality; for the object of sensation rouses the sense to activity, which hence necessarily is that which, before stimulation, it was potentially.

Now odour is a smoke-like fume and smoke-like fumes 25 originate from fire; hence the organ of smell is appropriately located in the regions around the brain, as the substrate of that which is cold is potentially hot.

The origin of the eyes is of the same fashion; they derive 30 their composition from the brain, the coldest and most watery of the bodily members.

The sense of touch is connected with earth; and taste is 439 a a species of touch. Hence the sensoria of both—taste as well as touch—are closely related to the heart, which has qualities contrary to those of the brain and is the warmest of the members.

5 περὶ μὲν τῶν αἰσθητικῶν τοῦ σώματος μορίων ἔστω τοῦτον τὸν τρόπον διωρισμένα.

III

Περὶ δὲ τῶν αἰσθητῶν τῶν καθ᾽ ἕκαστον αἰσθητήριον, οἷον λέγω χρώματος καὶ ψόφου καὶ ὀσμῆς καὶ χυμοῦ καὶ ἁφῆς, καθόλου μὲν εἴρηται ἐν τοῖς περὶ ψυχῆς, τί 10 τὸ ἔργον αὐτῶν καὶ τί τὸ ἐνεργεῖν καθ᾽ ἕκαστον τῶν αἰσθητηρίων. τί δέ ποτε δεῖ λέγειν ὁτιοῦν αὐτῶν, οἷον τί χρῶμα ἢ τί ψόφον ἢ τί ὀσμὴν ἢ χυμόν, ὁμοίως δὲ καὶ περὶ ἁφῆς, ἐπισκεπτέον, καὶ πρῶτον περὶ χρώματος. ἔστι μὲν οὖν ἕκαστον διχῶς λεγόμενον, τὸ μὲν ἐνεργείᾳ 15 τὸ δὲ δυνάμει. τὸ μὲν οὖν ἐνεργείᾳ χρῶμα καὶ ὁ ψόφος πῶς ἐστι τὸ αὐτὸ ἢ ἕτερον ταῖς κατ᾽ ἐνέργειαν αἰσθή-σεσιν, οἷον ὁράσει καὶ ἀκούσει, εἴρηται ἐν τοῖς περὶ ψυχῆς· τί δὲ ἕκαστον αὐτῶν ὂν ποιήσει τὴν αἴσθησιν καὶ τὴν ἐνέργειαν, νῦν λέγωμεν. ὥσπερ οὖν εἴρηται 20 περὶ φωτὸς ἐν ἐκείνοις, ὅτι ἐστὶ χρῶμα τοῦ διαφανοῦς κατὰ συμβεβηκός· ὅταν γὰρ ἐνῇ τι πυρῶδες ἐν διαφανεῖ, ἡ μὲν παρουσία φῶς, ἡ δὲ στέρησίς ἐστι σκότος· ὃ δὲ λέγομεν διαφανές, οὐκ ἔστιν ἴδιον ἀέρος ἢ ὕδατος οὐδ᾽ ἄλλου τῶν οὕτω λεγομένων σωμάτων, ἀλλά τις ἔστι 25 κοινὴ φύσις καὶ δύναμις, ἣ χωριστὴ μὲν οὐκ ἔστιν, ἐν τούτοις δ᾽ ἔστι, καὶ τοῖς ἄλλοις σώμασιν ἐνυπάρχει, τοῖς μὲν μᾶλλον τοῖς δ᾽ ἧττον· ὥσπερ οὖν καὶ τῶν σωμάτων ἀνάγκη τι εἶναι ἔσχατον, καὶ ταύτης· ἡ μὲν οὖν τοῦ φωτὸς φύσις ἐν ἀορίστῳ τῷ διαφανεῖ ἐστίν· 30 τοῦ δ᾽ ἐν τοῖς σώμασι διαφανοῦς τὸ ἔσχατον ὅτι μὲν εἴη ἄν τι, δῆλον, ὅτι δὲ τοῦτ᾽ ἐστὶ τὸ χρῶμα, ἐκ τῶν συμβαινόντων φανερόν. τὸ γὰρ χρῶμα ἢ ἐν τῷ πέρατί ἐστιν ἢ πέρας· διὸ καὶ οἱ Πυθαγόρειοι τὴν ἐπιφάνειαν χροιὰν ἐκάλουν· ἔστι μὲν γὰρ ἐν τῷ τοῦ σώματος πέρατι,

Let this be the way in which we discriminate the sensitive 5
organs of the body.

III

In the Psychology we have given a general account of the
objects corresponding to the particular sense-organs, to wit
colour, sound, smell, flavour, and touch ; we have stated what
their function is, and described the mode of their operation in 10
relation to the several sense-organs. But the nature we must
ascribe to any one of these objects we have still to consider ;
we must ask, for instance, what is colour, or sound, or odour,
or flavour? So, too, what is the object of touch? Let us
begin our inquiry with colour.

Now we can regard each of these sense objects in two
ways, as potentially or as actually existent. We have ex- 15
plained in the Psychology in what sense actual colour and
sound are identical with or different from actual sense experience, *e.g.* sight and hearing; but now we are to discuss
the nature of those sense objects in virtue of which they cause
sensation and its activity.

It was stated in the work quoted above when we treated
of light that it is the colour of the transparent medium con- 20
tingently determined ; for when anything of the nature of fire
is found in the transparent medium its presence constitutes
light, its absence darkness.

What we have spoken of as the transparent element is
nothing which is found exclusively in air or in water or in
any one of the substances of which transparency can be
predicated ; it is some sort of constitution and potency which
they have in common, and which, not being an independent 25
reality, finds its existence in these bodies and subsists in
varying degrees in the rest of material substances. Thus, in
so far as these bodies must have boundaries, this too must
have its limits.

Now it is in the transparent medium apart from its limits
that light has its being ; but it is clear that the boundary of
the transparent element which exists in bodies is something 30
real. That this is colour the facts make plain, for colour
either exists in the boundary or constitutes the boundary
of a thing, and hence (a corroborating circumstance) the
Pythagorean terminology identified the visible superficies
with colour. This was plausible, for colour exists in the

35 ἀλλ' οὔ τι τὸ τοῦ σώματος πέρας, ἀλλὰ τὴν αὐτὴν φύσιν
439 b δεῖ νομίζειν, ἥπερ καὶ ἔξω χρωματίζεται, ταύτην καὶ
ἐντός. φαίνεται δὲ καὶ ἀὴρ καὶ ὕδωρ χρωματιζόμενα·
καὶ γὰρ ἡ αὐγὴ τοιοῦτόν ἐστιν. ἀλλ' ἐκεῖ μὲν διὰ τὸ
ἐν ἀορίστῳ οὐ τὴν αὐτὴν ἐγγύθεν καὶ προσιοῦσι καὶ
5 πόρρωθεν ἔχει χροιὰν οὔθ' ὁ ἀὴρ οὔθ' ἡ θάλαττα· ἐν
δὲ τοῖς σώμασιν ἐὰν μὴ τὸ περιέχον ποιῇ τὸ μεταβάλλειν,
ὥρισται καὶ ἡ φαντασία τῆς χρόας. δῆλον ἄρα ὅτι τὸ
αὐτὸ κἀκεῖ κἀνθάδε δεκτικὸν τῆς χρόας ἐστίν. τὸ ἄρα
διαφανὲς καθ' ὅσον ὑπάρχει ἐν τοῖς σώμασιν (ὑπάρχει
10 δὲ μᾶλλον καὶ ἧττον ἐν πᾶσι) χρώματος ποιεῖ μετέχειν.
ἐπεὶ δ' ἐν πέρατι ἡ χρόα, τούτου ἂν ἐν πέρατι εἴη. ὥστε
χρῶμα ἂν εἴη τὸ τοῦ διαφανοῦς ἐν σώματι ὡρισμένῳ
πέρας. καὶ αὐτῶν δὲ τῶν διαφανῶν, οἷον ὕδατος καὶ
εἴ τι ἄλλο τοιοῦτον, καὶ ὅσοις φαίνεται χρῶμα ἴδιον
15 ὑπάρχειν κατὰ τὸ ἔσχατον, ὁμοίως πᾶσιν ὑπάρχει.
ἔστι μὲν οὖν ἐνεῖναι ἐν τῷ διαφανεῖ τοῦθ' ὅπερ καὶ ἐν
17 τῷ ἀέρι ποιεῖ φῶς, ἔστι δὲ μή, ἀλλ' ἐστερῆσθαι.
17
                                                Ὥσπερ οὖν
ἐκεῖ τὸ μὲν φῶς τὸ δὲ σκότος, οὕτως ἐν τοῖς σώμασιν
ἐγγίγνεται τὸ λευκὸν καὶ τὸ μέλαν. περὶ δὲ τῶν ἄλλων
20 χρωμάτων εἴδη διελομένους ποσαχῶς ἐνδέχεται γίγνεσθαι
λεκτέον. ἐνδέχεται μὲν γὰρ παρ' ἄλληλα τιθέμενα τὸ
λευκὸν καὶ τὸ μέλαν, ὥσθ' ἑκάτερον μὲν εἶναι ἀόρατον
διὰ σμικρότητα, τὸ δ' ἐξ ἀμφοῖν ὁρατόν, οὕτω γίγνεσθαι.
τοῦτο γὰρ οὔτε λευκὸν οἷόν τε φαίνεσθαι οὔτε μέλαν·
25 ἐπεὶ δ' ἀνάγκη μέν τι ἔχειν χρῶμα, τούτων δ' οὐδέτερον
δυνατόν, ἀνάγκη μικτόν τι εἶναι καὶ εἶδός τι χρόας
ἕτερον. ἔστι μὲν οὖν οὕτως ὑπολαβεῖν πλείους εἶναι
χρόας παρὰ τὸ λευκὸν καὶ τὸ μέλαν, πολλὰς δὲ τῷ
λόγῳ· τρία γὰρ πρὸς δύο, καὶ τρία πρὸς τέτταρα, καὶ
30 κατ' ἄλλους ἀριθμοὺς ἔστι παρ' ἄλληλα κεῖσθαι, τὰ δ'

439 b, 20 εἴδη conicio | ἤδη omn. codd. et edd.

boundary, but it by no means *is* the boundary of the body ; 35
nay, we must believe that internally there exists the same 439 b
constitution as externally displays colour. So both air and
water show tint ; the sheen they have is a phenomenon of
this kind ; but here, because it exists in something with no
definite boundaries, the colour both of the air and of the sea
is not the same when regarded from afar and from near at
hand.   In solid bodies, however, unless the surrounding 5
medium cause it to change, the coloured appearance remains,
equally with the surface, fixed.   It is therefore clear that in
both cases it is the same nature which is capable of being
endowed with colour : hence the transparent element in so
far as it is found in bodies (and it exists in all in varying
degrees) causes them to be endowed with colour.   But since 10
it is in a bounding surface that colour is found, it is in the
surface of this—the transparent element—that colour exists.
Colour then is the limit of the transparent element in a
determinately bounded body ; and it is found in all bodies
alike, both in transparent substances themselves, such as
water and anything similar to it, and in those which appear
to have a surface colour of their own.   Consequently, that, 15
which in air causes light, may be present in the transparent medium or it may not, *i.e.* may be awanting.

Thus, just as we can explain light and darkness respectively by the presence or absence of this cause in the
air, so in the case of solid bodies we can account for the
existence of black and white colour.   But the other colours
still await classification and an inquiry into the various ways 20
in which they may be produced.

Firstly, white and black may be juxtaposed in such a way
that by the minuteness of the division of its parts each is
invisible while their product is visible, and thus colour may
be produced.   This product can appear neither white nor
black, but, since it must have some colour and can have
neither of the above two, it must be a sort of compound and 25
a fresh kind of tint.   In this way, then, we may conceive that
numbers of colours over and above black and white may be
produced, and that their multiplicity is due to differences in
the proportion of their composition.   The juxtaposition may
be in the proportion of three of the one to two of the other,
or three to four or according to other ratios.   Others again 30

ὅλως κατὰ μὲν λόγον μηδένα, καθ᾽ ὑπεροχὴν δέ τινα
καὶ ἔλλειψιν ἀσύμμετρον, καὶ τὸν αὐτὸν δὴ τρόπον
ἔχειν ταῦτα ταῖς συμφωνίαις· τὰ μὲν γὰρ ἐν ἀριθμοῖς
εὐλογίστοις χρώματα, καθάπερ ἐκεῖ τὰς συμφωνίας, τὰ
440 a ἥδιστα τῶν χρωμάτων εἶναι δοκοῦντα, οἷον τὸ ἁλουργὸν
καὶ φοινικοῦν καὶ ὀλίγ᾽ ἄττα τοιαῦτα, δι᾽ ἥνπερ αἰτίαν
καὶ αἱ συμφωνίαι ὀλίγαι, τὰ δὲ μὴ ἐν ἀριθμοῖς τἆλλα
χρώματα, ἢ καὶ πάσας τὰς χρόας ἐν ἀριθμοῖς εἶναι, τὰς
5 μὲν τεταγμένας τὰς δὲ ἀτάκτους, καὶ αὐτὰς ταύτας, ὅταν
μὴ καθαραὶ ὦσι, διὰ τὸ μὴ ἐν ἀριθμοῖς εἶναι τοιαύτας
γίγνεσθαι. εἷς μὲν οὖν τρόπος τῆς γενέσεως τῶν χρωμάτων οὗτος, εἷς δὲ τὸ φαίνεσθαι δι᾽ ἀλλήλων, οἷον
ἐνίοτε οἱ γραφεῖς ποιοῦσιν, ἑτέραν χρόαν ἐφ᾽ ἑτέραν
10 ἐναργεστέραν ἐπαλείφουσιν, ὥσπερ ὅταν ἐν ὕδατί τι ἢ
ἐν ἀέρι βούλωνται ποιῆσαι φαινόμενον, καὶ οἷον ὁ ἥλιος
καθ᾽ αὑτὸν μὲν λευκὸς φαίνεται, διὰ δ᾽ ἀχλύος καὶ
καπνοῦ φοινικοῦς. πολλαὶ δὲ καὶ οὕτως ἔσονται χρόαι
τὸν αὐτὸν τρόπον τῷ πρότερον εἰρημένῳ· λόγος γὰρ ἂν
15 εἴη τις τῶν ἐπιπολῆς πρὸς τὰ ἐν βάθει, τὰ δὲ καὶ ὅλως
οὐκ ἐν λόγῳ. [τὸ μὲν οὖν, ὥσπερ καὶ οἱ ἀρχαῖοι, λέγειν
ἀπορροίας εἶναι τὰς χροίας καὶ ὁρᾶσθαι διὰ τοιαύτην
αἰτίαν ἄτοπον· πάντως γὰρ δι᾽ ἁφῆς ἀναγκαῖον αὐτοῖς
ποιεῖν τὴν αἴσθησιν, ὥστ᾽ εὐθὺς κρεῖττον φάναι τῷ
20 κινεῖσθαι τὸ μεταξὺ τῆς αἰσθήσεως ὑπὸ τοῦ αἰσθητοῦ
γίνεσθαι τὴν αἴσθησιν, ἁφῇ καὶ μὴ ταῖς ἀπορροίαις.]
ἐπὶ μὲν οὖν τῶν παρ᾽ ἄλληλα κειμένων ἀνάγκη ὥσπερ
καὶ μέγεθος λαμβάνειν ἀόρατον, οὕτω καὶ χρόνον ἀναίσθητον, ἵνα λάθωσιν αἱ κινήσεις ἀφικνούμεναι καὶ ἐν
25 δοκῇ εἶναι διὰ τὸ ἅμα φαίνεσθαι· ἐνταῦθα δὲ οὐδεμία
ἀνάγκη, ἀλλὰ τὸ ἐπιπολῆς χρῶμα ἀκίνητον ὂν καὶ κινούμενον ὑπὸ τοῦ ὑποκειμένου οὐχ ὁμοίαν ποιήσει τὴν

---

440 a, 21 interpositis vers. 16—21 contextum interrumpi recte iudicat Thurot,
cui assentitur Susemihl, Philol. 1855.

may be compounded in no commensurate proportion, with an excess of the one element and deficiency of the other which are incommensurable, and colours may, indeed, be analogous to harmonies. Thus, those compounded according to the simplest proportions, exactly as is the case in harmonies, will appear to be the most pleasant colours, *e.g.* purple, crimson, 440 a and a few similar species. (It is an exactly parallel reason that causes harmonies to be few in number.) Mixtures not in a calculable ratio will constitute the other colours. Or again, all tints may show a calculable proportion between their elements, but in some the scheme of composition may be regular, in others not, while when those of the latter class are themselves impure, this may be due to an absence of 5 calculable proportion in their composition.

This is one of the ways in which colours may be produced ; a second is effected by the shining of one colour through another. This we may illustrate by the practice sometimes adopted by painters when they give a wash of colour over another more vivid tint, when, for example, they wish to make a thing look 10 as though it were in the water or in the air. Again, we may illustrate by the sun, which in itself appears white, but looks red when seen through mist and smoke.

According to this account the multiplicity of the colours will be explained in the same way as in the theory mentioned before ; we should have to suppose there was some ratio between the superficial and the underlying tints in the case of some colours, while in others there would be an entire lack 15 of commensurate proportion.

[Thus we see that it is absurd to maintain, with the early philosophers, that colours are effluxes and that vision is effected by a cause of the efflux type. It was in every way binding on them to account for sensation by means of contact, and therefore it was obviously better to say that sensation was due to a movement set up by the sense object in the medium 20 of sensation, and thus account for it by contact without the instrumentality of effluxes.]

According to the theory of juxtaposition, just as we must assume that there are invisible spatial quanta, so must we postulate an imperceptible time to account for the imperceptibility of the diverse stimuli transmitted to the sense organ, which seem to be one because they appear to be simultaneous. But on the other theory there is no such 25 necessity ; the surface colour causes different motions in the medium when acted on and when not acted on by an under-

κίνησιν. διὸ καὶ ἕτερον φαίνεται καὶ οὔτε λευκὸν οὔτε
μέλαν. ὥστ᾽ εἰ μὴ ἐνδέχεται μηδὲν εἶναι μέγεθος
30 ἀόρατον, ἀλλὰ πᾶν ἔκ τινος ἀποστήματος ὁρατόν, καὶ
αὕτη τίς ἂν εἴη χρωμάτων μίξις; κἀκείνως δ᾽ οὐδὲν
κωλύει φαίνεσθαί τινα χρόαν κοινὴν τοῖς πόρρωθεν·
ὅτι γὰρ οὐκ ἔστιν οὐδὲν μέγεθος ἀόρατον, ἐν τοῖς
ὕστερον ἐπισκεπτέον. εἰ δ᾽ ἐστὶ μίξις τῶν σωμάτων
440 b μὴ μόνον τὸν τρόπον τοῦτον ὅνπερ οἴονταί τινες, παρ᾽
ἄλληλα τῶν ἐλαχίστων τιθεμένων, ἀδήλων δ᾽ ἡμῖν διὰ
τὴν αἴσθησιν, ἀλλ᾽ ὅλως πάντῃ πάντως, ὥσπερ ἐν τοῖς
περὶ μίξεως εἴρηται καθόλου περὶ πάντων· ἐκείνως μὲν
5 γὰρ μίγνυται ταῦτα μόνον ὅσα ἐνδέχεται διελεῖν εἰς τὰ
ἐλάχιστα, καθάπερ ἀνθρώπους ἵππους ἢ τὰ σπέρματα·
τῶν μὲν γὰρ ἀνθρώπων ἄνθρωπος ἐλάχιστος, τῶν δ᾽
ἵππων ἵππος· ὥστε τῇ τούτων παρ᾽ ἄλληλα θέσει τὸ
πλῆθος μέμικται τῶν συναμφοτέρων· ἄνθρωπον δὲ ἕνα
10 ἑνὶ ἵππῳ οὐ λέγομεν μεμῖχθαι· ὅσα δὲ μὴ διαιρεῖται εἰς
τὸ ἐλάχιστον, τούτων οὐκ ἐνδέχεται μίξιν γενέσθαι τὸν
τρόπον τοῦτον ἀλλὰ τῷ πάντῃ μεμῖχθαι, ἅπερ καὶ
μάλιστα μίγνυσθαι πέφυκεν· πῶς δὲ τοῦτο γίγνεσθαι
δυνατόν, ἐν τοῖς περὶ μίξεως εἴρηται πρότερον· ἀλλ᾽ ὅτι
15 ἀνάγκη μιγνυμένων καὶ τὰς χρόας μίγνυσθαι, δῆλον,
καὶ ταύτην τὴν αἰτίαν εἶναι κυρίαν τοῦ πολλὰς εἶναι
χροίας, ἀλλὰ μὴ τὴν ἐπιπόλασιν μηδὲ τὴν παρ᾽ ἄλληλα
θέσιν· οὐ γὰρ πόρρωθεν μὲν ἐγγύθεν δ᾽ οὐ φαίνεται
μία χρόα τῶν μεμιγμένων, ἀλλὰ πάντοθεν. πολλαὶ δ᾽
20 ἔσονται χρόαι διὰ τὸ πολλοῖς λόγοις ἐνδέχεσθαι μίγνυσθαι ἀλλήλοις τὰ μιγνύμενα, καὶ τὰ μὲν ἐν ἀριθμοῖς
τὰ δὲ καθ᾽ ὑπεροχὴν μόνον. καὶ τἆλλα δὴ τὸν αὐτὸν
τρόπον ὅνπερ ἐπὶ τῶν παρ᾽ ἄλληλα τιθεμένων χρωμάτων
ἢ ἐπιπολῆς, ἐνδέχεται λέγειν καὶ περὶ τῶν μιγνυμένων.

---

440 a, 31 τίς...μίξις; Simon | τις...μίξις. Biehl, Bek. et ceteri omnes.

lying tint. Thus it appears to be something different, and neither black nor white.

Therefore, if an invisible spatial quantity is an impossibility and every magnitude must be visible at some distance, we must dismiss the former theory and ask what sort of a colour 30 mixture this latter also is. But, on the former theory as well, there is nothing to prevent distant objects appearing to have a uniform colour ; for no magnitude is invisible, a problem to be discussed later on.

But let us premise that substances are mixed not merely 440 b in the way some people think—by a juxtaposition of their ultimate minute parts, which, however, are imperceptible to sense—but that they entirely interpenetrate each other in every part throughout ; how this happens in all cases was explained in general terms in our dissertation on mixture. The former theory accounts for the mixture only of those 5 things which can be resolved into ultimate least parts, *e.g.* men or horses or seeds. In a division of men, a man is the least part ; in the case of horses, a horse ; thus by the juxtaposition of these individuals the mixture produced is a mass consisting of both components, whereas we do not talk of mixing single man with single horse. On the other hand, 10 things which cannot be resolved into least parts, cannot be mingled in this way; they must entirely interpenetrate each other ; and these are the things which most naturally mix. We have already, in our treatment of mixture, explained how this is possible.

Now, all this being so, it is clear that when substances are 15 mixed their colours too must be commingled, and that this is the supreme reason why there is a plurality of colours ; neither superposition nor juxtaposition is the cause. In such mixtures the colour does not appear single when you are at a distance and diverse when you come near ; it is a single tint from all points of view. The reason for the multiplicity of colours will be the fact that things which mix can be mixed in many 20 different proportions, and some mixtures will show a numerical ratio, others only an incommensurable excess of one of the elements. So far indeed as other considerations go, the same account will apply to the juxtaposition or superposition of

25 διὰ τίνα δ᾽ αἰτίαν εἴδη τῶν χρωμάτων ἐστὶν ὡρισμένα
καὶ οὐκ ἄπειρα, καὶ χυμῶν καὶ ψόφων, ὕστερον ἐροῦμεν.

IV

Τί μὲν οὖν ἐστὶ χρῶμα καὶ διὰ τίν᾽ αἰτίαν πολλαὶ
χροιαί εἰσιν, εἴρηται· περὶ δὲ ψόφου καὶ φωνῆς εἴρηται
πρότερον ἐν τοῖς περὶ ψυχῆς· περὶ δὲ ὀσμῆς καὶ χυμοῦ
30 νῦν λεκτέον. σχεδὸν γάρ ἐστι τὸ αὐτὸ πάθος, οὐκ ἐν
τοῖς αὐτοῖς δ᾽ ἐστὶν ἑκάτερον αὐτῶν. ἐναργέστερον δ᾽
ἐστὶν ἡμῖν τὸ τῶν χυμῶν γένος ἢ τὸ τῆς ὀσμῆς. τούτου
441 a δ᾽ αἴτιον ὅτι χειρίστην ἔχομεν τῶν ἄλλων ζῴων τὴν
ὄσφρησιν καὶ τῶν ἐν ἡμῖν αὐτοῖς αἰσθήσεων, τὴν δ᾽
ἀφὴν ἀκριβεστάτην τῶν ἄλλων ζῴων. ἡ δὲ γεῦσις
4 ἀφή τις ἐστίν.

4 Ἡ μὲν οὖν τοῦ ὕδατος ψύσις βούλεται
5 ἄχυμος εἶναι· ἀνάγκη δ᾽ ἢ ἐν αὐτῷ τὸ ὕδωρ ἔχειν τὰ
γένη τῶν χυμῶν ἀναίσθητα διὰ μικρότητα, καθάπερ
Ἐμπεδοκλῆς φησίν, ἢ ὕλην τοιαύτην εἶναι οἷον πανσπερμίαν χυμῶν, καὶ ἅπαντα μὲν ἐξ ὕδατος γίγνεσθαι,
ἄλλα δ᾽ ἐξ ἄλλου μέρους, ἢ μηδεμίαν ἔχοντος διαφορὰν
10 τοῦ ὕδατος τὸ ποιοῦν αἴτιον εἶναι, οἷον εἰ τὸ θερμὸν
καὶ τὸν ἥλιον φαίη τις. τούτων δ᾽, ὡς μὲν Ἐμπεδοκλῆς
λέγει, λίαν εὐσύνοπτον τὸ ψεῦδος· ὁρῶμεν γὰρ μεταβάλλοντας ὑπὸ τοῦ θερμοῦ τοὺς χυμοὺς ἀφαιρουμένων
τῶν περικαρπίων εἰς τὸν ἥλιον καὶ πυρρουμένων, ὡς
15 οὐ τῷ ἐκ τοῦ ὕδατος ἕλκειν τοιούτους γιγνομένους, ἀλλ᾽
ἐν αὐτῷ τῷ περικαρπίῳ μεταβάλλοντας, καὶ ἐξικμαζο-
μένους δὲ καὶ κειμένους, διὰ τὸν χρόνον, αὐστηροὺς ἐκ
γλυκέων καὶ πικροὺς καὶ παντοδαποὺς γιγνομένους, καὶ
ἑψομένους εἰς πάντα τὰ γένη τῶν χυμῶν ὡς εἰπεῖν
20 μεταβάλλοντας. ὁμοίως δὲ καὶ τὸ πανσπερμίας εἶναι

---

441 a, 14 πυρρουμένων conicio | πυρουμένων Biehl, Bek. etc.

colours as to their mixture. The reason why they, and like- 25 wise tastes and sounds, have definite species limited in number, will be given later on.

IV

We have defined colour and accounted for the multiplicity of its tints, while sound and articulate utterance have been treated in the Psychology; we are now to discuss smell and taste.

While as subjective phenomena they are practically 30 identical, their vehicle is diverse ; and tastes as a class are more vividly presented to human perception than odours. The reason for this is that our sense of smell is inferior to that 441 a of other animals, and is the poorest of the human senses. In delicacy of touch, however, we excel all other animals; now taste is a sort of touch.

To proceed to our discussion—water is characteristically of a flavourless nature ; yet, either it must, tasteless as it is, 5 be the receptacle in which the various flavours reside in amounts too minute to be detected—the Empedoclean theory —or it must be a material adapted to be the matrix, as it were, for the germs of all tastes. In this case all tastes will originate out of water, but different ones will arise from different parts of the matrix. Or we may hold that water is entirely undifferentiated, and impute the causality to that which acts upon it, for instance heat or the sun. A glance 10 will suffice to show the falsity of the Empedoclean theory; for we can observe that the alteration in flavour is due to heat, when fruits are plucked, integument and all, and set in the sun and reddened. Their new flavour, then, cannot be extracted from water ; nay, the change must take place within the fruit- 15 covering itself. Through lying and drying fruits become, in time, harsh and bitter instead of sweet, and display all sorts of flavours; further, any kind of taste, so to speak, can be produced by subjecting them to the process of cooking.

Similarly water cannot possibly constitute the material of 20

τὸ ὕδωρ ὕλην ἀδύνατον· ἐκ τοῦ αὐτοῦ γὰρ ὁρῶμεν ὡς
τροφῆς γιγνομένους ἑτέρους χυμούς. λείπεται δὴ τῷ
πάσχειν τι τὸ ὕδωρ μεταβάλλειν. ὅτι μὲν τοίνυν οὐχ
ὑπὸ τῆς τοῦ θερμοῦ δυνάμεως λαμβάνει ταύτην τὴν
25 δύναμιν ἣν καλοῦμεν χυμόν, φανερόν· λεπτότατον γὰρ
τῶν πάντων ὑγρῶν τὸ ὕδωρ ἐστί, καὶ αὐτοῦ τοῦ ἐλαίου·
ἀλλ' ἐπεκτείνεται ἐπὶ πλεῖον τοῦ ὕδατος τὸ ἔλαιον διὰ
τὴν γλισχρότητα· τὸ δ' ὕδωρ ψαθυρόν ἐστι· διὸ καὶ
χαλεπώτερον φυλάξαι ἐν τῇ χειρὶ τὸ ὕδωρ ἤπερ ἔλαιον.
30 ἐπεὶ δὲ θερμαινόμενον οὐδὲν φαίνεται παχυνόμενον τὸ
ὕδωρ αὐτὸ μόνον, δῆλον ὅτι ἑτέρα τις ἂν εἴη αἰτία·
οἱ γὰρ χυμοὶ πάντες πάχος ἔχουσι μᾶλλον· τὸ δὲ
θερμὸν συναίτιον. φαίνονται δ' οἱ χυμοὶ ὅσοιπερ καὶ
441 b ἐν τοῖς περικαρπίοις, οὗτοι ὑπάρχοντες καὶ ἐν τῇ γῇ.
διὸ καὶ πολλοί φασι τῶν ἀρχαίων φυσιολόγων τοιοῦτον
εἶναι τὸ ὕδωρ δι' οἵας ἂν γῆς πορεύηται. καὶ τοῦτο
δῆλόν ἐστιν ἐπὶ τῶν ἁλμυρῶν ὑδάτων μάλιστα· οἱ γὰρ
5 ἅλες γῆς τι εἶδός εἰσιν. καὶ τὰ διὰ τῆς τέφρας διηθού-
μενα πικρᾶς οὔσης πικρὸν ποιεῖ τὸν χυμόν. εἰσί τε
κρῆναι πολλαὶ αἱ μὲν πικραί, αἱ δ' ὀξεῖαι, αἱ δὲ παντοδαποὺς ἔχουσαι χυμοὺς ἄλλους. διὸ εὐλόγως ἐν τοῖς
φυομένοις τὸ τῶν χυμῶν γίγνεται γένος μάλιστα. πά-
10 σχειν γὰρ πέφυκε τὸ ὑγρόν, ὥσπερ καὶ τἆλλα, ὑπὸ
τοῦ ἐναντίου· ἐναντίον δὲ τὸ ξηρόν. διὸ καὶ ὑπὸ τοῦ
πυρὸς πάσχει τι· ξηρὰ γὰρ ἡ τοῦ πυρὸς φύσις. ἀλλ'
ἴδιον τοῦ πυρὸς τὸ θερμόν ἐστι, γῆς δὲ τὸ ξηρόν,
ὥσπερ εἴρηται ἐν τοῖς περὶ στοιχείων. ᾗ μὲν οὖν πῦρ
15 καὶ ᾗ γῆ, οὐδὲν πέφυκε ποιεῖν καὶ πάσχειν, οὐδ' ἄλλο
οὐδέν· ᾗ δ' ὑπάρχει ἐναντιότης ἐν ἑκάστῳ, ταύτῃ πάντα
καὶ ποιοῦσι καὶ πάσχουσιν. ὥσπερ οὖν οἱ ἐναποπλύνοντες ἐν τῷ ὑγρῷ τὰ χρώματα καὶ τοὺς χυμοὺς τοιοῦτον
ἔχειν ποιοῦσι τὸ ὕδωρ, οὕτως καὶ ἡ φύσις τὸ ξηρὸν

---

441 b, 8 διὸ εὐλόγως L S U | εὐλόγως δ' Biehl et Bek.

a universal matrix of flavours. It is a matter of observation that out of the very same water taken as nutriment, plants develop different flavours.

True, this leaves us with the theory that the water is acted on in some way, and changes in consequence. Now, plainly, it is not owing to the power resident in heat that it acquires the potency we call flavour; water is the thinnest of all liquids, 25 thinner even than oil, though oil on the other hand spreads out more than water on account of its viscosity. Water, however, is non-cohesive, and hence is more difficult to keep in the hand without spilling than oil.

Since water by itself is the only substance which shows no 30 thickening under the influence of heat, clearly something else must be the cause of the phenomenon in question, for all flavours tend to exhibit density. The heat is the cooperating cause.

It is a conspicuous fact that all the savours found in fruits exist also in the soil. Hence many of the early physical 441 b philosophers allege that water takes its character from the soil through which it passes. This is clearly so in the case of saline waters, for salt is a species of earth. Filtration through 5 ash—a bitter substance—makes the taste bitter, and there are many springs, some of which are bitter, some acid, and others possessing manifold other tastes. Hence, as one would expect, it is principally in plants that flavours as a class develop.

The reason for this acquisition of a specific character by water is—it is the nature of humidity, as of everything else, to be acted on by its opposite; now its opposite is dryness. 10 Hence fire too has an effect upon it, for fire by constitution is dry. But of fire heat is a peculiar property, of earth dryness, as we explained in discussing the elements.

Now, by constitution, fire *quâ* fire and earth *quâ* earth do not display activity and passivity, nor do any of the other 15 elements *per se*; it is in so far as they have opposing qualities that the elements one and all react on each other. Thus, just as men by dissolving colours or savours in water communicate those qualities to the water, so nature acts upon that which is dry and earthy in character; by the aid of heat it causes liquid

20 καὶ τὸ γεῶδες, καὶ διὰ τοῦ ξηροῦ καὶ γεώδους διηθοῦσα
καὶ κινοῦσα τῷ θερμῷ ποιόν τι τὸ ὑγρὸν παρασκευάζει.
καὶ ἔστι τοῦτο χυμὸς τὸ γιγνόμενον ὑπὸ τοῦ εἰρημένου
ξηροῦ πάθος ἐν τῷ ὑγρῷ τῆς γεύσεως τῆς κατὰ δύναμιν
ἀλλοιωτικὸν εἰς ἐνέργειαν· ἄγει γὰρ τὸ αἰσθητικὸν εἰς
25 τοῦτο δυνάμει προϋπάρχον· οὐ γὰρ κατὰ τὸ μανθάνειν
ἀλλὰ κατὰ τὸ θεωρεῖν ἐστι τὸ αἰσθάνεσθαι. ὅτι δ' οὐ
παντὸς ξηροῦ ἀλλὰ τοῦ τροφίμου οἱ χυμοὶ ἢ πάθος
εἰσὶν ἢ στέρησις, δεῖ λαβεῖν ἐντεῦθεν, ὅτι οὔτε τὸ ξηρὸν
ἄνευ τοῦ ὑγροῦ οὔτε τὸ ὑγρὸν ἄνευ τοῦ ξηροῦ· τροφὴ
30 γὰρ οὐχ ἓν μόνον τοῖς ζῴοις, ἀλλὰ τὸ μεμιγμένον. καὶ
ἔστι τῆς προσφερομένης τροφῆς τοῖς ζῴοις τὰ μὲν ἁπτὰ
τῶν αἰσθητῶν αὔξησιν ποιοῦντα καὶ φθίσιν· τούτων
μὲν γὰρ αἴτιον ᾗ θερμὸν καὶ ψυχρὸν τὸ προσφερόμενον·
442 a ταῦτα γὰρ ποιεῖ καὶ αὔξησιν καὶ φθίσιν· τρέφει δὲ ᾗ
γευστὸν τὸ προσφερόμενον· πάντα γὰρ τρέφεται τῷ
γλυκεῖ, ἢ ἁπλῶς ἢ μεμιγμένως. δεῖ μὲν οὖν διορίζειν
περὶ τούτων ἐν τοῖς περὶ γενέσεως, νῦν δ' ὅσον ἀναγκαῖον
5 ἅψασθαι αὐτῶν. τὸ γὰρ θερμὸν αὐξάνει καὶ δημιουργεῖ
τὴν τροφήν, καὶ τὸ μὲν κοῦφον ἕλκει, τὸ δ' ἁλμυρὸν
καὶ πικρὸν καταλείπει διὰ βάρος. ὃ δὴ ἐν τοῖς ἔξω
σώμασι ποιεῖ τὸ ἔξω θερμόν, τοῦτο τὸ ἐν τῇ φύσει
τῶν ζῴων καὶ φυτῶν· διὸ τρέφεται τῷ γλυκεῖ. συμμί-
10 γνυνται δ' οἱ ἄλλοι χυμοὶ εἰς τὴν τροφὴν τὸν αὐτὸν
τρόπον τῷ ἁλμυρῷ καὶ ὀξεῖ, ἀντὶ ἡδύσματος. ταῦτα
δὲ διὰ τὸ ἀντὶ πάντων λίαν τρόφιμον εἶναι τὸ γλυκὺ
13 καὶ ἐπιπολαστικόν.
13   ὥσπερ δὲ τὰ χρώματα ἐκ λευκοῦ καὶ
μέλανος μίξεώς ἐστιν, οὕτως οἱ χυμοὶ ἐκ γλυκέος καὶ
15 πικροῖ. καὶ κατὰ λόγον δὴ τῷ μᾶλλον καὶ ἧττον
ἕκαστοί εἰσιν, εἴτε κατ' ἀριθμούς τινας τῆς μίξεως καὶ

441 b, 30 οὐχ ἓν μόνον | οὐδὲν αὐτῶν Biehl.
442 a, 12 ἀντὶ πάντων Biehl | ἀντισπᾶν τῷ Bek. et reliqui edd.

to percolate and pass through dry and earthy substance, and 20 thus gives it a definite quality. This is flavour, the modification which the said dry element produces in liquids, and which is capable of stimulating the sense of taste existing as a potentiality into active operation. This effect which it produces upon the sense-faculty has already potential existence in the sense-faculty, for sensation is parallel, not to learning, but to the exercise of knowledge.

It is not of all dry substance but of that which is nutritive 25 that flavours are a modification positive or negative. The fact that neither does the dry apart from the humid nor liquidity apart from dryness yield savour, supplies us with a proof of this, for neither of these alone, but their mixture, furnishes nutriment to animals. In the food of animals it is 30 the objects of tactual sensation that cause growth and decay; it is *quâ* hot or cold that the food they eat is responsible for these phenomena, as heat and cold cause growth and decay. 442 a On the other hand it is in so far as it affects the taste that what is given to animals nourishes them, for they all thrive on that which is sweet, either pure or mixed with something else.

The full discussion of these facts which is entailed will be found in the work *On Generation*; at present we must touch on them only so far as is necessary. Heat causes growth; it 5 is the active cause in the preparation of food, making the light elements rise and allowing the saline and bitter to fall on account of their weight. In fact, in plants and animals, their native heat performs the same function as that fulfilled by external heat in the case of external bodies; hence it is by sweet things that they are nourished. Other tastes are commingled with food for the same reason as the saline and acid; 10 they serve as seasoning. This is necessary because the sweet is, in comparison with all other things, excessively nutritive, and tends to rise in the stomach.

Just as colours arise from a mixture of black and white, so tastes are a product of the sweet and the bitter. Proportion it is—a difference in the quantity of their components, that 15 gives them individuality; and either the mixture and conse-

κινήσεως, εἴτε καὶ ἀορίστως. οἱ δὲ τὴν ἡδονὴν ποιοῦντες μιγνύμενοι, οὗτοι ἐν ἀριθμοῖς. μόνος μὲν οὖν λιπαρὸς ὁ τοῦ γλυκέος ἐστὶ χυμός, τὸ δ' ἁλμυρὸν καὶ πικρὸν 20 σχεδὸν τὸ αὐτό, ὁ δὲ αὐστηρὸς καὶ δριμὺς καὶ στρυφνὸς καὶ ὀξὺς ἀνὰ μέσον. σχεδὸν γὰρ ἴσα καὶ τὰ τῶν χυμῶν εἴδη καὶ τὰ τῶν χρωμάτων ἐστίν. ἑπτὰ γὰρ ἀμφοτέρων εἴδη, ἄν τις τιθῇ, ὥσπερ εὔλογον, τὸ φαιὸν μέλαν τι εἶναι· λείπεται γὰρ τὸ ξανθὸν μὲν τοῦ λευκοῦ εἶναι 25 ὥσπερ τὸ λιπαρὸν τοῦ γλυκέος, τὸ φοινικοῦν δὲ καὶ ἁλουργὸν καὶ πράσινον καὶ κυανοῦν ἀνὰ μέσον τοῦ λευκοῦ καὶ μέλανος, τὰ δ' ἄλλα μικτὰ ἐκ τούτων. καὶ ὥσπερ τὸ μέλαν στέρησις ἐν τῷ διαφανεῖ τοῦ λευκοῦ, οὕτω τὸ ἁλμυρὸν καὶ πικρὸν τοῦ γλυκέος ἐν τῷ τροφίμῳ 30 ὑγρῷ. διὸ καὶ ἡ τέφρα τῶν καομένων πικρὰ πάντων· 31 ἐξίκμασται γὰρ τὸ πότιμον ἐξ αὐτῶν.

31   Δημόκριτος δὲ καὶ οἱ πλεῖστοι τῶν φυσιολόγων, ὅσοι λέγουσι περὶ αἰσθήσεως, 442 b ἀτοπώτατόν τι ποιοῦσιν· πάντα γὰρ τὰ αἰσθητὰ ἁπτὰ ποιοῦσιν. καίτοι εἰ καὶ τοῦτο οὕτως ἔχει, δῆλον ὡς καὶ τῶν ἄλλων αἰσθήσεων ἑκάστη ἁφή τις ἐστίν· τοῦτο δ' ὅτι ἀδύνατον, οὐ χαλεπὸν συνιδεῖν. ἔτι δὲ τοῖς κοινοῖς 5 τῶν αἰσθήσεων πασῶν χρῶνται ὡς ἰδίοις· μέγεθος γὰρ καὶ σχῆμα καὶ τὸ τραχὺ καὶ τὸ λεῖον, ἔτι δὲ τὸ ὀξὺ καὶ τὸ ἀμβλὺ τὸ ἐν τοῖς ὄγκοις κοινὰ τῶν αἰσθήσεών ἐστιν, εἰ δὲ μὴ πασῶν, ἀλλ' ὄψεώς γε καὶ ἁφῆς. διὸ καὶ περὶ μὲν τούτων ἀπατῶνται, περὶ δὲ τῶν ἰδίων οὐκ 10 ἀπατῶνται, οἷον ἡ ὄψις περὶ χρώματος καὶ ἡ ἀκοὴ περὶ ψόφων. οἱ δὲ τὰ ἴδια εἰς ταῦτα ἀνάγουσιν, ὥσπερ Δημόκριτος τὸ λευκὸν καὶ τὸ μέλαν· τὸ μὲν γὰρ τραχύ φησιν εἶναι τὸ δὲ λεῖον, εἰς δὲ τὰ σχήματα ἀνάγει τοὺς χυμούς. καίτοι ἢ οὐδεμιᾶς ἢ μᾶλλον τῆς ὄψεως τὰ 15 κοινὰ γνωρίζειν. εἰ δ' ἄρα τῆς γεύσεως μᾶλλον, τὰ

---

442 a, 22 ἑπτὰ] ἒξ volunt legi Biehl et Susemihl, Philol. 1885.

quent stimulus is in terms of some numerical ratio, or it varies
indefinitely.

The mixtures, however, which produce pleasure are in a
calculable proportion. Sweet flavours alone are oily ; saline
and bitter are practically the same ; but sour, pungent, 20
astringent, and acid occupy an intermediate position. The
species of tastes and colours are practically equal in number.
If, as is reasonable, one reckons grey to be a kind of black,
there are seven of each, for there remain yellow—to be
referred to white, as oily was to sweet—with crimson, purple, 25
green, and blue intermediate between black and white ; and
all other colours are got by combining these. Just as black
is absence of white in the transparent medium so salinity and
bitterness are a deficiency of sweetness in nutritive liquid.
Consequently the ashes of things which have been burned 30
are bitter, for the scorching they have received has expelled
their palatable fluid qualities.

Democritus and most of the physical philosophers who
treat of sensation commit a most senseless blunder. They 442 b
identify all sense qualities with the tactual. It is clear
that if this were true each of the other senses would be
a sort of touch ; but it is not difficult to see that this is
impossible.

In addition they treat the common sensibles as though
they were the objects of a special sense ; but this is erroneous,
for magnitude, figure, roughness, and smoothness, as well as 5
the sharpness and bluntness found in material bodies, are
generic objects of sensation which, if not discerned by all the
senses, are common to sight and touch at least. Hence we
can explain the fact that we can make mistakes in perceiving
the latter, but are never deceived as to the special sensibles ;
sight, for instance, makes no mistakes about colour, nor does 10
hearing err in the matter of sounds.

These philosophers, however, reduce the special to the
common, following the example of Democritus in the case of
black and white. He identifies the one with the rough, the
other with the smooth, and he reduces flavours to geometrical
figures. But it falls to sight first, if to any sense, to discriminate 15

γοῦν ἐλάχιστα τῆς ἀκριβεστάτης ἐστὶν αἰσθήσεως διακρίνειν περὶ ἕκαστον γένος, ὥστε ἐχρῆν τὴν γεῦσιν
καὶ τῶν ἄλλων κοινῶν αἰσθάνεσθαι μάλιστα καὶ τῶν
σχημάτων εἶναι κριτικωτάτην. ἔτι τὰ μὲν αἰσθητὰ
20 πάντα ἔχει ἐναντίωσιν, οἷον ἐν χρώματι τῷ μέλανι τὸ
λευκὸν καὶ ἐν χυμοῖς τῷ γλυκεῖ τὸ πικρόν· σχῆμα δὲ
σχήματι οὐ δοκεῖ εἶναι ἐναντίον· τίνι γὰρ τῶν πολυ-
γώνων τὸ περιφερὲς ἐναντίον; ἔτι ἀπείρων ὄντων τῶν
σχημάτων ἀναγκαῖον καὶ τοὺς χυμοὺς εἶναι ἀπείρους·
25 διὰ τί γὰρ ὁ μὲν ἂν ποιήσειεν αἴσθησιν, ὁ δ᾽ οὐκ ἂν
ποιήσειεν; καὶ περὶ μὲν τοῦ γευστοῦ καὶ χυμοῦ εἴρηται·
τὰ γὰρ ἄλλα πάθη τῶν χυμῶν οἰκείαν ἔχει τὴν σκέψιν
ἐν τῇ φυσιολογίᾳ τῇ περὶ τῶν φυτῶν.

V

Τὸν αὐτὸν δὲ τρόπον δεῖ νοῆσαι καὶ περὶ τὰς ὀσμάς·
30 ὅπερ γὰρ ποιεῖ ἐν τῷ ὑγρῷ τὸ ξηρόν, τοῦτο ποιεῖ ἐν
ἄλλῳ γένει τὸ ἔγχυμον ὑγρόν, ἐν ἀέρι καὶ ὕδατι ὁμοίως.
κοινὸν δὲ κατὰ τούτων νῦν μὲν λέγομεν τὸ διαφανές,
443 a ἔστι δ᾽ ὀσφραντὸν οὐχ ᾗ διαφανές, ἀλλ᾽ ᾗ πλυντικὸν ἢ
ῥυπτικὸν ἐγχύμου ξηρότητος· οὐ γὰρ μόνον ἐν ἀέρι
ἀλλὰ καὶ ἐν ὕδατι τὸ τῆς ὀσφρήσεώς ἐστιν. δῆλον δ᾽
ἐπὶ τῶν ἰχθύων καὶ τῶν ὀστρακοδέρμων· φαίνονται γὰρ
5 ὀσφραινόμενα οὔτε ἀέρος ὄντος ἐν τῷ ὕδατι (ἐπιπολάζει
γὰρ ὁ ἀήρ, ὅταν ἐγγένηται) οὔτ᾽ αὐτὰ ἀναπνέοντα. εἰ
οὖν τις θείη καὶ τὸν ἀέρα καὶ τὸ ὕδωρ ἄμφω ὑγρά,
εἴη ἂν ἡ ἐν ὑγρῷ τοῦ ἐγχύμου ξηροῦ φύσις ὀσμή, καὶ
ὀσφραντὸν τὸ τοιοῦτον. ὅτι δ᾽ ἀπ᾽ ἐγχύμου ἐστὶ τὸ
10 πάθος, δῆλον ἐκ τῶν ἐχόντων καὶ μὴ ἐχόντων ὀσμήν·
τά τε γὰρ στοιχεῖα ἄοσμα, οἷον πῦρ ἀὴρ γῆ ὕδωρ, διὰ
τὸ τά τε ὑγρὰ καὶ ξηρὰ αὐτῶν ἄχυμα εἶναι, ἂν μή τι
μιγνύμενον ποιῇ. διὸ καὶ ἡ θάλαττα ἔχει ὀσμήν· ἔχει

the common sensibles ; it is, at any rate, the function of the most delicate sense to discern the finest differences in its particular domain, and so, if it fall to taste first to perceive the common sensibles, taste would need to possess the finest discrimination of figure and be as well the best means of perceiving the other common sensibles.

A further objection is, that the objects of special sense all show contrariety in their determinations; for example, in 20 colour black and white are opposed, in taste sweet and bitter. But there seems to be no opposition between one figure and another. To which of the polygons is the circle a contrary? Again, as figures are infinite in number, there must be an infinitude of tastes also, for why should one figure produce a 25 taste and not another?

This is our account of flavour and its effect on taste. The other qualities which flavours present find their special treatment in the Natural History of Plants.

V

The theory to be accepted about odour also is the same as that about flavour. Precisely as dry substance produces 30 an effect in liquid, liquid impregnated with flavour acts in a new field, operating in air and water alike.

We have just said that the transparent element is common to these two substances, but it is not *quâ* transparent that 443 a they affect the sense of smell ; they do this in so far as they dissolve and absorb by erosion dry substance which possesses flavour ; both substances form a medium for this sense, for smell is exercised not only in air but in water also. The case of the fishes and the testacea makes this plain ; they evidently employ the sense of smell and yet neither is there 5 air in the water (for it rises to the surface if ever it gets in) nor do these animals breathe.

Premising, then, the fact that air and water are both moist, we might define odour as the nature dry substance possessing flavour assumes in the moist, and the object of the sense of smell will be anything so qualified.

That this phenomenon issues from the possession of flavour, is clear on a review of those substances that are and 10 those that are not odorous. The elements have no odour, to wit—fire, air, earth, and water, since they are flavourless— both those of them which are moist and those which are dry—except when forming a combination. Hence the sea too smells, for it has a taste and contains dry substance.

γὰρ χυμὸν καὶ ξηρότητα. καὶ ἅλες μᾶλλον νίτρου
15 ὀσμώδεις· δηλοῖ δὲ τὸ ἐξικμάζον ἐξ αὐτῶν ἔλαιον· τὸ
δὲ νίτρον γῆς ἐστὶ μᾶλλον. ἔτι λίθος μὲν ἄοσμον,
ἄχυμον γάρ, τὰ δὲ ξύλα ὀσμώδη, ἔγχυμα γάρ· καὶ
τούτων τὰ ὑδατώδη ἧττον. ἔτι ἐπὶ τῶν μεταλλευομένων
χρυσὸς ἄοσμον, ἄχυμον γάρ, ὁ δὲ χαλκὸς καὶ ὁ σίδηρος
20 ὀσμώδη. ὅταν δ' ἐκκαυθῇ τὸ ὑγρόν, ἀοσμότεραι αἱ
σκωρίαι γίγνονται πάντων. ἄργυρος δὲ καὶ καττίτερος
τῶν μὲν μᾶλλον ὀσμώδη τῶν δ' ἧττον· ὑδατώδη γάρ.
δοκεῖ δ' ἐνίοις ἡ καπνώδης ἀναθυμίασις εἶναι ὀσμή,
οὖσα κοινὴ γῆς τε καὶ ἀέρος. [καὶ πάντες ἐπιφέρονται
25 ἐπὶ τοῦτο περὶ ὀσμῆς·] διὸ καὶ Ἡράκλειτος οὕτως
εἴρηκεν, ὡς εἰ πάντα τὰ ὄντα καπνὸς γίγνοιτο, ὅτι ῥῖνες
ἂν διαγνοῖεν. ἐπεὶ δὲ τὴν ὀσμὴν πάντες ἐπιφέρονται
<ἐπὶ τοῦτο>, οἱ μὲν ὡς ἀτμίδα, οἱ δ' ὡς ἀναθυμίασιν,
οἱ δ' ὡς ἄμφω ταῦτα· ἔστι δ' ἡ μὲν ἀτμὶς ὑγρότης τις,
30 ἡ δὲ καπνώδης ἀναθυμίασις, ὥσπερ εἴρηται, κοινὸν ἀέρος
καὶ γῆς· καὶ συνίσταται ἐκ μὲν ἐκείνης ὕδωρ, ἐκ δὲ
ταύτης γῆς τι εἶδος· ἀλλ' οὐδέτερον τούτων ἔοικεν· ἡ
μὲν γὰρ ἀτμίς ἐστιν ὕδατος, ἡ δὲ καπνώδης ἀναθυμίασις
ἀδύνατος ἐν ὕδατι γενέσθαι· ὀσμᾶται δὲ καὶ τὰ ἐν τῷ
443 b ὕδατι, ὥσπερ εἴρηται πρότερον· ἔτι ἡ ἀναθυμίασις
ὁμοίως λέγεται ταῖς ἀπορροίαις· εἰ οὖν μηδ' ἐκείνη
καλῶς, οὐδ' αὕτη καλῶς. ὅτι μὲν οὖν ἐνδέχεται ἀπο-
λαύειν τὸ ὑγρὸν καὶ τὸ ἐν τῷ πνεύματι καὶ τὸ ἐν τῷ
5 ὕδατι καὶ πάσχειν τι ὑπὸ τῆς ἐγχύμου ξηρότητος, οὐκ
ἄδηλον· καὶ γὰρ ὁ ἀὴρ ὑγρὸν τὴν φύσιν ἐστίν. ἔτι δ'
εἴπερ ὁμοίως ἐν τοῖς ὑγροῖς ποιεῖ καὶ ἐν τῷ ἀέρι οἷον
ἀποπλυνόμενον τὸ ξηρόν, φανερὸν ὅτι δεῖ ἀνάλογον εἶναι
τὰς ὀσμὰς τοῖς χυμοῖς. ἀλλὰ μὴν τοῦτό γε ἐπ' ἐνίων
10 συμβέβηκεν· καὶ γὰρ δριμεῖαι καὶ γλυκεῖαί εἰσιν ὀσμαὶ
καὶ αὐστηραὶ καὶ στρυφναὶ καὶ λιπαραί, καὶ τοῖς πικροῖς

443 a, 24 καὶ...ὀσμῆς 25 damnat Thurot.   28 ἐπὶ τοῦτο om. codd. et edd.,
addidit Christ probat etiam Biehl.

Salt smells more than natron, as the oil extracted from it 15
proves, while natron is more of the nature of earth. Moreover, stone is odourless, since flavourless; but woods, being
possessed of taste, are scented, the watery ones less so.
Again, among metals gold is odourless, having no taste;
bronze and iron have a smell. The dross left, when the 20
fluid element is smelted out of these metals, in every case
possesses less odour than the ore itself. Silver and tin smell
more than the one class and less than the other; for they are
aqueous.

Some people think that the smoky variety of fume
constitutes odour, since it is a joint product of earth and
air. [All ascribe odour to this.] Hence too the saying of 25
Heraclitus that "if all things were turned into smoke the
nostrils would distinguish them." Now all ascribe odour to
this phenomenon, some taking it to be steam, others a fume,
while some again ascribe it to both.

Steam is a sort of moisture, and smoke-like fume is a
joint product of air and earth, as has been said; out of the 30
former water condenses, out of the latter some species of
earth. But neither of these seems to be odour; for steam
may be classed as water, while again smoke-like fumes
cannot exist in water; but creatures living in water do
employ the sense of smell, as already said. Further the 443 b
theory of fumes is similar to that of effluxes and, if that
theory was erroneous, so is this.

It is clear that moisture, both as it exists in the atmosphere and as it exists in water, can derive something from
and be modified by dry substance which possesses flavour, 5
for air too has moisture in its constitution. Moreover if the
effect of the dry substance in liquids and in air, when it is, as
it were, dissolved in them, is similar to its previous action in
liquid alone, manifestly odours and tastes must be analogous
to each other. Indeed in several cases this correspondence
occurs; odours are pungent and sweet, harsh, astringent and 10

τὰς σαπρὰς ἄν τις ἀνάλογον εἴποι. διὸ ὥσπερ ἐκεῖνα
δυσκατάποτα, τὰ σαπρὰ δυσανάπνευστά ἐστιν. δῆλον
ἄρα ὅτι ὅπερ ἐν τῷ ὕδατι ὁ χυμός, τοῦτ᾽ ἐν τῷ ἀέρι καὶ
15 ὕδατι ἡ ὀσμή. καὶ διὰ τοῦτο τὸ ψυχρὸν καὶ ἡ πῆξις
καὶ τοὺς χυμοὺς ἀμβλύνει καὶ τὰς ὀσμὰς ἀφανίζει· τὸ
γὰρ θερμὸν τὸ κινοῦν καὶ δημιουργοῦν ἀφανίζουσιν ἡ
ψύξις καὶ ἡ πῆξις.

Εἴδη δὲ τοῦ ὀσφραντοῦ δύο ἐστίν· οὐ γὰρ ὥσπερ
20 τινές φασιν, οὐκ ἔστιν εἴδη τοῦ ὀσφραντοῦ, ἀλλ᾽ ἔστιν.
διοριστέον δὲ πῶς ἔστι καὶ πῶς οὐκ ἔστιν· τὸ μὲν γάρ
ἐστι κατὰ τοὺς χυμοὺς τεταγμένον αὐτῶν, ὥσπερ εἴπομεν,
καὶ τὸ ἡδὺ καὶ τὸ λυπηρὸν κατὰ συμβεβηκὸς ἔχουσιν·
διὰ γὰρ τὸ θρεπτικοῦ πάθη εἶναι, ἐπιθυμούντων μὲν
25 ἡδεῖαι αἱ ὀσμαὶ τούτων εἰσί, πεπληρωμένοις δὲ καὶ
μηδὲν δεομένοις οὐχ ἡδεῖαι, οὐδ᾽ ὅσοις μὴ καὶ ἡ τροφὴ
ἡ ἔχουσα τὰς ὀσμὰς ἡδεῖα, οὐδὲ τούτοις. ὥστε αὗται
μέν, καθάπερ εἴπομεν, κατὰ συμβεβηκὸς ἔχουσι τὸ ἡδὺ
καὶ λυπηρόν, διὸ καὶ πάντων εἰσὶ κοιναὶ τῶν ζῴων· αἱ
30 δὲ καθ᾽ αὑτὰς ἡδεῖαι τῶν ὀσμῶν εἰσίν, οἷον αἱ τῶν
ἀνθῶν· οὐδὲν γὰρ μᾶλλον οὐδ᾽ ἧττον πρὸς τὴν τροφὴν
παρακαλοῦσιν, οὐδὲ συμβάλλονται πρὸς ἐπιθυμίαν οὐδέν,
ἀλλὰ τοὐναντίον μᾶλλον· ἀληθὲς γὰρ ὅπερ Εὐριπίδην
σκώπτων εἶπε Στράττις, "ὅταν φακῆν ἕψητε, μὴ ᾽πιχεῖν
444 a μύρον." οἱ δὲ νῦν μιγνύντες εἰς τὰ πόματα τὰς τοιαύτας
δυνάμεις βιάζονται τῇ συνηθείᾳ τὴν ἡδονήν, ἕως ἂν ἐκ
δύ᾽ αἰσθήσεων γένηται τὸ ἡδὺ ὡς ἂν καὶ ἀπὸ μιᾶς.
τοῦτο μὲν οὖν τὸ ὀσφραντὸν ἴδιον τῶν ἀνθρώπων ἐστίν,
5 ἡ δὲ κατὰ τοὺς χυμοὺς τεταγμένη καὶ τῶν ἄλλων ζῴων,
ὥσπερ εἴρηται πρότερον· κἀκείνων μέν, διὰ τὸ κατὰ
συμβεβηκὸς ἔχειν τὸ ἡδύ, διήρηται τὰ εἴδη κατὰ τοὺς
χυμούς, ταύτης δ᾽ οὐκέτι, διὰ τὸ τὴν φύσιν αὐτῆς εἶναι
καθ᾽ αὑτὴν ἡδεῖαν ἢ λυπηράν. αἴτιον δὲ τοῦ ἴδιον εἶναι
10 ἀνθρώπου τὴν τοιαύτην ὀσμὴν διὰ τὴν ἕξιν τὴν περὶ

oily, and we might regard fetid odours as corresponding to bitter tastes; this would explain the parallel unpalatability of the latter and noisomeness of the former. Thus it is clear that smell is in air and water precisely what flavour is in water.

It is for this reason that cold and frost blunt flavours 15 and reduce odours to non-existence, for the heat which is the active and creative cause is nullified by the cooling and congelation.

There are two sorts of odorous qualities; it is not the case, as some allege, that there are not different species of 20 odour. They do exist; but we must determine in what sense they are authentic and in what sense not.

The one set are in order parallel to the various flavours as we have explained. Their pleasantness and unpleasantness belong to them contingently, for, since they are qualities of that which forms our food, these smells are pleasant when we are hungry, but when we are sated and not requiring to eat, 25 they are not pleasant; neither are they pleasant to those who dislike the food of which they are the odour. Hence, as we said, their pleasantness and unpleasantness are contingent and hence too they are common to all animals. But the other class of smells are *per se* pleasant, for example the scents of 30 flowers. They have no influence either great or small in attracting us to our food nor do they contribute anything to the longing for it. Their effect is rather the opposite; there is a truth contained in Strattis's jibe at Euripides— "Pray perfume not the good pea-soup." Those who do as a 444 a fact mix such elixirs with their drink get a forced pleasure by accustoming themselves to it, so that the pleasantness arising from the two sensations becomes apparently the result of one. This sort of odorous quality is thus peculiarly the object of human sense, but that coordinate with the varieties of flavour is proper to the other animals as well, 5 as said before. Those odours, because their pleasantness is contingently attached to them, are classified in species which correspond to the several flavours, but in the other group this feature disappears, as there agreeableness and the reverse attach to the essential nature of the odour.

The cause of the restriction of odour of this kind to human sense comes from the constitution of the body in the 10

τὸν ἐγκέφαλον. ψυχροῦ γὰρ ὄντος τὴν φύσιν τοῦ ἐγκεφάλου, καὶ τοῦ αἵματος τοῦ περὶ αὐτὸν ἐν τοῖς φλεβίοις
ὄντος λεπτοῦ μὲν καὶ καθαροῦ, εὐψύκτου δέ (διὸ καὶ
ἡ τῆς τροφῆς ἀναθυμίασις ψυχομένη διὰ τὸν τόπον τὰ
15 νοσηματικὰ ῥεύματα ποιεῖ), τοῖς ἀνθρώποις πρὸς βοήθειαν ὑγιείας γέγονε τὸ τοιοῦτον εἶδος τῆς ὀσμῆς· οὐδὲν
γὰρ ἄλλο ἔργον ἐστὶν αὐτῆς [ἢ τοῦτο]. τοῦτο δὲ ποιεῖ
φανερῶς· ἡ μὲν γὰρ τροφὴ ἡδεῖα οὖσα, καὶ ξηρὰ καὶ
ὑγρά, πολλάκις νοσώδης ἐστίν, ἡ δ' ἀπὸ τοῦ εὐώδους
20 ὀσμὴ ἡ καθ' αὑτὴν <ἡδεῖα> ὁπωσοῦν ἔχουσιν ὠφέλιμος
ὡς εἰπεῖν ἀεί. καὶ διὰ τοῦτο γίγνεται διὰ τῆς ἀναπνοῆς,
οὐ πᾶσιν ἀλλὰ τοῖς ἀνθρώποις καὶ τῶν ἐναίμων οἷον
τοῖς τετράποσι καὶ ὅσα μετέχει μᾶλλον τῆς τοῦ ἀέρος
φύσεως· ἀναφερομένων γὰρ τῶν ὀσμῶν πρὸς τὸν ἐγκέ-
25 φαλον διὰ τὴν ἐν αὐταῖς τῆς θερμότητος κουφότητα
ὑγιεινοτέρως ἔχει τὰ περὶ τὸν τόπον τοῦτον· ἡ γὰρ
τῆς ὀσμῆς δύναμις θερμὴ τὴν φύσιν ἐστίν. κατακέχρηται δ' ἡ φύσις τῇ ἀναπνοῇ ἐπὶ δύο, ὡς ἔργῳ μὲν
ἐπὶ τὴν εἰς τὸν θώρακα βοήθειαν, ὡς παρέργῳ δ' ἐπὶ
30 τὴν ὀσμήν· ἀναπνέοντος γὰρ ὥσπερ ἐκ παρόδου ποιεῖται
διὰ τῶν μυκτήρων τὴν κίνησιν. ἴδιον δὲ τῆς τοῦ ἀνθρώπου φύσεώς ἐστι τὸ τῆς ὀσμῆς τῆς τοιαύτης γένος
διὰ τὸ πλεῖστον ἐγκέφαλον καὶ ὑγρότατον ἔχειν τῶν
ἄλλων ζῴων ὡς κατὰ μέγεθος· διὰ γὰρ τοῦτο καὶ μόνον
35 ὡς εἰπεῖν αἰσθάνεται τῶν ζῴων ἄνθρωπος καὶ χαίρει ταῖς
τῶν ἀνθῶν καὶ ταῖς τῶν τοιούτων ὀσμαῖς· σύμμετρος γὰρ
444 b αὐτῶν ἡ θερμότης καὶ ἡ κίνησις πρὸς τὴν ὑπερβολὴν
τῆς ἐν τῷ τόπῳ ὑγρότητος καὶ ψυχρότητός ἐστιν. τοῖς
δ' ἄλλοις ὅσα πλεύμονα ἔχει διὰ τοῦ ἀναπνεῖν τοῦ ἑτέρου
γένους τῆς ὀσμῆς τὴν αἴσθησιν ἀποδέδωκεν ἡ φύσις,

444 a, 17 ἢ τοῦτο leg. L S U Alex. vet. tr. et omnes edd. excepto Biehl.
18 ἡ ante ξηρὰ et ante ὑγρὰ legunt exceptis E M Y et Biehl omnes codd. et edd.
19 et 20 ἡ δ' ἀπὸ τῆς ὀσμῆς τῆς καθ' αὑτὴν (ἑαυτὴν L P U) εὐώδους (quibus verbis
ἡδεῖα addunt L S U) habent omnes codd. et edd., text. recept. omisso ἡδεῖα Biehl.
444 b, 3 τὸ ἀναπνεῖν edd., τοῦ P U et Wilson.

region of the brain. The brain is of a cold nature and the blood around it in the veins is thin and pure and is easily chilled (this explains why the upward ascending fumes from food on turning cold owing to the nature of that region cause a morbid flow of rheum). Hence it is for man's benefit, for 15 the preservation of his health, that this species of odour has come into existence. This is its only function and it evidently fulfils it. Food, though sweet, being both dry and moist, is frequently unhealthy; but the odour, *per se* pleasant, of a 20 fragrant perfume, is beneficial to us in whatever state we are. It is for this reason that it is by means of respiration that smell takes place, if not in all animals, yet in man and, among sanguineous animals, in the quadrupeds and such as participate more largely in an aerial constitution. When scents are carried up to the brain, owing to the lightness of the 25 warm element contained in them, the parts in this region have a healthier tone; this takes place because the power in odour to produce an effect is constituted by heat.

Nature employs respiration for two purposes; its chief function is to maintain the action of the chest, its secondary one subserves the ends of smell, secondary, for the passage 30 of the breath through the nostrils is, as it were, a cursory contrivance.

The reason why the class of odours of this description is restricted to man, is, that his brain is larger and more humid than that of all other animals in proportion to his size. This is why he alone, so to speak, among the animals, perceives 35 and also enjoys the odours of flowers and similar scented objects; they are pleasant because their heat and activity 444 b are proportionate to the excess of humidity and cold in that part of the body.

Among other animals, in those which have lungs, breathing is the means which nature has bestowed upon them for the

5 ὅπως μὴ αἰσθητήρια δύο ποιῇ· ἀπόχρη γὰρ καὶ ἀναπνέουσιν, ὥσπερ τοῖς ἀνθρώποις ἀμφοτέρων τῶν ὀσφραντῶν,
τούτοις τῶν ἑτέρων μόνων ὑπάρχουσα ἡ αἴσθησις. τὰ
δὲ μὴ ἀναπνέοντα ὅτι μὲν ἔχει αἴσθησιν τοῦ ὀσφραντοῦ,
φανερόν· καὶ γὰρ ἰχθύες καὶ τὸ τῶν ἐντόμων γένος πᾶν
10 ἀκριβῶς καὶ πόρρωθεν αἰσθάνεται, διὰ τὸ θρεπτικὸν
εἶδος τῆς ὀσμῆς, ἀπέχοντα πολὺ τῆς οἰκείας τροφῆς,
οἷον αἵ τε μέλιτται καὶ τὸ τῶν μικρῶν μυρμήκων γένος,
οὓς καλοῦσί τινες κνίπας, καὶ τῶν θαλαττίων αἱ πορφύραι, καὶ πολλὰ τῶν ἄλλων τῶν τοιούτων ζῴων ὀξέως
15 αἰσθάνεται τῆς τροφῆς διὰ τὴν ὀσμήν. ὅτῳ δὲ αἰσθάνεται, οὐχ ὁμοίως φανερόν. διὸ κἂν ἀπορήσειέ τις τίνι
αἰσθάνεται τῆς ὀσμῆς, εἴπερ ἀναπνέουσι μὲν γίνεται
τὸ ὀσμᾶσθαι μοναχῶς (τοῦτο γὰρ φαίνεται ἐπὶ τῶν
ἀναπνεόντων συμβαῖνον πάντων), ἐκείνων δ᾽ οὐθὲν ἀνα-
20 πνεῖ, αἰσθάνεται μέντοι, εἰ μή τις παρὰ τὰς πέντε
αἰσθήσεις ἑτέρα. τοῦτο δ᾽ ἀδύνατον· τοῦ γὰρ ὀσφραντοῦ
ὄσφρησις, ἐκεῖνα δὲ τούτου αἰσθάνεται, ἀλλ᾽ οὐ τὸν
αὐτὸν ἴσως τρόπον, ἀλλὰ τοῖς μὲν ἀναπνέουσι τὸ πνεῦμα
ἀφαιρεῖ τὸ ἐπικείμενον ὥσπερ πῶμά τι (διὸ οὐκ αἰσθά-
25 νεται μὴ ἀναπνέοντα), τοῖς δὲ μὴ ἀναπνέουσιν ἀφῄρηται
τοῦτο, καθάπερ ἐπὶ τῶν ὀφθαλμῶν τὰ μὲν ἔχει βλέφαρα
τῶν ζῴων, ὧν μὴ ἀνακαλυφθέντων οὐ δύναται ὁρᾶν, τὰ
δὲ σκληρόφθαλμα οὐκ ἔχει, διόπερ οὐ προσδεῖται οὐδενὸς
τοῦ ἀνακαλύψοντος, ἀλλ᾽ ὁρᾷ ἐκ τοῦ δυνατοῦ ὄντος αὐτοῦ
30 εὐθύς. ὁμοίως δὲ καὶ τῶν ἄλλων ζῴων ὁτιοῦν οὐδὲν
δυσχεραίνει τῶν καθ᾽ αὐτὰ δυσωδῶν τὴν ὀσμήν, ἂν μή
τι τύχῃ φθαρτικὸν ὄν. ὑπὸ τούτων δ᾽ ὁμοίως φθείρεται
καθάπερ καὶ οἱ ἄνθρωποι ὑπὸ τῆς τῶν ἀνθράκων ἀτμίδος
καρηβαροῦσι καὶ φθείρονται πολλάκις· οὕτως ὑπὸ τῆς

---

444 b, 5 ἐπείπερ καὶ ὡς ἀναπν. leg. exceptis E M Y et Biehl reliqui omnes et
scripti et impressi, etiam Alex. et vet. tr.   29 ὄντος Biehl | ὁρᾶν L S U Alex.
et omnes edd., "a facultate existente" vet. tr. | αὑτοῦ E M Y Biehl, αὑτῷ reliqui
et scripti et impressi.

perception of the other genus of odour. This was to avoid
creating two sense-organs ; for if creatures merely breathe, 5
the sense of smell is sufficiently well provided for, in the case
of the animals the perception of the one class of odorous
qualities, the only one possessed by them, just as it is in man
who perceives both kinds.

That non-respiring animals perceive odorous quality is a
matter of observation. Fishes and the insect-tribe perceive 10
quite accurately and at a distance by means of the species of
odour connected with nutriment, even when they are far away
from the things that form their special food. For example
bees and the kind of small ants called *knipes* and, among
marine creatures, the purple-murex and many similar animals,
have a very acute perception of food by means of smell.

But the organ of perception is not so obvious and so one 15
might raise a difficulty and ask, "what is the organ with
which these animals perceive smell, if in all respiring animals
the sensation occurs in one way only, viz. by respiration (as
is evidently the case in all creatures that breathe), and none
of these breathe but yet do perceive odour? Perhaps they 20
do not smell but have a new sense over and above the five."

This, however, is impossible ; it is smell that is the sense
of that which smells and this they perceive. Yet perhaps
the manner of perception is not the same ; perhaps in the
case of respiring animals the breath displaces a superficial
structure which serves in a way like a lid to cover the sense-
organ ; (this will explain why when we do not inhale the
breath we do not smell ;) but in the non-respiring animals 25
this is entirely lacking. A parallel for this is the eye ; some
animals have eyelids and, unless these are open, they cannot
see ; but hard-eyed animals, not possessing them, do not
require anything to open them, but see an object directly
out of the organ which itself has the capacity of vision.

Similarly in accordance with our previous distinction we 30
must notice that none of the other animals are distressed by
the smell of things *per se* malodorous, unless any of these
chance to be destructive to life. These noxious odours have
a destructive effect upon them, just as they have upon men
too, in whom the gas arising from coal causes headache and
frequently death. So too, sulphurous and bituminous fumes

35 τοῦ θείου δυνάμεως καὶ τῶν ἀσφαλτωδῶν φθείρεται
445 a τἆλλα ζῷα, καὶ φεύγει διὰ τὸ πάθος. αὐτῆς δὲ καθ᾽
αὑτὴν τῆς δυσωδίας οὐδὲν φροντίζουσιν, καίτοι πολλὰ
τῶν φυομένων δυσώδεις ἔχει τὰς ὀσμάς, ἐὰν μή τι
συμβάλληται πρὸς τὴν γεῦσιν ἢ τὴν ἐδωδὴν αὐτοῖς.
5 ἔοικε δ᾽ ἡ αἴσθησις ἡ τοῦ ὀσφραίνεσθαι περιττῶν οὐσῶν
τῶν αἰσθήσεων καὶ τοῦ ἀριθμοῦ ἔχοντος μέσον τοῦ
περιττοῦ καὶ αὐτὴ μέση εἶναι τῶν τε ἁπτικῶν, οἷον
ἀφῆς καὶ γεύσεως, καὶ τῶν δι᾽ ἄλλου αἰσθητικῶν, οἷον
ὄψεως καὶ ἀκοῆς. διὸ καὶ τὸ ὀσφραντὸν τῶν θρεπτικῶν
10 ἐστὶ πάθος τι (ταῦτα δ᾽ ἐν τῷ ἁπτῷ γένει) καὶ τοῦ
ἀκουστοῦ δὲ καὶ τοῦ ὁρατοῦ, διὸ καὶ ἐν ἀέρι καὶ ἐν
ὕδατι ὀσμῶνται. ὥστ᾽ ἐστὶ τὸ ὀσφραντὸν κοινόν τι
τούτων ἀμφοτέρων, καὶ τῷ τε ἁπτῷ ὑπάρχει καὶ τῷ
ἀκουστῷ καὶ διαφανεῖ· διὸ εὐλόγως παρείκασται ξηρό-
15 τητος ἐν ὑγρῷ καὶ χυτῷ οἷον βαφή τις εἶναι καὶ
πλύσις. πῶς μὲν οὖν εἴδη δεῖ λέγειν καὶ πῶς οὐ δεῖ
17 τοῦ ὀσφραντοῦ, ἐπὶ τοσοῦτον εἰρήσθω.

17　　　Ὃ δὲ λέγουσί τινες
τῶν Πυθαγορείων, οὐκ ἔστιν εὔλογον· τρέφεσθαι γάρ
φασιν ἔνια ζῷα ταῖς ὀσμαῖς. πρῶτον μὲν γὰρ ὁρῶμεν
20 ὅτι τὴν τροφὴν δεῖ εἶναι συνθέτην· καὶ γὰρ τὰ τρεφόμενα
οὐχ ἁπλᾶ ἐστίν, διὸ καὶ περίττωμα γίνεται τῆς τροφῆς,
ὃ μὲν ἐν αὐτοῖς ὃ δὲ ἔξω, ὥσπερ τοῖς φυτοῖς. ἔτι δ᾽
οὐδὲ τὸ ὕδωρ ἐθέλει αὐτὸ μόνον ἄμικτον ὂν τρέφειν·
σωματῶδες γάρ τι δεῖ εἶναι τὸ συστησόμενον. ἔτι
25 πολὺ ἧττον εὔλογον τὸν ἀέρα σωματοῦσθαι. πρὸς δὲ
τούτοις, ὅτι πᾶσίν ἐστι τοῖς ζῴοις τόπος δεκτικὸς τῆς
τροφῆς, ἐξ οὗ ὅταν εἰσέλθῃ λαμβάνει τὸ σῶμα· τοῦ
δ᾽ ὀσφραντοῦ ἐν τῇ κεφαλῇ τὸ αἰσθητήριον, καὶ μετὰ
πνευματώδους εἰσέρχεται ἀναθυμιάσεως, ὥστ᾽ εἰς τὸν
30 ἀναπνευστικὸν βαδίζοι ἂν τόπον. ὅτι μὲν οὖν οὐ
συμβάλλεται εἰς τροφὴν τὸ ὀσφραντόν, ᾗ ὀσφραντόν,

have the power of causing death in the other animals and are 35
shunned by them in consequence. But they reck not at all 445 a
of the essential unpleasantness of the smell (though many
plants are malodorous) unless it make some difference to the
taste and to eating.

The number of the senses is uneven and the sense of 5
smell, since an uneven number has a middle term, seems
itself to occupy the intermediate position between the senses
which require contact, viz. touch and taste, and those where
the perception is mediated by something else, to wit, sight
and hearing. For this reason also odour is a quality both of
that which is nutritive (which falls within the class of things 10
tangible) and of the audible and the visible, and hence the
sense of smell is exercised both in air and in water. Thus
the object of smell is something common to both of these
and is found in things tangible, things audible and things
transparent.

We had, therefore, good reason in comparing it to an
infusion and solution of dry substance in that which is liquid 15
and fluid. This is the sum of our account of the sense in
which it is correct and that in which it is incorrect to talk
of species in odour.

The theory held by certain Pythagoreans that some
animals live on odours is an irrational doctrine.

In the first place, food must be a composite substance;
the creatures that it nourishes are themselves not simple in
structure. Hence from food a waste residue is developed 20
which in some is internal, in others — plants, external;
secondly, water by itself alone and unmixed has no nutritive
tendency; food which is to form a concrete body must have
solidity. Much less reason is there for supposing that air
can be solidified. Furthermore, in all animals there is a 25
receptacle for food and out of this the body is supplied upon
the entrance of nutriment. But the organ for perceiving
smell is in the head; odour enters the body along with the
waft of the air we breathe and so must pass into the organs
of breathing.

It is clear, then, that the object of the sense of smell has, 30

δῆλον· ὅτι μέντοι εἰς ὑγίειαν, καὶ ἐκ τῆς αἰσθήσεως
καὶ ἐκ τῶν εἰρημένων φανερόν, ὥστε ὅπερ ὁ χυμὸς ἐν
τῷ θρεπτικῷ καὶ πρὸς τὰ τρεφόμενα, τοῦτ᾽ ἐστὶ πρὸς
445 b ὑγίειαν τὸ ὀσφραντόν. καθ᾽ ἕκαστον μὲν οὖν αἰσθητήριον διωρίσθω τὸν τρόπον τοῦτον.

VI

Ἀπορήσειε δ᾽ ἄν τις, εἰ πᾶν σῶμα εἰς ἄπειρα διαιρεῖται, ἆρα καὶ τὰ παθήματα τὰ αἰσθητά, οἷον χρῶμα
5 καὶ χυμὸς καὶ ὀσμὴ καὶ ψόφος καὶ βάρος καὶ ψυχρὸν
καὶ θερμὸν καὶ κοῦφον καὶ σκληρὸν καὶ μαλακόν; ἢ
ἀδύνατον· ποιητικὸν γάρ ἐστιν ἕκαστον αὐτῶν τῆς
αἰσθήσεως· τῷ δύνασθαι γὰρ κινεῖν αὐτὴν λέγεται
πάντα. ὥστ᾽ ἀνάγκη τήν τε αἴσθησιν εἰς ἄπειρα διαι-
10 ρεῖσθαι καὶ πᾶν εἶναι μέγεθος αἰσθητόν· ἀδύνατον γὰρ
λευκὸν μὲν ὁρᾶν, μὴ ποσὸν δέ. εἰ γὰρ μὴ οὕτως,
ἐνδέχοιτ᾽ ἂν εἶναί τι σῶμα μηδὲν ἔχον χρῶμα μηδὲ
βάρος μηδ᾽ ἄλλο τι τοιοῦτον πάθος. ὥστ᾽ οὐδ᾽ αἰσθητὸν
ὅλως· ταῦτα γὰρ τὰ αἰσθητά. τὸ ἄρ᾽ αἰσθητὸν ἔσται
15 συγκείμενον οὐκ ἐξ αἰσθητῶν. ἀλλ᾽ ἀναγκαῖον· οὐ γὰρ
δὴ ἔκ γε τῶν μαθηματικῶν. ἔτι τίνι κρινοῦμεν ταῦτα
ἢ γνωσόμεθα; ἢ τῷ νῷ. ἀλλ᾽ οὐ νοητά, οὐδὲ νοεῖ ὁ
νοῦς τὰ ἐκτὸς μὴ μετ᾽ αἰσθήσεως. ἅμα δ᾽ εἰ ταῦτ᾽ ἔχει
οὕτως, ἔοικε μαρτυρεῖν τοῖς τὰ ἄτομα ποιοῦσι μεγέθη·
20 οὕτω γὰρ ἂν λύοιτο ὁ λόγος. ἀλλ᾽ ἀδύνατα· εἴρηται δὲ
περὶ αὐτῶν ἐν τοῖς λόγοις τοῖς περὶ κινήσεως. περὶ δὲ
τῆς λύσεως αὐτῶν ἅμα δῆλον ἔσται καὶ διὰ τί πεπέρανται
τὰ εἴδη καὶ χρώματος καὶ χυμοῦ καὶ φθόγγων καὶ τῶν
ἄλλων αἰσθητῶν. ὧν μὲν γάρ ἐστιν ἔσχατα, ἀναγκαῖον
25 πεπεράνθαι τὰ ἐντός· τὰ δ᾽ ἐναντία ἔσχατα. πᾶν δὲ
τὸ αἰσθητὸν ἔχει ἐναντίωσιν, οἷον ἐν χρώματι τὸ λευκὸν

per se, nothing to do with nourishment. That it makes a difference to health is, however, obvious ; both the experience of the sensation itself and our argument prove it. Hence we may conclude that odour has precisely the same office in relation to health as flavour has in food and in relation to the creatures that food nourishes.

This finishes our account of the objects relative to the 445 several sense-organs.

VI

The question might be raised whether, if all bodies are infinitely divisible, the same is the case with their sensuous qualities also, *e.g.* colour, flavour, odour, sound, weight, cold, 5 heat, lightness, hardness and softness. Or is this impossible ? Each of those phenomena is able to cause sensation ; they are all styled sense-qualities owing to their power of stimulating the sense. Consequently, on the former alternative sensation will be capable of infinite subdivision and, as well, every magnitude will be perceptible, since it is impossible to 10 perceive anything white which is not a quantum.

If this were not so, body might exist which was totally without colour or weight or any other similar attribute. Consequently it would be totally imperceptible, for the above form the list of the sense-qualities. The object of sensation must then be composed of things which are imperceptible. But it must be composed of constituents which are sen- 15 sible ; for it certainly cannot consist of mathematical entities. Further how should we distinguish them or be aware of them ? By means of thought ? But they are not objects of thought ; thought does not think external objects unless sense cooperates.

At the same time also, this, if true, seems to give evidence in support of the theory of atomic magnitudes, since that would furnish a solution of the problem. But atomic magni- 20 tudes are impossible, as was explained in our treatment of motion.

The solution of this problem and the reason why the species of colour, taste, sound, etc. are limited in number, will become apparent at the same time.

Where extremes exist the internal parts must be determinate. Now contraries are extremes and every object of 25 sense exhibits contrariety, *e.g.* in colour black and white,

καὶ τὸ μέλαν, ἐν χυμῷ γλυκὺ καὶ πικρόν· καὶ ἐν τοῖς
ἄλλοις δὴ πᾶσίν ἐστιν ἔσχατα τὰ ἐναντία. τὸ μὲν οὖν
συνεχὲς εἰς ἄπειρα τέμνεται ἄνισα, εἰς δ᾽ ἴσα πεπε-
30 ρασμένα· τὸ δὲ μὴ καθ᾽ αὑτὸ συνεχὲς εἰς πεπερασμένα
εἴδη. ἐπεὶ οὖν τὰ μὲν πάθη ὡς εἴδη λεκτέον, ὑπάρχει
δὲ συνέχεια ἀεὶ ἐν τούτοις, ληπτέον ὅτι τὸ δυνάμει καὶ
τὸ ἐνεργείᾳ ἕτερον· καὶ διὰ τοῦτο τὸ μυριοστημόριον
446 a λανθάνει τῆς κέγχρου ὁρωμένης, καίτοι ἡ ὄψις ἐπελήλυθεν, καὶ ὁ ἐν τῇ διέσει φθόγγος λανθάνει, καίτοι
συνεχοῦς ὄντος ἀκούει τοῦ μέλους παντός. τὸ δὲ διάστημα τὸ τοῦ μεταξὺ πρὸς τοὺς ἐσχάτους λανθάνει.
5 ὁμοίως δὲ καὶ ἐν τοῖς ἄλλοις αἰσθητοῖς τὰ μικρὰ πάμπαν·
δυνάμει γὰρ ὁρατά, ἐνεργείᾳ δ᾽ οὔ, ὅταν μὴ χωρὶς ᾖ· καὶ
γὰρ ἐνυπάρχει δυνάμει ἡ ποδιαία τῇ δίποδι, ἐνεργείᾳ
δ᾽ ἤδη διαιρεθεῖσα. χωριζόμεναι δ᾽ αἱ τηλικαῦται ὑπε-
ροχαὶ εὐλόγως μὲν ἂν καὶ διαλύοιντο εἰς τὰ περιέχοντα,
10 ὥσπερ καὶ ἀκαριαῖος χυμὸς εἰς τὴν θάλατταν ἐκχυθείς.
οὐ μὴν ἀλλ᾽ ἐπειδὴ οὐδ᾽ ἡ τῆς αἰσθήσεως ὑπεροχὴ καθ᾽
αὑτὴν αἰσθητὴ οὐδὲ χωριστή (δυνάμει γὰρ ἐνυπάρχει
ἐν τῇ ἀκριβεστέρᾳ ἡ ὑπεροχή), οὐδὲ τὸ τηλικοῦτον
αἰσθητὸν χωριστὸν ἔσται ἐνεργείᾳ αἰσθάνεσθαι, ἀλλ᾽
15 ὅμως ἔσται αἰσθητόν· δυνάμει τε γάρ ἐστιν ἤδη, καὶ
ἐνεργείᾳ ἔσται προσγενόμενον. ὅτι μὲν οὖν ἔνια μεγέθη
καὶ πάθη λανθάνει, καὶ διὰ τίν᾽ αἰτίαν, καὶ πῶς αἰσθητὰ
καὶ πῶς οὔ, εἴρηται. ὅταν δὲ δὴ ἐνυπάρχοντα οὕτω
ἤδη πρὸς αὑτὰ ᾖ ὥστε καὶ ἐνεργείᾳ αἰσθητὰ εἶναι, καὶ
20 μὴ μόνον ὅτι ἐν τῷ ὅλῳ ἀλλὰ καὶ χωρίς, πεπερασμένα
ἀνάγκη εἶναι τὸν ἀριθμὸν καὶ χρώματα καὶ χυμοὺς
22 καὶ φθόγγους.

22   Ἀπορήσειε δ᾽ ἄν τις, ἆρ᾽ ἀφικνοῦνται ἢ τὰ
αἰσθητὰ ἢ αἱ κινήσεις αἱ ἀπὸ τῶν αἰσθητῶν, ὁποτέρως

---

446 a, 6 μὴ χωρὶς ᾖ] μὴ χωρὶς ᾖ E M Y vet. tr., χωρισθῇ Biehl, Bek.   7 τῇ
δίποδι] τῷ ποδὶ E M Y   18 ἐνυπάρχῃ τούτῳ τοσαῦτα L S U Alex., ἐνυπάρχοντα
οὕτω πως ἅττα ᾖ P vet. tr. Bek. Didot text. recept. Biehl.

in taste sweet and bitter, and in the others every one the contrary qualities form extremes.

Now continuous quantity when divided falls into an infinite number of unequal parts but into a finite number of equal parts. On the other hand that which is not *per se* 30 continuous, falls into a finite number of species. Thus, while on the one hand sense-qualities must be considered as species, but on the other hand universally present the aspect of continuity, we must, to solve the difficulty, bring in the distinction between potential and actual. It is by this means that we explain why the ten thousandth part of a visible 446 a grain of millet escapes notice although the sight has encountered it, and why a sound within a quarter-tone escapes detection, although the whole series of notes in which it exists, being continuous, is heard ; the interval between the mean point and extremes is not discernible and so too 5 it is with very minute fractions in other objects of sense ; they are potentially perceptible but not actually so unless they be isolated. So even the one-foot measure has but potential existence in the two-foot rule but, from the moment bisection takes place, it is something actual.

But it is reasonable to believe that, when fractions so excessively minute are isolated, they are moreover resolved into the surrounding medium, just as a tiny drop of flavouring 10 is lost when spilled in the ocean, and so escapes perception. However that may be, since not even in the perception of minute objects is the excessively minute sensation in its individuality appreciable or isolable (it has a potential existence in that which is more accurately discriminated), neither will it be possible to have actual perception of the similarly minute object of sense in its separateness. Nevertheless perceptible it is ; for it already is so potentially and, when 15 taken in union with the whole, it becomes actually perceptible. Thus certain magnitudes and their qualities escape detection ; this is our account of them and of the reason why that is so and of the senses in which they are and are not perceptible. But when the constituents of anything are already so related among themselves as to be also actually perceptible and perceptible not merely in the whole but 20 individually as well, the determinations of colour and flavour and sound must be finite in number.

It may be asked—Do the objects of sense or the motions which issue from sense-objects (whichever of the two theories perception involves), when acting on us penetrate the medium through which they pass, prior to causing sensation ? This is

ποτὲ γίνεται ἡ αἴσθησις, ὅταν ἐνεργῶσιν, εἰς τὸ μέσον
25 πρῶτον, οἷον ἥ τε ὀσμὴ φαίνεται ποιοῦσα καὶ ὁ ψόφος·
πρότερον γὰρ ὁ ἐγγὺς αἰσθάνεται τῆς ὀσμῆς, καὶ ὁ
ψόφος ὕστερον ἀφικνεῖται τῆς πληγῆς. ἆρ᾽ οὖν οὕτω
καὶ τὸ ὁρώμενον καὶ τὸ φῶς; καθάπερ καὶ Ἐμπεδοκλῆς
φησὶν ἀφικνεῖσθαι πρότερον τὸ ἀπὸ τοῦ ἡλίου φῶς εἰς
30 τὸ μεταξὺ πρὶν πρὸς τὴν ὄψιν ἢ ἐπὶ τὴν γῆν. δόξειε
δ᾽ ἂν εὐλόγως τοῦτο συμβαίνειν· τὸ γὰρ κινούμενον
κινεῖταί ποθέν ποι, ὥστ᾽ ἀνάγκη εἶναί τινα καὶ χρόνον
446 b ἐν ᾧ κινεῖται ἐκ θατέρου πρὸς θάτερον· ὁ δὲ χρόνος πᾶς
διαιρετός, ὥστε ἦν ὅτε οὔπω ἑωρᾶτο ἀλλ᾽ ἔτ᾽ ἐφέρετο
ἡ ἀκτὶς ἐν τῷ μεταξύ. καὶ εἰ ἅπαν ἅμα ἀκούει καὶ
ἀκήκοε καὶ ὅλως αἰσθάνεται καὶ ᾔσθηται, καὶ μή ἐστι
5 γένεσις αὐτῶν, ἀλλ᾽ εἰσὶν ἄνευ τοῦ γίγνεσθαι ὅμως οὐδὲν
ἧττον, ὥσπερ ὁ ψόφος ἤδη γεγενημένης τῆς πληγῆς οὔπω
πρὸς τῇ ἀκοῇ. δηλοῖ δὲ τοῦτο καὶ ἡ τῶν γραμμάτων
μετασχημάτισις, ὡς γιγνομένης τῆς φορᾶς ἐν τῷ μεταξύ·
οὐ γὰρ τὸ λεχθὲν φαίνονται ἀκηκοότες διὰ τὸ μετα-
10 σχηματίζεσθαι φερόμενον τὸν ἀέρα. ἆρ᾽ οὖν οὕτω καὶ
τὸ χρῶμα καὶ τὸ φῶς; οὐ γὰρ δὴ τῷ πως ἔχειν τὸ μὲν
ὁρᾷ τὸ δ᾽ ὁρᾶται, ὥσπερ ἴσα ἐστίν· οὐθὲν γὰρ ἂν ἔδει
που ἑκάτερον εἶναι· τοῖς γὰρ ἴσοις γιγνομένοις οὐδὲν
διαφέρει ἢ ἐγγὺς ἢ πόρρω ἀλλήλων εἶναι. ἢ περὶ μὲν
15 τὸν ψόφον καὶ τὴν ὀσμὴν τοῦτο συμβαίνειν εὔλογον·
ὥσπερ γὰρ ὁ ἀὴρ καὶ τὸ ὕδωρ, συνεχῆ μέν, μεμέρισται
δ᾽ ἀμφοτέρων ἡ κίνησις. διὸ καὶ ἔστι μὲν ὡς τὸ αὐτὸ
ἀκούει ὁ πρῶτος καὶ ὁ ὕστερος καὶ ὀσφραίνεται, ἔστι
δ᾽ ὡς οὔ. δοκεῖ δέ τισιν εἶναι ἀπορία καὶ περὶ τούτων·
20 ἀδύνατον γάρ φασί τινες ἄλλον ἄλλῳ τὸ αὐτὸ ἀκούειν
καὶ ὁρᾶν καὶ ὀσφραίνεσθαι· οὐ γὰρ οἷόν τ᾽ εἶναι πολλοὺς
καὶ χωρὶς ὄντας ἀκούειν καὶ ὀσφραίνεσθαι· τὸ γὰρ ἓν
χωρὶς ἂν αὐτὸ αὑτοῦ εἶναι. ἢ τοῦ μὲν κινήσαντος
πρώτου, οἷον τῆς κώδωνος ἢ λιβανωτοῦ ἢ πυρός, τοῦ

evidently the case, *e.g.*, with odour and sound ; he who stands 25
nearer perceives the odour earlier, and a sound reaches the
ear after the blow is struck.   Is the same thing true of the
object of vision and light?   Empedocles too had the very same
theory ; he says that the light coming from the sun penetrates
the medium first before meeting our sight or reaching the earth.
This looks like a reasonable account of the phenomenon, for 30
when a thing moves it moves from starting point to terminus
and hence there must be some lapse of time as well while it
passes from the one point to the other.   Now every lapse of 446 b
time is divisible and so there was a moment when as yet the
ray of light was not perceived but was still on its passage
through the medium.   Though, in every act, hearing and
perception generally are complete as soon as exercised and
there is no process in the establishment of the content of
sense, yet sensation is not devoid of process on this account
nor possesses it any the less ; take for example the case of 5
sound which does not meet the ear simultaneously with the
striking of the blow.   This is shown too by the distortion
of the letters of a word when uttered, which is explained by
their passage through the medium ; we appear not to hear
what has actually been said because the air in moving gets
distorted.   Does the same lapse of time in transmission occur
in the case of colour and light?   It is not, certainly, in virtue 10
of some such modal determination as constitutes the relation
of equality that subject and object in vision are related.   If
it were, they would not require both to be in a definite place ;
when things are equal it makes no difference to their equality
whether they are near or far apart.   In the case of sound and
odour it is reasonable that this lapse of time during transmission should occur.   Like the air and the water they are 15
continuous, yet in both cases the motion of transmission falls
into a number of parts.   Hence too there is a sense in which
it is the same thing which is heard by the person who stands
nearest and by him who is farthest away and the same thing
which is smelled by both ; and there is a sense in which it is
not.   This seems to constitute a difficulty for some people ;
they say it is impossible that what is identical should be
heard or seen or smelt by different persons and that they 20
cannot hear and smell it because they are many and apart ;
if they could, what is one thing would itself become separated
from itself.

The solution is, that all do perceive the numerically
identical and self-same thing which is the originating cause
of the movement, *e.g.* the bell, the frankincense, or the fire,

25 αὐτοῦ καὶ ἑνὸς ἀριθμῷ αἰσθάνονται πάντες, τοῦ δὲ δὴ
ἰδίου ἑτέρου ἀριθμῷ, εἴδει δὲ τοῦ αὐτοῦ, διὸ καὶ ἅμα
πολλοὶ ὁρῶσι καὶ ὀσμῶνται καὶ ἀκούουσιν. ἔστι δ᾽
οὔτε σώματα ταῦτα, ἀλλὰ πάθος καὶ κίνησίς τις (οὐ
γὰρ ἂν τοῦτο συνέβαινεν), οὐδ᾽ ἄνευ σώματος. περὶ δὲ
30 τοῦ φωτὸς ἄλλος λόγος· τῷ ἐνεῖναι γάρ τι φῶς ἐστίν,
ἀλλ᾽ οὐ κίνησις. ὅλως δὲ οὐδὲ ὁμοίως ἐπί τε ἀλλοιώσεως ἔχει καὶ φορᾶς· αἱ μὲν γὰρ φοραὶ εὐλόγως εἰς
τὸ μεταξὺ πρῶτον ἀφικνοῦνται (δοκεῖ δ᾽ ὁ ψόφος εἶναι
447 a φερομένου τινὸς κίνησις), ὅσα δ᾽ ἀλλοιοῦται, οὐκέτι
ὁμοίως· ἐνδέχεται γὰρ ἀθρόον ἀλλοιοῦσθαι, καὶ μὴ τὸ
ἥμισυ πρότερον, οἷον τὸ ὕδωρ ἅμα πᾶν πήγνυσθαι. οὐ
μὴν ἀλλ᾽ ἂν ᾖ πολὺ τὸ θερμαινόμενον ἢ πηγνύμενον,
5 τὸ ἐχόμενον ὑπὸ τοῦ ἐχομένου πάσχει, τὸ δὲ πρῶτον
ὑπ᾽ αὐτοῦ τοῦ ἀλλοιοῦντος μεταβάλλει, καὶ οὐκ ἀνάγκη
ἅμα ἀλλοιοῦσθαι καὶ ἀθρόον. ἦν δ᾽ ἂν καὶ τὸ γεύεσθαι
ὥσπερ ἡ ὀσμή, εἰ ἐν ὑγρῷ ἦμεν καὶ πορρωτέρω πρὶν
θιγεῖν αὐτοῦ ᾐσθανόμεθα. εὐλόγως δ᾽ ὧν ἐστὶ μεταξὺ
10 τοῦ αἰσθητηρίου, οὐχ ἅμα πάντα πάσχει, πλὴν ἐπὶ τοῦ
φωτὸς διὰ τὸ εἰρημένον. διὰ τὸ αὐτὸ δὲ καὶ ἐπὶ τοῦ
ὁρᾶν· τὸ γὰρ φῶς ποιεῖ τὸ ὁρᾶν.

VII

Ἔστι δέ τις ἀπορία καὶ ἄλλη τοιάδε περὶ αἰσθήσεως,
πότερον ἐνδέχεται δυεῖν ἅμα δύνασθαι αἰσθάνεσθαι ἐν
15 τῷ αὐτῷ καὶ ἀτόμῳ χρόνῳ, ἢ οὔ, εἰ δὴ ἀεὶ ἡ μείζων
κίνησις τὴν ἐλάττω ἐκκρούει· διὸ τὸ ἐπιφερόμενον ἐπὶ
τὰ ὄμματα οὐκ αἰσθάνονται, ἐὰν τύχωσι σφόδρα τι
ἐννοοῦντες ἢ φοβούμενοι ἢ ἀκούοντες πολὺν ψόφον. τοῦτο
δὲ δὴ ὑποκείσθω, καὶ ὅτι ἑκάστου μᾶλλον ἔστιν αἰσθά-

446 b, 30 τῷ ἐνεῖναι Alex., εἶναι Biehl et codd.

but yet the stimulus peculiar to each is numerically different 25 though specifically the same. We can hence explain how many people may see and smell and hear the same thing and do this at the same time too. Here we are dealing not with bodies, but qualities and motions (if this were not so the latter phenomenon could not occur), though they do not exist apart from body.

About light a different account must be given. Light is due to the presence of something but is not a motion. 30 Universally speaking there is not even similarity between qualitative alteration and spatial transference; motions of translation, as one would expect, penetrate the medium first before reaching us (sound seems to be a motion of something which travels). On the other hand with things that suffer 447 a alteration this ceases to be true; they may be altered in one mass, and not one half before the other; for example water freezes all at one time. However if what is heated or frozen is great in bulk, one part is acted on by that which is contiguous to it, the change in the first being due to the 5 agent itself which is the cause of the alteration; and the alteration does not necessarily take place at the same time and over the whole. Taste would be like odour if we lived in water and perceived things at a distance before touching them. It is reasonable to believe that in those cases where the organ of perception employs a medium the effects are not 10 all simultaneously produced; but we except the case of light for the reason given and, on the very same account, sight too, for it is light which causes vision.

VII

There is a certain other problem also connected with perception—Can we perceive two things in the same individual moment of time, or can we not? Not, if it is the case that a 15 stronger stimulus displaces one which is more feeble. This is the reason why one does not see things that directly meet the eyes, when one is in a state of profound meditation or of terror or when hearkening to a loud sound.

Let us posit this as true, and likewise the fact that any

20 νεσθαι ἁπλοῦ ὄντος ἢ κεκραμένου, οἷον οἴνου ἀκράτου
ἢ κεκραμένου, καὶ μέλιτος, καὶ χρόας, καὶ τῆς νήτης
μόνης ἢ ἐν τῷ διὰ πασῶν, διὰ τὸ ἀφανίζειν ἄλληλα.
τοῦτο δὲ ποιεῖ ἐξ ὧν ἕν τι γίνεται. εἰ δὴ ἡ μείζων τὴν
ἐλάττω κίνησιν ἐκκρούει, ἀνάγκη, ἂν ἅμα ὦσι, καὶ
25 αὐτὴν ἧττον αἰσθητὴν εἶναι ἢ εἰ μόνη ἦν· ἀφήρηται
γάρ τι ἡ ἐλάττων μιγνυμένη, εἴπερ ἅπαντα τὰ ἁπλᾶ
μᾶλλον αἰσθητά ἐστιν. ἐὰν ἄρα ἴσαι ὦσιν ἕτεραι οὖσαι,
οὐδετέρας ἔσται αἴσθησις· ἀφανιεῖ γὰρ ἡ ἑτέρα ὁμοίως
τὴν ἑτέραν. ἁπλῆς δ' οὐκ ἔστιν αἰσθάνεσθαι. ὥστε
30 ἢ οὐδεμία ἔσται αἴσθησις ἢ ἄλλη ἐξ ἀμφοῖν. ὅπερ καὶ
γίγνεσθαι δοκεῖ ἐκ τῶν κεραννυμένων ἐν ᾧ ἂν μιχθῶσιν.
ἐπεὶ οὖν ἐκ μὲν ἐνίων γίνεταί τι, ἐκ δ' ἐνίων οὐ γίνεται,
447 b τοιαῦτα δὲ τὰ ὑφ' ἑτέραν αἴσθησιν (μίγνυνται γὰρ ὧν
τὰ ἔσχατα ἐναντία· οὐκ ἔστι δ' ἐκ λευκοῦ καὶ ὀξέος ἓν
γενέσθαι ἀλλ' ἢ κατὰ συμβεβηκός, ἀλλ' οὐχ ὡς ἐξ
ὀξέος καὶ βαρέος συμφωνία)· οὐκ ἄρα οὐδ' αἰσθάνεσθαι
5 ἐνδέχεται αὐτῶν ἅμα. ἴσαι μὲν γὰρ οὖσαι αἱ κινήσεις
ἀφανιοῦσιν ἀλλήλας, ἐπεὶ μία οὐ γίνεται ἐξ αὐτῶν· ἂν
δ' ἄνισοι, ἡ κρείττων αἴσθησιν ποιεῖ, ἐπεὶ μᾶλλον ἅμα
δυεῖν αἴσθοιτ' ἂν ἡ ψυχὴ τῇ μιᾷ αἰσθήσει ὧν μία
αἴσθησις, οἷον ὀξέος καὶ βαρέος· μᾶλλον γὰρ ἅμα ἡ
10 κίνησις τῆς μιᾶς ταύτης ἢ τοῖν δυοῖν, οἷον ὄψεως καὶ
ἀκοῆς. τῇ μιᾷ δὲ ἅμα δυοῖν οὐκ ἔστιν αἰσθάνεσθαι
ἂν μὴ μιχθῇ· τὸ γὰρ μῖγμα ἓν βούλεται εἶναι, τοῦ δ'
ἑνὸς μία αἴσθησις, ἡ δὲ μία ἅμα αὐτῇ. ὥστ' ἐξ ἀνάγκης
τῶν μεμιγμένων ἅμα αἰσθάνεται, ὅτι μιᾷ αἰσθήσει κατ'
15 ἐνέργειαν αἰσθάνεται· ἑνὸς μὲν γὰρ ἀριθμῷ ἡ κατ'
ἐνέργειαν μία, εἴδει δὲ ἡ κατὰ δύναμιν μία. καὶ εἰ
μία τοίνυν ἡ αἴσθησις ἡ κατ' ἐνέργειαν, ἓν ἐκεῖνα ἐρεῖ.
μεμῖχθαι ἄρα ἀνάγκη αὐτά. ὅταν ἄρα μὴ ᾖ μεμιγμένα,

---

447 a, 31　ἐν ᾧ, fort. ἐφ' ᾧ.

single thing is more perceptible by itself than when in a 20
compound. For example, a wine is more readily distinguished
when pure than when mixed; so with honey and tint, and the
tonic is more distinctly perceived when alone than when it is
sounded along with the octave, as the two when together annul
each other.

This result is produced by things out of which a unity
is formed. If it is the case that the stronger stimulus
displaces the weaker, it must, if they are simultaneous, itself
be less distinct to sense than if it were alone, having suffered 25
diminution to some extent by the admixture of the weaker,
if the pure is always the more perceptible. So if two different
stimuli are equal, neither will be perceived; either will annul
the other to an equal extent. But they cannot be perceived
as pure; hence either no sensation will result or another one 30
derived from both, precisely as things when mingled yield
something fresh so long as it is true mixture that takes place.

Thus in certain cases of the simultaneous presentation of
sensation something derivative results, but in certain cases
not, and such are instances of objects falling under diverse 447 b
senses. (Mixture occurs with objects when their most extreme
divergences of quality are related as contraries; white and
shrill do not yield anything unitary except *per accidens*, but,
quite otherwise, low and high yield a concord.) Since then
this is so, neither will it be possible to perceive them together.
If they are equal in intensity the stimuli will cancel each 5
other, since no unitary sensation is derived from them, while
if they are unequal the stronger will produce sensation, and
both will not be perceptible, since consciousness would more
readily distinguish two objects by a single sense and if they
both belonged to a single sense, *e.g.* high and low, than it
would these, for the stimuli are more closely located in the
case of this selfsame sense than when we have two different 10
senses, *e.g.* sight and hearing.

But by a single sense we cannot perceive two objects
simultaneously unless they combine with each other. For
the combination requires to be something unitary, and of a
unitary object the perception is single and a single sensation
is one possessing internal simultaneity. Consequently things
in combination must be simultaneously perceived, because
apprehended by a single act of perception. It is of what is 15
numerically one that the explicit perception is single while it
is of the specifically one that the implicit perception is unitary.
Hence also, if the explicit perception is single it pronounces
those objects to be numerically one. Hence they must have
entered into combination, and so, when they are not combined,

δύο ἔσονται αἰσθήσεις αἱ κατ᾽ ἐνέργειαν. ἀλλὰ κατὰ
20 μίαν δύναμιν καὶ ἄτομον χρόνον μίαν ἀνάγκη εἶναι τὴν
ἐνέργειαν· μιᾶς γὰρ εἰσάπαξ μία κίνησις καὶ χρῆσις,
μία δὲ ἡ δύναμις. οὐκ ἄρα ἐνδέχεται δυεῖν ἅμα αἰσθάνεσθαι τῇ μιᾷ αἰσθήσει. ἀλλὰ μὴν εἰ τὰ ὑπὸ τὴν αὐτὴν
αἴσθησιν ἅμα ἀδύνατον, ἐὰν ᾖ δύο, δῆλον ὅτι ἧττον ἔτι
25 τὰ κατὰ δύο αἰσθήσεις ἐνδέχεται ἅμα αἰσθάνεσθαι, οἷον
λευκὸν καὶ γλυκύ. φαίνεται γὰρ τὸ μὲν τῷ ἀριθμῷ ἓν
ἡ ψυχὴ οὐδενὶ ἑτέρῳ λέγειν ἀλλ᾽ ἢ τῷ ἅμα, τὸ δὲ τῷ
εἴδει ἓν τῇ κρινούσῃ αἰσθήσει καὶ τῷ τρόπῳ. λέγω
δὲ τοῦτο, ὅτι ἴσως τὸ λευκὸν καὶ τὸ μέλαν, ἕτερον τῷ
30 εἴδει ὄν, ἡ αὐτὴ κρίνει, καὶ τὸ γλυκὺ καὶ τὸ πικρόν, ἡ
αὐτὴ μὲν ἑαυτῇ, ἐκείνης δ᾽ ἄλλη, ἀλλ᾽ ἑτέρως ἑκάτερον
τῶν ἐναντίων, ὡς δ᾽ αὕτως ἑαυταῖς τὰ σύστοιχα, οἷον
448a ὡς ἡ γεῦσις τὸ γλυκύ, οὕτως ἡ ὄψις τὸ λευκόν· ὡς δ᾽
αὕτη τὸ μέλαν, οὕτως ἐκείνη τὸ πικρόν. ἔτι εἰ αἱ τῶν
ἐναντίων κινήσεις ἐναντίαι, ἅμα δὲ τὰ ἐναντία ἐν τῷ
αὐτῷ καὶ ἀτόμῳ οὐκ ἐνδέχεται ὑπάρχειν, ὑπὸ δὲ τὴν
5 αἴσθησιν τὴν μίαν ἐναντία ἐστίν, οἷον γλυκὺ πικρῷ,
οὐκ ἂν ἐνδέχοιτο αἰσθάνεσθαι ἅμα. ὁμοίως δὲ δῆλον
ὅτι οὐδὲ τὰ μὴ ἐναντία· τὰ μὲν γὰρ τοῦ λευκοῦ τὰ δὲ
τοῦ μέλανός ἐστιν, καὶ ἐν τοῖς ἄλλοις ὁμοίως, οἷον τῶν
χυμῶν οἱ μὲν τοῦ γλυκέος οἱ δὲ τοῦ πικροῦ. οὐδὲ τὰ
10 μεμιγμένα ἅμα· λόγοι γάρ εἰσιν ἀντικειμένων, οἷον τὸ
διὰ πασῶν καὶ τὸ διὰ πέντε, ἂν μὴ ὡς ἓν αἰσθάνηται.
οὕτως δ᾽ εἷς λόγος ὁ τῶν ἄκρων γίνεται, ἄλλως δ᾽ οὔ·
ἔσται γὰρ ἅμα ὁ μὲν πολλοῦ πρὸς ὀλίγον ἢ περιττοῦ
πρὸς ἄρτιον, ὁ δ᾽ ὀλίγου πρὸς πολὺ ἢ ἀρτίου πρὸς
15 περιττόν. εἰ οὖν πλεῖον ἔτι ἀπέχει ἀλλήλων καὶ διαφέρει
τὰ συστοίχως μὲν λεγόμενα ἐν ἄλλῳ δὲ γένει τῶν ἐν τῷ
αὐτῷ γένει λεγομένων (οἷον τὸ γλυκὺ καὶ τὸ λευκὸν ἀλλ᾽
ὡς σύστοιχα, γένει δ᾽ ἕτερα), τὸ γλυκὺ δὲ τοῦ μέλανος
πλεῖον ἔτι τῷ εἴδει διαφέρει ἢ τοῦ λευκοῦ, ἔτι ἂν ἧττον

448a, 19 τοῦ λευκοῦ LSU Alex. Ald. Bus., τὸ λευκόν reliqui codd. Sylb.
Bek. Didot, Torst. coni. 18 τοῦ λευκοῦ et 19 ἢ τὸ μέλαν p. 169, cui assentitur
Thurot; τῷ εἴδει 19 deleri volunt Torst. et Biehl.

there will be two explicit sensations. But when the faculty is single and the time individual, the activity of sense must be nu- 20 merically one ; the stimulation and exercise of a single faculty at a unitary time must be single ; and the faculty *is* single.

Thus it is impossible to perceive two things simultaneously by a single sense. But certainly, when objects of the same sense, if dual, cannot be simultaneously perceived, it is clear that still less will this be possible in the case of objects of two 25 different senses, *e.g.* white and sweet.

Consciousness appears to recognize numerical identity not otherwise than by the simultaneity of the perception, while specific unity is given by the unity of the sense which discriminates it and the manner in which the perception occurs. By this I mean that, though supposing it be black and white, objects specifically distinct, which the same sense discriminates, 30 and sweet and bitter, which a sense that is self-identical, though different from the former, distinguishes, yet there is a diverse manner in which it perceives either contrary, and it is in the same manner as each other that the senses apprehend corresponding members of different pairs of opposites ; *e.g.* sight perceives white in the same manner as taste does sweet- 448 a ness, and the former perceives black as the latter does bitter.

Further, if contrary sensibles give contrary stimuli and contraries cannot coexist in anything identical and individual, but under a single sense we find things opposed to each other, 5 as, for example, sweet is opposed to bitter, it is impossible to perceive them simultaneously. Similarly it is clear that neither will things that are not opposites be simultaneously intuitable. Some of them fall within the province of white and others of black, and in the same way in other cases, *e.g.* flavours, some are assignable to sweet, others to bitter. Neither can composites be simultaneously perceived unless as forming a unity, 10 for they are proportionate combinations of opposites, *e.g.* chords of the octave and of the fifth. If they *are* apprehended as one, a single ratio prevails between the extremes, but otherwise not, for that would require the simultaneous apprehension of the ratio of greater to less or odd to even on the one hand, and on the other that of less to greater or even to odd.

The consequence of all this is that, if there is a still greater 15 remoteness and diversity between qualities which, though occupying corresponding positions in their respective genera, yet are heterogeneous, than between those ascribed to the same genus, *e.g.* sweet and white, which, though corresponding to each other, nevertheless are heterogeneous, and if sweet differs still more from black than from white in kind, then they, sweet and black, are still less capable of being

20 ἅμα ἐνδέχοιτο αὐτὰ αἰσθάνεσθαι ἢ τὰ τῷ γένει ταὐτά.
21 ὥστ᾽ εἰ μὴ ταῦτα, οὐδ᾽ ἐκεῖνα.

21 　　　　　ᵃὋ δὲ λέγουσί τινες τῶν περὶ
τὰς συμφωνίας, ὅτι οὐχ ἅμα μὲν ἀφικνοῦνται οἱ ψόφοι,
φαίνονται δέ, καὶ λανθάνει, ὅταν ὁ χρόνος ᾖ ἀναίσθητος,
πότερον ὀρθῶς λέγεται ἢ οὔ; τάχα γὰρ ἂν φαίη τις καὶ
25 νῦν παρὰ τοῦτο δοκεῖν ἅμα ὁρᾶν καὶ ἀκούειν, ὅτι οἱ
μεταξὺ χρόνοι λανθάνουσιν. ἢ τοῦτ᾽ οὐκ ἀληθές, οὐδ᾽
ἐνδέχεται χρόνον εἶναι ἀναίσθητον ἢ οὐδένα λανθάνειν,
ἀλλὰ παντὸς ἐνδέχεται αἰσθάνεσθαι. εἰ γὰρ ὅτε αὐτὸς
αὐτοῦ τις αἰσθάνεται ἢ ἄλλου ἐν συνεχεῖ χρόνῳ, μὴ
30 ἐνδέχεται τότε λανθάνειν ὅτι ἐστίν, ἔστι δέ τις ἐν τῷ
συνεχεῖ καὶ τοσοῦτος ὅσος ὅλως ἀναίσθητός ἐστι, δῆλον
ὅτι τότε λανθάνοι ἂν εἰ ἔστιν αὐτὸς αὐτόν καὶ εἰ ὁρᾷ
448 b καὶ αἰσθάνεται· καὶ εἰ αἰσθάνεται ἔτι, οὐκ ἂν εἴη οὔτε
χρόνος οὔτε πρᾶγμα οὐδὲν ὃ αἰσθάνεται ἢ ἐν ᾧ, εἰ μὴ
οὕτως, ὅτι ἐν τούτου τινὶ ἢ ὅτι τούτου τι ὁρᾷ, εἴπερ
ἔστι τι μέγεθος καὶ χρόνου καὶ πράγματος ἀναίσθητον
5 ὅλως διὰ μικρότητα· εἰ γὰρ τὴν ὅλην ὁρᾷ, καὶ αἰσθάνεται τὸν αὐτὸν συνεχῶς χρόνον, οὐ τῶν νῦν τούτων
τινί. ἀφῃρήσθω ἡ [τὸ] ΓΒ, ἐν ᾗ οὐκ ᾐσθάνετο. οὐκοῦν
ἐν ταύτης τινὶ ἢ ταύτης τι, ὥσπερ τὴν γῆν ὁρᾷ ὅλην,
ὅτι τοδὶ αὐτῆς, καὶ ἐν τῷ ἐνιαυτῷ βαδίζει, ὅτι ἐν τῳδὶ
10 τῷ μέρει αὐτοῦ. ἀλλὰ μὴν ἐν τῷ ΒΓ οὐδὲν αἰσθάνεται.
τῷ ἄρα ἐν τούτου τινὶ τοῦ ΑΒ αἰσθάνεσθαι λέγεται τοῦ
ὅλου αἰσθάνεσθαι καὶ τὴν ὅλην. ὁ δ᾽ αὐτὸς λόγος καὶ
ἐπὶ τῆς ΑΓ· ἀεὶ γὰρ ἐν τινὶ καὶ τινός, ὅλου δ᾽ οὐκ
ἔστιν αἰσθάνεσθαι. ἅπαντα μὲν οὖν αἰσθητά ἐστιν,
15 ἀλλ᾽ οὐ φαίνεται ὅσα ἐστίν· τοῦ γὰρ ἡλίου τὸ μέγεθος
ὁρᾷ καὶ τὸ τετράπηχυ πόρρωθεν, ἀλλ᾽ οὐ φαίνεται ὅσον,
ἀλλ᾽ ἐνίοτε ἀδιαίρετον, ὁρᾷ δ᾽ οὐκ ἀδιαίρετον. ἡ δ᾽ αἰτία
εἴρηται ἐν τοῖς ἔμπροσθεν περὶ τούτου. ὅτι μὲν οὖν
19 οὐθείς ἐστι χρόνος ἀναίσθητος, ἐκ τούτων φανερόν·

19　　　　　　　　　　　　　　　　　　　Περὶ δὲ

448 b 7　ἤ] τὸ omisso ἤ L S U Alex.

simultaneously perceived than members of the same genus; 20
hence, if in the latter case this is impossible, neither can it
occur with the former.

There is a theory mooted by certain people about concords,
that the sounds, though not arriving simultaneously, yet appear
to do so, their lack of simultaneity being undetected, when the
time between them is imperceptible.

Is this correct, or is it not? If true, one might readily
assert that we also apparently see and hear at the same time 25
because the intervening moments are undetected.

We answer that it is not true, and there can be no imperceptible time, none that escapes us; every moment can be
perceived. For if, when one has consciousness of one's self
or of another person during a continuous period of time, one
cannot at that time be unaware that one exists, but there is 30
within the continuous time a section of such minute size as to
be wholly imperceptible, clearly one would then be unaware
whether one was one's self and whether one saw or perceived;
if one still perceived, there would be neither time in which 448 b
nor thing of which one could be conscious except thus—by
being percipient during part of the time or perceiving part of
the thing, if there are magnitudes both in time and in things
which their minuteness makes imperceptible. But this is not
so, for if one sees a whole line and perceives a time continuously 5
identical, one does not do so by means of one of the particular
" now's " contained in it. Subtract, from AB the whole line, a
part CB in which there is no sensation; then perception in
one part of this whole or of one part of it gives consciousness
of the whole, which is like seeing the whole earth because one
sees this particular part of it, or walking a whole year because
one walks during this part of it. Remember, in BC there is 10
no consciousness; hence, by being conscious in part of this
whole, AB, one is said to be conscious of the whole time and
see the whole extent.

The same reasoning will hold with the part AC, for perception is always in a part and of a part, and it is impossible to
perceive anything in its entirety. Hence, the above conclusion
being absurd, everything is perceptible though its size is not
apparent; we see the extension of the sun or a four-cubit 15
measure from afar, though the determinate size is not apparent, and sometimes things seem not to have size but to
be indivisible.

We cannot, however, see the indivisible; the reason for
this was stated before. Hence from these considerations it
is clear that no part of time is imperceptible.

But we have to discuss the problem raised before—whether

20 τῆς πρότερον λεχθείσης ἀπορίας σκεπτέον, πότερον
ἐνδέχεται ἅμα πλειόνων αἰσθάνεσθαι ἢ οὐκ ἐνδέχεται.
τὸ δ᾽ ἅμα λέγω ἐν ἑνὶ καὶ ἀτόμῳ χρόνῳ πρὸς ἄλληλα. πρῶτον μὲν οὖν ἆρ᾽ ὧδ᾽ ἐνδέχεται, ἅμα μέν, ἑτέρῳ
δὲ τῆς ψυχῆς αἰσθάνεσθαι, καὶ οὐ τῷ ἀτόμῳ, οὕτω
25 δ᾽ ἀτόμῳ ὡς παντὶ ὄντι συνεχεῖ; ἢ ὅτι πρῶτον μὲν τὰ
κατὰ τὴν μίαν αἴσθησιν, οἷον λέγω ὄψιν, εἰ ἔσται ἄλλῳ
αἰσθανομένη ἄλλου καὶ ἄλλου χρώματος, πλείω γε μέρη
ἕξει εἴδει ταῦτα; καὶ γὰρ αἰσθάνεται πάλιν τῷ αὐτῷ
γένει. εἰ δὲ ὅτι ὡς δύο ὄμματα φαίη τις, οὐδὲν κωλύει,
30 οὕτω καὶ ἐν τῇ ψυχῇ, ὅτι ἴσως ἐκ μὲν τούτων ἕν τι
γίνεται καὶ μία ἡ ἐνέργεια αὐτῶν· εἴδει δὲ ᾗ μὲν ἓν
τὸ ἐξ ἀμφοῖν, ἓν καὶ τὸ αἰσθανόμενον ἔσται, εἰ δὲ
χωρίς, οὐχ ὁμοίως ἕξει. ἔτι αἰσθήσεις αἱ αὐταὶ πλείους
449 a ἔσονται, ὥσπερ εἴ τις ἐπιστήμας διαφόρους φαίη· οὔτε
γὰρ ἡ ἐνέργεια ἄνευ τῆς καθ᾽ αὑτὴν ἔσται δυνάμεως,
οὔτ᾽ ἄνευ ταύτης ἔσται αἴσθησις. εἰ δὲ τούτων ἐν ἑνὶ
καὶ ἀτόμῳ ⟨μὴ⟩ αἰσθάνεται, δῆλον ὅτι καὶ τῶν ἄλλων·
5 μᾶλλον γὰρ ἐνεδέχετο τούτων ἅμα πλειόνων ἢ τῶν τῷ
γένει ἑτέρων. εἰ δὲ δὴ ἄλλῳ μὲν γλυκέος ἄλλῳ δὲ λευκοῦ
αἰσθάνεται ἡ ψυχὴ μέρει, ἤτοι τὸ ἐκ τούτων ἕν τί ἐστιν
ἢ οὐχ ἕν. ἀλλ᾽ ἀνάγκη ἕν· ἓν γάρ τι τὸ αἰσθητικόν
ἐστι μέρος. τίνος οὖν ἐκεῖνο ἑνός; οὐδὲν γὰρ ἐκ τούτων

---

448 b, 24 οὐ τῷ ἀτόμῳ et mox δ᾽ om. L S U et Alex., qui autem pro οὕτω
δέ habet καὶ οὕτως, quam Alexandri lectionem genuinam esse putant Thurot et
Bäumker (Jahrb. für Philol. 1886), praeterquam quod pro καὶ Thurot καὶ ἐν vult
poni, Bäumker autem κᾶν, sed nihil eorum satisfacit; legendum videtur: οὐ τῷ
ἀτόμῳ, η οὕτω ἀτόμῳ; vertit vet. tr.: et non indivisibili, sic autem indivisibili, ut
omni existenti continuo. | οὕτω δὲ ἀτόμον E Y, ἄτομα pro ἀτόμῳ M.   28 ταῦτα
E M et Biehl, ταὐτά reliqui omnes et scripti et edd. | γὰρ] γὰρ ᾶ L S U P et edd.
except. Biehl | πάλιν E M Y, ἐν rel. et edd. except. Biehl.   29 γένει ἐστὶν L S U P
et edd. except. Biehl. | κωλύει E Y, κωλύειν reliqui codd., etiam Alex. Ald. Basil.,
κωλύει Sylb.   31 αὐτῶι E Y | εἴδει δὲ ᾗ conicio, εἰ δὲ ᾗ E Biehl, εἰ δὲ ἡ M Y,
ἐκεῖ δὲ εἰ reliqui codd. et edd. etiam Alex. et vet. tr.   32 ἓν καὶ Biehl, ἐκεῖνο
L S U P Alex. vet. tr. et omnes reliqui edd. except. Biehl.   449 a, 1 ἀδιαφόρους
P vet. tr.   4 μὴ iam Alex. desiderat, probant Biehl, Thurot, Bäumker,
Neuhäuser, Poppelreuter.   7 ἐκ om. Biehl.

it is possible or not to perceive several things simultaneously. 20 By simultaneously I mean, in a time which, for the various things relatively to each other, is one and atomic.

Firstly, then, is the following solution possible—that they are indeed simultaneously perceived but by different psychical organs, not by an individual organ, though by one which is individual in the sense of forming a continuous whole? Or 25 is it the case that if so, in a single sense, for instance sight, which will perceive different colours by something different in each case, these partitions will assuredly form a plurality specifically various? This is so, for it, again, perceives by means of generic identity.

If some one were to allege that there is no difficulty in the psychical faculties being like the two eyes, specifically alike, 30 we may reply that perhaps in the case of the eyes there is a single product and the exercise of their function is unitary, and, so far as they yield a unitary result, specifically the sense-organs are also single, but when the sensations are diverse the case is different.

Further identical senses will be rendered multiple and distinct in the same sense as one talks of distinct sciences; 449 a for neither is there activity apart from its appropriate potentiality, nor without activity does sensation exist.

But if these contentions are correct and hence these qualities cannot be perceived in a single individual moment by means of a division in the organ of perception, it is clear that no other qualities can, for there was a better possibility of these in their severalness being simultaneously perceived 5 than of qualities generically different. If it is really the case that the mind perceives sweet with one part, white with another, the product of these must be either one or not one. But it must be a unity because the sentient organ is a unity. What is the unity then which that perceives? There is no such unitary product.

R.   7

10 ἕν. ἀνάγκη ἄρα ἕν τι εἶναι τῆς ψυχῆς, ᾧ ἅπαντα αἰσθάνεται, καθάπερ εἴρηται πρότερον, ἄλλο δὲ γένος δι᾽ ἄλλου.
ἆρ᾽ οὖν ᾗ μὲν ἀδιαίρετόν ἐστι κατ᾽ ἐνέργειαν, ἕν τί ἐστι
τὸ αἰσθητικὸν γλυκέος καὶ λευκοῦ, ὅταν δὲ διαιρετὸν
γένηται κατ᾽ ἐνέργειαν, ἕτερον; ἢ ὥσπερ ἐπὶ τῶν πραγ-
15 μάτων αὐτῶν ἐνδέχεται, οὕτως καὶ ἐπὶ τῆς ψυχῆς. τὸ
γὰρ αὐτὸ καὶ ἓν ἀριθμῷ λευκὸν καὶ γλυκύ ἐστι, καὶ
ἄλλα πολλά, εἰ μὴ χωριστὰ τὰ πάθη ἀλλήλων, ἀλλὰ
τὸ εἶναι ἕτερον ἑκάστῳ. ὁμοίως τοίνυν θετέον καὶ ἐπὶ
τῆς ψυχῆς τὸ αὐτὸ καὶ ἓν εἶναι ἀριθμῷ τὸ αἰσθητικὸν
20 πάντων, τῷ μέντοι εἶναι ἕτερον καὶ ἕτερον τῶν μὲν γένει
τῶν δὲ εἴδει. ὥστε καὶ αἰσθάνοιτ᾽ ἂν ἅμα τῷ αὐτῷ καὶ
22 ἑνί, λόγῳ δ᾽ οὐ τῷ αὐτῷ.

22 ὅτι δὲ τὸ αἰσθητὸν πᾶν ἐστὶ μέ-
γεθος καὶ οὐκ ἔστιν ἀδιαίρετον αἰσθάνεσθαι, δῆλον.
ἔστι γὰρ ὅθεν μὲν οὐκ ἂν ὀφθείη, ἄπειρον τὸ ἀπόστημα,
25 ὅθεν δὲ ὁρᾶται, πεπερασμένον· ὁμοίως δὲ καὶ τὸ ὀσφραντὸν καὶ ἀκουστὸν καὶ ὅσων μὴ αὐτῶν ἁπτόμενοι
αἰσθάνονται. ἔστι δέ τι ἔσχατον τοῦ ἀποστήματος ὅθεν
οὐχ ὁρᾶται, καὶ πρῶτον ὅθεν ὁρᾶται. τοῦτο δὴ ἀνάγκη
ἀδιαίρετον εἶναι, οὗ ἐν μὲν τῷ ἐπέκεινα οὐκ ἐνδέχεται
30 αἰσθάνεσθαι ὄντος, ἐν δὲ τῷ ἐπὶ ταδὶ ἀνάγκη αἰσθάνεσθαι. εἰ δή τί ἐστιν ἀδιαίρετον αἰσθητόν, ὅταν τεθῇ
ἐπὶ τῷ ἐσχάτῳ ὅθεν ἐστὶν ὕστατον μὲν οὐκ αἰσθητὸν
πρῶτον δ᾽ αἰσθητόν, ἅμα συμβήσεται ὁρατὸν εἶναι καὶ
ἀόρατον· τοῦτο δ᾽ ἀδύνατον.

449 b περὶ μὲν οὖν τῶν αἰσθητηρίων καὶ τῶν αἰσθητῶν
τίνα τρόπον ἔχει καὶ κοινῇ καὶ καθ᾽ ἕκαστον αἰσθητήριον
εἴρηται· τῶν δὲ λοιπῶν πρῶτον σκεπτέον περὶ μνήμης
4 καὶ τοῦ μνημονεύειν.

Hence there must be some unity in the soul by which we 10 perceive all things, as before stated, though different genera are perceived by different organs. Is that, therefore, which apprehends sweet and white, a unit so far as it is actually indivisible, but diverse in so far as it is actually divisible? We answer that in the case of the soul it is the same as with things. An identical and numerically single thing can be 15 sweet and white and have many other qualities, so long as its properties are not disunited from one another, though in aspect of existence each is diverse. Accordingly we must in the same way affirm that with the soul too, that, which is percipient of everything, is self-identical and numerically single, though, in apprehending objects now generically now in species 20 different, it has a corresponding diversity in the aspect of its existence. Hence the mind may perceive things simultaneously by means of something selfsame and unitary though not notionally the same.

That every object is a magnitude and that the indivisible cannot be perceived, is clear. The distances from which an object cannot be seen are infinite in number, but the range from which it is visible is limited, and this holds true also for 25 the objects of smell and hearing and all things perceived without actual contact. But there is a point which terminates the range from which vision is impossible and is the first from which the thing becomes visible. That indeed must be indivisible which, when at a distance beyond this 30 point, cannot be seen, but must be seen when nearer. If, then, there is really anything indivisible which is an object of perception, when placed at the terminal point which, while the last at which it is not perceptible, is yet the first at which it is perceptible, it will turn out to be both visible and invisible at the same time, which is impossible.

This is our account of the sensoria and the objects of 449 b sense and the manner of their existence both generally and relatively to each sense-organ. Of the remaining subjects let us consider first memory and the act of remembering.

I

4   Περὶ δὲ μνήμης καὶ τοῦ μνημονεύειν
5 λεκτέον τί ἐστι καὶ διὰ τίν᾽ αἰτίαν γίγνεται καὶ τίνι
τῶν τῆς ψυχῆς μορίων συμβαίνει τοῦτο τὸ πάθος καὶ
τὸ ἀναμιμνήσκεσθαι· οὐ γὰρ οἱ αὐτοί εἰσι μνημονικοὶ
καὶ ἀναμνηστικοί, ἀλλ᾽ ὡς ἐπὶ τὸ πολὺ μνημονικοὶ μὲν
οἱ βραδεῖς, ἀναμνηστικώτεροι δὲ οἱ ταχεῖς καὶ εὐμαθεῖς.
10 πρῶτον μὲν οὖν ληπτέον ποῖά ἐστι τὰ μνημονευτά·
πολλάκις γὰρ ἐξαπατᾶται τοῦτο. οὔτε γὰρ τὸ μέλλον
ἐνδέχεται μνημονεύειν, ἀλλ᾽ ἔστι δοξαστὸν καὶ ἐλπιστόν
(εἴη δ᾽ ἂν καὶ ἐπιστήμη τις ἐλπιστική, καθάπερ τινές
φασι τὴν μαντικήν), οὔτε τοῦ παρόντος, ἀλλ᾽ αἴσθησις·
15 ταύτῃ γὰρ οὔτε τὸ μέλλον οὔτε τὸ γενόμενον γνωρίζομεν,
ἀλλὰ τὸ παρὸν μόνον. ἡ δὲ μνήμη τοῦ γενομένου· τὸ δὲ
παρὸν ὅτι πάρεστιν, οἷον τοδὶ τὸ λευκὸν ὅτε ὁρᾷ, οὐδεὶς
ἂν φαίη μνημονεύειν, οὐδὲ τὸ θεωρούμενον, ὅτε θεωρῶν
τυγχάνει καὶ ἐννοῶν· ἀλλὰ τὸ μὲν αἰσθάνεσθαί φησι,
20 τὸ δ᾽ ἐπίστασθαι μόνον· ὅταν δ᾽ ἄνευ τῶν ἐνεργειῶν
ἔχῃ τὴν ἐπιστήμην καὶ τὴν αἴσθησιν, οὕτω μέμνηται
[τὰς τοῦ τριγώνου ὅτι δύο ὀρθαῖς ἴσαι], τὸ μὲν ὅτι
ἔμαθεν ἢ ἐθεώρησεν, τὸ δὲ ὅτι ἤκουσεν ἢ εἶδεν ἢ ὅ τι
τοιοῦτον· δεῖ γὰρ ὅταν ἐνεργῇ κατὰ τὸ μνημονεύειν,
25 οὕτως ἐν τῇ ψυχῇ λέγειν, ὅτι πρότερον τοῦτο ἤκουσεν
ἢ ᾔσθετο ἢ ἐνόησεν. ἔστι μὲν οὖν ἡ μνήμη οὔτε
αἴσθησις οὔτε ὑπόληψις, ἀλλὰ τούτων τινὸς ἕξις ἢ

---

449 b, 22   τὰς...ἴσαι recte volunt deleri Biehl et Freudenthal.

I

We must define and account for memory and the act of remembrance and assign the psychical faculty which provides 5 for this phenomenon and for the act of recollection. The two phenomena are not identical, for it is not the same people who have good memories and who have good powers of recollection; as a rule those people remember well who are slow-witted, while on the other hand those excel in powers of recall who are clever and quick at learning.

Hence as a preliminary to our argument the question 10 arises—how are the objects of memory characterised? Mistakes are often made about this. Now the future cannot be remembered; it is rather the object of opinion and hope. (There might be a science which belonged to the province of hope; some people say that prophecy is such a science.) Nor does memory regard the present; it is perception which is concerned with this, for by perception we apprehend neither 15 the future nor the past but the present only. Memory concerns the past; no one would say that he remembers that the present is present, *e.g.* this particular white object, when he is looking at it. Nor would he say that he remembers that the object of thought is present whensoever he chances to be engaged in thought or contemplation; in the one case he says he perceives, in the other merely that he knows. But when 20 knowledge or perception is present without actual experience of the real objects, in those circumstances one remembers in the one case that he learned something or thought of something, in the other that he heard, or saw, or had some similar sense-experience. When one actually remembers, he must recognize in consciousness that previously he had heard or 25 perceived or thought of the thing remembered.

Hence memory is neither perception nor conceptual

πάθος, ὅταν γένηται χρόνος. τοῦ δὲ νῦν ἐν τῷ νῦν οὐκ
ἔστι μνήμη, καθάπερ εἴρηται καὶ πρότερον, ἀλλὰ τοῦ
30 μὲν παρόντος αἴσθησις, τοῦ δὲ μέλλοντος ἐλπίς, τοῦ δὲ
γενομένου μνήμη. διὸ μετὰ χρόνου πᾶσα μνήμη. ὥσθ᾽
ὅσα χρόνου αἰσθάνεται, ταῦτα μόνα τῶν ζῴων μνημονεύει,
καὶ τούτῳ ᾧ αἰσθάνεται. ἐπεὶ δὲ περὶ φαντασίας εἴρηται
πρότερον ἐν τοῖς περὶ ψυχῆς, καὶ νοεῖν οὐκ ἔστιν ἄνευ
450 a φαντάσματος· συμβαίνει γὰρ τὸ αὐτὸ πάθος ἐν τῷ νοεῖν
ὅπερ καὶ ἐν τῷ διαγράφειν· ἐκεῖ τε γὰρ οὐθὲν προσχρώ-
μενοι τῷ τὸ ποσὸν ὡρισμένον εἶναι τοῦ τριγώνου, ὅμως
γράφομεν ὡρισμένον κατὰ τὸ ποσόν· καὶ ὁ νοῶν ὡσαύ-
5 τως, κἂν μὴ ποσὸν νοῇ, τίθεται πρὸ ὀμμάτων ποσόν,
νοεῖ δ᾽ οὐχ ᾗ ποσόν· ἂν δ᾽ ἡ φύσις ᾖ τῶν ποσῶν,
ἀορίστων δέ, τίθεται μὲν ποσὸν ὡρισμένον, νοεῖ δ᾽ ᾗ
ποσὸν μόνον· διὰ τίνα μὲν οὖν αἰτίαν οὐκ ἐνδέχεται
νοεῖν οὐδὲν ἄνευ τοῦ συνεχοῦς, οὐδ᾽ ἄνευ χρόνου τὰ μὴ
10 ἐν χρόνῳ ὄντα, λόγος ἄλλος· μέγεθος δ᾽ ἀναγκαῖον
γνωρίζειν καὶ κίνησιν ᾧ καὶ χρόνον· καὶ τὸ φάντασμα
τῆς κοινῆς αἰσθήσεως πάθος ἐστίν· ὥστε τοῦτο φανερὸν
ὅτι τῷ πρώτῳ αἰσθητικῷ τούτων ἡ γνῶσίς ἐστιν· ἡ δὲ
μνήμη καὶ ἡ τῶν νοητῶν οὐκ ἄνευ φαντάσματός ἐστιν·
15 ὥστε τοῦ νοητικοῦ κατὰ συμβεβηκὸς ἂν εἴη, καθ᾽ αὑτὸ
δὲ τοῦ πρώτου αἰσθητικοῦ. διὸ καὶ ἑτέροις τισὶν ὑπάρχει
τῶν ζῴων, καὶ οὐ μόνον ἀνθρώποις καὶ τοῖς ἔχουσι δόξαν
ἢ φρόνησιν. εἰ δὲ τῶν νοητικῶν τι μορίων ἦν, οὐκ ἂν
ὑπῆρχε πολλοῖς τῶν ἄλλων ζῴων, ἴσως δ᾽ οὐδενὶ τῶν
20 θνητῶν, ἐπεὶ οὐδὲ νῦν πᾶσι διὰ τὸ μὴ πάντα χρόνου
αἴσθησιν ἔχειν· ἀεὶ γὰρ ὅταν ἐνεργῇ τῇ μνήμῃ, καθάπερ
καὶ πρότερον εἴπομεν, ὅτι εἶδε τοῦτο ἢ ἤκουσεν ἢ ἔμαθε,
προσαισθάνεται ὅτι πρότερον· τὸ δὲ πρότερον καὶ

---

449 b 29 καὶ πρότερον om. L S U M Them. vet. tr., deleri volunt Freudenthal
et Biehl.

450 a, 20 θνητῶν] θηρίων Rassow et Biehl.

thought, but some permanent condition or modification attaching to them dependent upon lapse of time. What is now present we do not now in present time remember, as has been said before; with the present perception is employed, 30 with the future hope, with the past memory. Hence all remembering implies lapse of time; and so, those that have a sense of time are the only animals that remember, and the organ of memory is that which enables us to perceive time.

Imagination has been already discussed in the Psychology. We cannot think without imagery, for the same phenomenon 450 a occurs in thinking as is found in the construction of geometrical figures; there, though we do not employ as a supplementary requirement of our proof a determinateness in the size of the triangle, yet when we draw it we make it of a determinate size. Similarly in thinking also, though we do not think of 5 the size, yet we present the object visually to ourselves as a quantum, though we do not think of it as a quantum. If the nature of the object be quantitative but indeterminate, our presentation is of a determinate quantity, though we think of it as quantitative merely.

The reason why we can think of nothing apart from continuity and cannot think of objects not in time apart from time, belongs to a different inquiry from this, but we must 10 apprehend magnitude and change by the same means as that by which we are conscious of time. Imagery is a phenomenon belonging to the common sense; so this is clear, that the apprehension of these determinations belongs to the primary organ of sensation: and memory, even the memory of concepts, cannot exist apart from imagery.

Hence since all this is so, indirectly it belongs to the 15 noëtic faculty, but in its essential nature to the primary principle of sensation. This is the reason why it is found in several of the other animals and not only in man or those possessing the power of entertaining opinions and endowed with intelligence. If it belonged to the conceptual faculties it would not be found in many of the other animals and perhaps in none that are mortal, since, as facts are, all living beings do 20 not possess it, because not all have a sense of time. Always, when in the act of memory, as already said, we remember that we have heard or seen or learned this thing, we are conscious also that it was prior; now prior and posterior are distinctions in time.

ὕστερον ἐν χρόνῳ ἐστίν. τίνος μὲν οὖν τῶν τῆς ψυχῆς
25 ἐστὶν ἡ μνήμη, φανερόν, ὅτι οὗπερ καὶ ἡ φαντασία· καὶ
ἔστι μνημονευτὰ καθ᾽ αὑτὰ μὲν ὅσα ἐστὶ φανταστά, κατὰ
27 συμβεβηκὸς δὲ ὅσα μὴ ἄνευ φαντασίας.

27   ἀπορήσειε δ᾽ ἄν
τις πῶς ποτὲ τοῦ μὲν πάθους παρόντος τοῦ δὲ πράγματος
ἀπόντος μνημονεύεται τὸ μὴ παρόν. δῆλον γὰρ ὅτι δεῖ
30 νοῆσαι τοιοῦτον τὸ γιγνόμενον διὰ τῆς αἰσθήσεως ἐν τῇ
ψυχῇ καὶ τῷ μορίῳ τοῦ σώματος τῷ ἔχοντι αὐτήν, οἷον
ζωγράφημά τι τὸ πάθος, οὗ φαμὲν τὴν ἕξιν μνήμην εἶναι·
ἡ γὰρ γιγνομένη κίνησις ἐνσημαίνεται οἷον τύπον τινὰ
τοῦ αἰσθήματος, καθάπερ οἱ σφραγιζόμενοι τοῖς δακτυ-
450 b λίοις.   διὸ καὶ τοῖς μὲν ἐν κινήσει πολλῇ διὰ πάθος ἢ
δι᾽ ἡλικίαν οὖσιν οὐ γίγνεται μνήμη, καθάπερ ἂν εἰς
ὕδωρ ῥέον ἐμπιπτούσης τῆς κινήσεως καὶ τῆς σφραγῖδος·
τοῖς δὲ διὰ τὸ ψήχεσθαι, καθάπερ τὰ παλαιὰ τῶν οἰκο-
5 δομημάτων, καὶ διὰ σκληρότητα τοῦ δεχομένου τὸ πάθος
οὐκ ἐγγίγνεται ὁ τύπος.   διόπερ οἵ τε σφόδρα νέοι καὶ
οἱ γέροντες ἀμνήμονές εἰσιν· ῥέουσι γὰρ οἱ μὲν διὰ τὴν
αὔξησιν, οἱ δὲ διὰ τὴν φθίσιν. ὁμοίως δὲ καὶ οἱ λίαν
ταχεῖς καὶ οἱ λίαν βραδεῖς οὐδέτεροι φαίνονται μνήμονες·
10 οἱ μὲν γάρ εἰσιν ὑγρότεροι τοῦ δέοντος, οἱ δὲ σκληρό-
τεροι· τοῖς μὲν οὖν οὐ μένει τὸ φάντασμα ἐν τῇ ψυχῇ,
τῶν δ᾽ οὐχ ἅπτεται. ἀλλ᾽ εἰ δὴ τοιοῦτόν ἐστι τὸ συμβαῖνον περὶ τὴν μνήμην, πότερον τοῦτο μνημονεύει τὸ
πάθος, ἢ ἐκεῖνο ἀφ᾽ οὗ ἐγένετο; εἰ μὲν γὰρ τοῦτο, τῶν
15 ἀπόντων οὐδὲν ἂν μνημονεύοιμεν· εἰ δ᾽ ἐκεῖνο, πῶς
αἰσθανόμενοι τούτου μνημονεύομεν, οὗ μὴ αἰσθανόμεθα,
τὸ ἀπόν; εἴ τ᾽ ἐστὶν ὅμοιον ὥσπερ τύπος ἢ γραφὴ ἐν
ἡμῖν, τούτου αὐτοῦ ἡ αἴσθησις διὰ τί ἂν εἴη μνήμη
ἑτέρου, ἀλλ᾽ οὐκ αὐτοῦ τούτου; ὁ γὰρ ἐνεργῶν τῇ μνήμῃ
20 θεωρεῖ τὸ πάθος τοῦτο καὶ αἰσθάνεται τούτου.   πῶς οὖν
τὸ μὴ παρὸν μνημονεύει; εἴη γὰρ ἂν καὶ ὁρᾶν τὸ μὴ

Hence it is clear to what psychic faculty memory belongs; it belongs to that to which imagination must be assigned. 25 To the class of objects of memory *per se* belong all things that can be imagined; to the indirect, all that cannot be divorced from imagination.

A difficulty might be raised as to how it can ever come about that, though contemporaneously with our present mental modification the real object is not present, yet it is the absent object which is remembered. But this is no impossibility, for it is clear that we must regard the modification arising from 30 sensation in the soul and in that bodily part where sense resides, as if it were a picture of the real thing, and memory we call the permanent existence of this modification. When a stimulus occurs it imprints as it were a mould of the sense-affection exactly as a seal-ring acts in stamping.

This is the reason why memory does not occur in those 450 b who are in a rapid state of transition, whether owing to some perturbing experience or their period of life; it is as if this stimulus, like the seal, were stamped on running water. Again in others their worn out condition—like that of old buildings—and the hardness of the receptive structure, pre- 5 vent the sense-affection from leaving an impression. Hence we explain why the very young and the aged have no memory; in the former growth, in the latter decay, cause rapid transition. For like reasons, neither very quick-witted nor very slow people seem to have good memories; in the one class there 10 is too much fluidity, in the other too much density, and hence the former do not retain the image in the mind, while in the latter it never gets fixed.

If these are indeed the facts with regard to memory, whether do we remember this resultant modification or that which caused it? If the former, there would be no such thing as memory of things absent. On the other hand, if it is the 15 latter we remember, how, though perceiving the former, do we remember the absent object which we do not perceive? Once more, if what is retained is like the original in the fashion of an impression or copy, why is the perception of this very thing the memory of some other thing and not of it itself? It is this modification of consciousness which one engaged in remembering has present to his mind, and it is this that he perceives. How then can one remember what is 20

παρὸν καὶ ἀκούειν. ἢ ἔστιν ὡς ἐνδέχεται καὶ συμβαίνει
τοῦτο; οἷον γὰρ τὸ ἐν τῷ πίνακι γεγραμμένον ζῷον καὶ
ζῷόν ἐστι καὶ εἰκών, καὶ τὸ αὐτὸ καὶ ἓν τοῦτ' ἐστὶν ἄμφω,
25 τὸ μέντοι εἶναι οὐ ταὐτόν ἐστιν ἀμφοῖν, καὶ ἔστι θεωρεῖν
καὶ ὡς ζῷον καὶ ὡς εἰκόνα, οὕτω καὶ τὸ ἐν ἡμῖν φάντασμα
δεῖ ὑπολαβεῖν καὶ αὐτὸ καθ' ἑαυτὸ εἶναι θεώρημα καὶ
ἄλλου φάντασμα. ᾗ μὲν οὖν καθ' ἑαυτό, θεώρημα ἢ
φάντασμά ἐστιν, ᾗ δ' ἄλλου, οἷον εἰκὼν καὶ μνημόνευμα.
30 ὥστε καὶ ὅταν ἐνεργῇ ἡ κίνησις αὐτοῦ, ἂν μέν, ᾗ καθ'
αὐτό ἐστι, ταύτῃ αἰσθηται ἡ ψυχὴ αὐτοῦ, οἷον νόημά
τι ἢ φάντασμα φαίνεται ἐπελθεῖν· ἂν δ' ᾗ ἄλλου, ὥσπερ
ἐν τῇ γραφῇ ὡς εἰκόνα θεωρεῖ, καὶ μὴ ἑωρακὼς τὸν
Κορίσκον ὡς Κορίσκου· ἐνταῦθά τε ἄλλο τὸ πάθος τῆς
451a θεωρίας ταύτης καὶ ὅταν ὡς ζῷον γεγραμμένον θεωρῇ,
ἔν τε τῇ ψυχῇ τὸ μὲν γίγνεται ὥσπερ νόημα μόνον, τὸ
δ' ὡς ἐκεῖ ὅτι εἰκών, μνημόνευμα. καὶ διὰ τοῦτο ἐνίοτ'
οὐκ ἴσμεν, ἐγγινομένων ἡμῖν ἐν τῇ ψυχῇ τοιούτων κινή-
5 σεων ἀπὸ τοῦ αἰσθέσθαι πρότερον, εἰ κατὰ τὸ ᾐσθῆσθαι
συμβαίνει, καὶ εἰ ἔστι μνήμη ἢ οὔ διστάζομεν· ὁτὲ δὲ
συμβαίνει ἐννοῆσαι καὶ ἀναμνησθῆναι ὅτι ἠκούσαμέν
τι πρότερον ἢ εἴδομεν. τοῦτο δὲ συμβαίνει, ὅταν θεωρῶν
ὡς αὐτὸ μεταβάλῃ καὶ θεωρῇ ὡς ἄλλου. γίγνεται δὲ
10 καὶ τοὐναντίον, οἷον συνέβη Ἀντιφέροντι τῷ Ὠρείτῃ
καὶ ἄλλοις ἐξισταμένοις· τὰ γὰρ φαντάσματα ἔλεγον
ὡς γενόμενα καὶ ὡς μνημονεύοντες. τοῦτο δὲ γίγνεται,
ὅταν τις τὴν μὴ εἰκόνα ὡς εἰκόνα θεωρῇ. αἱ δὲ μελέται
τὴν μνήμην σῴζουσι τῷ ἐπαναμιμνήσκειν· τοῦτο δ' ἐστὶν
15 οὐδὲν ἕτερον ἢ τὸ θεωρεῖν πολλάκις ὡς εἰκόνα καὶ μὴ ὡς
καθ' αὐτό. τί μὲν οὖν ἐστι μνήμη καὶ τὸ μνημονεύειν,
εἴρηται, ὅτι φαντάσματος, ὡς εἰκόνος οὗ φάντασμα, ἕξις,
καὶ τίνος μορίου τῶν ἐν ἡμῖν, ὅτι τοῦ πρώτου αἰσθητικοῦ
καὶ ᾧ χρόνου αἰσθανόμεθα.

450 b, 27 αὐτὸ καθ' ἑαυτὸ E Y αὐτό τι καθ' αὐτὸ Biehl | om. θεώρημα L S U
Them. vet. tr. Biehl, θεώρ. et φάντασμα deleri vult Freudth.

not present to one? One might as well see or hear what is not present.

But perhaps there is a way in which this can occur and it does really come about? That is so, for, as the animal depicted on the panel is both animal and representation, and, while remaining one self-identical thing, is yet both of these, though in aspect of existence the two are not the same, and we can 25 regard it both as animal and as copy, so too the image in us must be considered as being both an object of direct consciousness in itself and relatively to something else an image; in its own nature it is an object of direct inspection or an image, so far as it represents something else it is a copy and a souvenir.

Hence when the change connected with it is actually 30 experienced, if the mind perceives it in terms of its own proper nature, it appears to present itself to consciousness in the guise of an object of thought or an image; but when it is perceived as referring to something else, we regard it as the copy in the painting and as the picture of Coriscus although we have not then beheld him. Here this way of regarding the thing is an experience different from what occurs when 451 a we regard the object as an animal in chalk merely; in the latter case the psychical modification occurs merely as an object of thought, in the former as a memory, because there it is viewed as a representation.

Hence sometimes we do not know, when those psychical changes due to previous perception take place in us, if it is 5 as connected with a previous perception that they occur, and we are in doubt whether it is a memory or not. Sometimes it chances that on reflection we recollect that we have heard or seen the thing previously; this takes place when, after regarding the object of consciousness in its own nature, we change and refer it to something else. The reverse of this also occurs, as befell in the case of Antipheron of Oreos and 10 other ecstatics; they took their mental images to be objective and said they remembered the occurrences. This comes about when we take what is not a representation as though it were one. But exercise strengthens the memory through the repeated performance of the act of recollection, which is merely to view the image frequently as a copy and not in its 15 own nature.

This is our account of memory and the act of remembering; it is the permanence of an image regarded as the copy of the thing it images, and the member in us to which it appertains is the primary seat of sensation and the organ employed in the perception of time.

II

20 Περὶ δὲ τοῦ ἀναμιμνήσκεσθαι λοιπὸν εἰπεῖν. πρῶτον
μὲν οὖν ὅσα ἐν τοῖς ἐπιχειρηματικοῖς λόγοις ἐστὶν ἀληθῆ,
δεῖ τίθεσθαι ὡς ὑπάρχοντα. οὔτε γὰρ μνήμης ἐστὶν
ἀνάληψις ἡ ἀνάμνησις οὔτε λῆψις· ὅταν γὰρ τὸ πρῶτον
μάθῃ ἢ πάθῃ, οὔτ᾽ ἀναλαμβάνει μνήμην οὐδεμίαν (οὐ-
25 δεμία γὰρ προγέγονεν) οὔτ᾽ ἐξ ἀρχῆς λαμβάνει· ὅταν
δὲ ἐγγένηται ἡ ἕξις καὶ τὸ πάθος, τότε ἡ μνήμη ἐστίν.
ὥστε μετὰ τοῦ πάθους ἐγγινομένου οὐκ ἐγγίνεται. ἔτι δ᾽
ὅτε τὸ πρῶτον ἐγγέγονε τῷ ἀτόμῳ καὶ ἐσχάτῳ, τὸ μὲν
πάθος ἐνυπάρχει ἤδη τῷ παθόντι καὶ ἡ ἐπιστήμη, εἰ δεῖ
30 καλεῖν ἐπιστήμην τὴν ἕξιν ἢ τὸ πάθος (οὐθὲν δὲ κωλύει
κατὰ συμβεβηκὸς καὶ μνημονεύειν ἔνια ὧν ἐπιστάμεθα)·
τὸ δὲ μνημονεύειν καθ᾽ αὑτὸ οὐχ ὑπάρξει πρὶν χρονισθῆ-
ναι· μνημονεύει γὰρ νῦν ὃ εἶδεν ἢ ἔπαθε πρότερον, οὐχ
451 b ὃ νῦν ἔπαθε, νῦν μνημονεύει. ἔτι δὲ φανερὸν ὅτι μνημονεύειν ἔστι μὴ νῦν ἀναμνησθέντα, ἀλλ᾽ ἐξ ἀρχῆς
αἰσθόμενον ἢ παθόντα. ἀλλ᾽ ὅταν ἀναλαμβάνῃ ἣν
πρότερον εἶχεν ἐπιστήμην ἢ αἴσθησιν ἢ οὗ ποτὲ τὴν
5 ἕξιν ἐλέγομεν μνήμην, τοῦτ᾽ ἐστὶ καὶ τότε τὸ ἀναμιμνήσκεσθαι τῶν εἰρημένων τι. τὸ δὲ μνημονεύειν συμβαίνει
καὶ ἡ μνήμη ἀκολουθεῖ. οὐδὲ δὴ ταῦτα ἁπλῶς, ἐὰν
ἔμπροσθεν ὑπάρξαντα πάλιν ἐγγένηται, ἀλλ᾽ ἔστιν ὡς,
ἔστι δ᾽ ὡς οὔ. δὶς γὰρ μαθεῖν καὶ εὑρεῖν ἐνδέχεται τὸν
10 αὐτὸν τὸ αὐτό· δεῖ οὖν διαφέρειν τὸ ἀναμιμνήσκεσθαι
τούτων, καὶ ἐνούσης πλείονος ἀρχῆς ἢ ἐξ ἧς μανθάνουσιν
12 ἀναμιμνήσκεσθαι.

12 συμβαίνουσι δ᾽ αἱ ἀναμνήσεις, ἐπειδὴ
πέφυκεν ἡ κίνησις ἥδε γενέσθαι μετὰ τήνδε· εἰ μὲν
ἐξ ἀνάγκης, δῆλον ὡς ὅταν ἐκείνη κινηθῇ, τήνδε τὴν

451 a, 28   τι post ἐγγέγονε inseri vult Freudenthal.

II

Recollection remains to be dealt with. First of all we 20 must posit as fact all the conclusions come to in our " Tentative Reasonings " which were correct. Recollection is neither the recovery nor the acquirement of memory.

When, on the first occasion, one learns or experiences something, he neither reacquires a memory, for none has previously existed, nor does he acquire it initially then. But when a disposition as well as the experience has once been 25 produced then memory is found; hence it does not come into being in conjunction with the origination of the experience in us.

Further, when memory first has been produced in the individual and ultimate organ of sensation, the experience and the knowledge in question (if it is proper to call the disposition or experience knowledge ; but there is nothing to 30 prevent our having indirectly remembrance also of some of the objects of knowledge) have already existence in the experiencing subject. But memory in the proper sense will not exist till after the lapse of time. We remember in present time what we have previously seen or heard, we do not now remember what we have now experienced. But further, 451 b clearly, we may remember, not in virtue of a present act of recollection, but by being conscious or feeling the experience from the start. On the other hand, when we reacquire the knowledge or perception or whatever it was, the permanence of which we called memory, here and now we have recollection 5 of any of these. As a result we remember them and memory ensues; not that that can be said without restriction in all cases when previous experiences are repeated in consciousness; in some cases it is so but in others not, for the same man may learn or discover the same thing twice. Recollection then 10 must differ from the latter operations; it requires a more considerable basis to start from than in the case of learning.

The occurrence of an act of recollection is due to the natural tendency of one particular change to follow another. If the sequence is necessary, it is clear that, on the former

15 κίνησιν κινηθήσεται· εἰ δὲ μὴ ἐξ ἀνάγκης ἀλλ' ἔθει,
ὡς ἐπὶ τὸ πολὺ κινηθήσεται. συμβαίνει δ' ἐνίους ἅπαξ
ἐθισθῆναι μᾶλλον ἢ ἄλλους πολλάκις κινουμένους· διὸ
ἔνια ἅπαξ ἰδόντες μᾶλλον μνημονεύομεν ἢ ἔτεροι πολλάκις. ὅταν οὖν ἀναμιμνησκώμεθα, κινούμεθα τῶν
20 προτέρων τινὰ κινήσεων, ἕως ἂν κινηθῶμεν μεθ' ἣν
ἐκείνη εἴωθεν. διὸ καὶ τὸ ἐφεξῆς θηρεύομεν νοήσαντες
ἀπὸ τοῦ νῦν ἢ ἄλλου τινός, καὶ ἀφ' ὁμοίου ἢ ἐναντίου
ἢ τοῦ σύνεγγυς. διὰ τοῦτο γίνεται ἡ ἀνάμνησις· αἱ
γὰρ κινήσεις τούτων τῶν μὲν αἱ αὐταί, τῶν δ' ἅμα, τῶν
25 δὲ μέρος ἔχουσιν, ὥστε τὸ λοιπὸν μικρὸν ὃ ἐκινήθη
μετ' ἐκεῖνο. ζητοῦσι μὲν οὖν οὕτω, καὶ μὴ ζητοῦντες
δ' οὕτως ἀναμιμνήσκονται, ὅταν μεθ' ἑτέραν κίνησιν
ἐκείνη γένηται· ὡς δὲ τὰ πολλὰ ἑτέρων γενομένων
κινήσεων οἵων εἴπομεν, ἐγένετο ἐκείνη. οὐδὲν δὲ δεῖ
30 σκοπεῖν τὰ πόρρω, πῶς μεμνήμεθα, ἀλλὰ τὰ σύνεγγυς·
δῆλον γὰρ ὅτι ὁ αὐτός ἐστι τρόπος. λέγω δὲ τὸ ἐφεξῆς
οὐ προζητήσας οὐδ' ἀναμνησθείς. τῷ γὰρ ἔθει ἀκολουθοῦσιν αἱ κινήσεις ἀλλήλαις, ἥδε μετὰ τήνδε. καὶ ὅταν
τοίνυν ἀναμιμνήσκεσθαι βούληται, τοῦτο ποιήσει· ζητή-
35 σει λαβεῖν ἀρχὴν κινήσεως, μεθ' ἣν ἐκείνη ἔσται. διὸ
452 a τάχιστα καὶ κάλλιστα γίνονται ἀπ' ἀρχῆς αἱ ἀναμνήσεις·
ὡς γὰρ ἔχουσι τὰ πράγματα πρὸς ἄλληλα τῷ ἐφεξῆς,
οὕτω καὶ αἱ κινήσεις. καὶ ἔστιν εὐμνημόνευτα ὅσα
τάξιν τινὰ ἔχει, ὥσπερ τὰ μαθήματα· τὰ δὲ φαῦλα
5 χαλεπῶς. καὶ τούτῳ διαφέρει τὸ ἀναμιμνήσκεσθαι τοῦ
πάλιν μανθάνειν, ὅτι δυνήσεταί πως δι' αὐτοῦ κινηθῆναι
ἐπὶ τὸ μετὰ τὴν ἀρχήν. ὅταν δὲ μή, ἀλλὰ δι' ἄλλου,
οὐκέτι μέμνηται. πολλάκις δ' ἤδη μὲν ἀδυνατεῖ ἀνα-

change occurring, the second will be summoned into activity;
when, however, the connection is not necessary but due to 15
custom, the occurrence of the second process will take place
only in most cases. It so happens that some people receive
a greater bent from a single experience than others in whom
the sequence has frequently taken place, and hence, in some
instances, after seeing the things once, we remember them
better than others who have seen them frequently. Thus,
when we recollect, one of our previous psychic changes is 20
stimulated which leads to the stimulation of that one, after
which the experience to be recollected is wont to occur.
Consequently we hunt for the next in the series, starting our
train of thought from what is now present or from something
else, and from something similar or contrary or contiguous to
it. This is the means of effecting recollection; the change in
those cases is now identical, now concomitant with, and now
partially inclusive of the idea to be recalled, and hence the 25
remainder formerly occurring subsequently to the rest is but
small.

This is the way in which the search for the idea not
present is carried out, and, even when there is no search, it
is in this way that recollection occurs, when the one process
occurs after the other; and in general it is after experience of
other changes such as we have described that the process in
question occurs. We must consider, not how we remember
things remotely connected but those that are close to each 30
other, for it is clear that the method is the same in both
cases. I use the expression "next in order" without implying
a prior search or act of recollection; for it is owing to the
custom of their being experienced in sequence that one particular process follows another. Hence, when one wishes to
recall something, this is what he does—he tries to find the
starting point of a process after which the one in question 35
will recur. This is why the swiftest and best way of recol- 452 a
lecting is to start from the beginning; the subjective changes
are related to each other in the same way as the facts
remembered stand to each other in virtue of their place in
the series. Those things are easily recalled which have an
orderly arrangement such as we find in mathematics; but
things wanting in exactitude are with difficulty remembered.
To recollect and to learn a second time differ in this, that he 5
who recalls a thing will be able by his own agency to pass to
the process succeeding the starting point; when this is not so
and the instrumentality of someone else is required, it is no
longer a case of remembering.

Often when as yet unable to recollect, by searching one

μνησθῆναι, ζητῶν δὲ δύναται καὶ εὑρίσκει. τοῦτο δὲ
10 γίνεται κινοῦντι πολλά, ἕως ἂν τοιαύτην κινήσῃ κίνησιν
ᾗ ἀκολουθήσει τὸ πρᾶγμα. τὸ γὰρ μεμνῆσθαί ἐστι τὸ
ἐνεῖναι δυνάμει τὴν κινοῦσαν· τοῦτο δέ, ὥστ᾽ ἐξ αὐτοῦ
καὶ ὧν ἔχει κινήσεων κινηθῆναι, ὥσπερ εἴρηται. δεῖ
δὲ λαβέσθαι ἀρχῆς. διὸ ἀπὸ τόπων δοκοῦσιν ἀναμιμνή-
15 σκεσθαι ἐνίοτε. τὸ δ᾽ αἴτιον ὅτι ταχὺ ἀπ᾽ ἄλλου ἐπ᾽
ἄλλο ἔρχονται, οἷον ἀπὸ γάλακτος ἐπὶ λευκόν, ἀπὸ λευκοῦ
δ᾽ ἐπ᾽ ἀέρα, καὶ ἀπὸ τούτου ἐφ᾽ ὑγρόν, ἀφ᾽ οὗ ἐμνήσθη
μετοπώρου, ταύτην ἐπιζητῶν τὴν ὥραν. ἔοικε δὴ καθόλου
ἀρχῇ καὶ τὸ μέσον πάντων· εἰ γὰρ μὴ πρότερον, ὅταν
20 ἐπὶ τοῦτο ἔλθῃ, μνησθήσεται, ἢ οὐκέτ᾽ οὐδὲ ἄλλοθεν,
οἷον εἴ τις νοήσειεν ἐφ᾽ ὧν Α Β Γ Δ Ε Ζ Η Θ· εἰ γὰρ μὴ
22 ἐπὶ τοῦ <Θ ἐμνήσθη, ἐπὶ τοῦ Ε μέμνηται, εἰ τὸ Η ἢ
22 τὸ Ζ ἐπιζητεῖ>· ἐντεῦθεν γὰρ ἐπ᾽ ἄμφω κινηθῆναι ἐνδέχεται, καὶ ἐπὶ τὸ Δ καὶ ἐπὶ τὸ Ζ. εἰ δὲ μὴ τούτων τι
ἐζήτει, ἐπὶ τὸ Γ ἐλθὼν μνησθήσεται, [εἰ τὸ Η ἢ τὸ Ζ
25 ἐπιζητεῖ]· εἰ δὲ μή, ἐπὶ τὸ Α· καὶ οὕτως ἀεί. τοῦ δ᾽
ἀπὸ τοῦ αὐτοῦ ἐνίοτε μὲν μνησθῆναι ἐνίοτε δὲ μή, αἴτιον
τὸ ἐπὶ πλεῖον ἐνδέχεσθαι κινηθῆναι ἀπὸ τῆς αὐτῆς ἀρχῆς,
οἷον ἀπὸ τοῦ Γ ἐπὶ τὸ Ζ ᾖ τὸ Δ. ἐὰν οὖν δι᾽ ἃ πάλαι οὐ
κινηθῇ, ἐπὶ τὸ συνηθέστερον κινεῖται· ὥσπερ γὰρ φύσις
30 ἤδη τὸ ἔθος. διὸ πολλάκις ἃ ἐννοοῦμεν, ταχὺ ἀναμιμνη-
σκόμεθα· ὥσπερ γὰρ φύσει τόδε μετὰ τόδε ἐστίν, οὕτω
452 b καὶ ἐνεργείᾳ· τὸ δὲ πολλάκις φύσιν ποιεῖ. ἐπεὶ δ᾽ ἐν
τοῖς φύσει γίγνεται καὶ παρὰ φύσιν καὶ ἀπὸ τύχης,
ἔτι μᾶλλον ἐν τοῖς δι᾽ ἔθος, οἷς ἡ φύσις γε μὴ ὁμοίως

452 a, 21–25 text. recept. habet Biehl, primus scripsit Freudth., Rh. Mus.
XXIV. et Archiv für Gesch. d. Philos. II. 1889. 21 vulgo legitur·: εἰ γὰρ μὴ
ἐπὶ τοῦ Ε μέμνηται, ἐπὶ τοῦ Ε Θ ἐμνήσθη, sed ἐπὶ τοῦ Ε μέμνηται om. Ε Μ Υ, pro
Ε Θ habet ν θ Ε, η θ Υ, θ L Them. Mich. Didot. 23 Δ] a Ε Μ. | pro Ζ vulgo
Ε, Ζ etiam vet. tr. 24 ἐζήτει Biehl, ἐπιζητεῖ S et reliqui edd., etiam Freudth.,
ἐπεζήτει L | Ζ] θ Ε Υ. 25 ἐπιζητεῖ habet etiam Ε (Bus.) | Α] δ Υ. 28 Ε
pro Γ legi vult Freudth. | ἐὰν οὖν δι᾽ ἃ πάλαι οὐ Biehl, ἐὰν οὖν μὴ L S U Y et
omnes reliqui edd. | διὰ παλαιοῦ L S U M Them. Mich. vet. tr. et omnes reliqui
edd., δι᾽ ἃ πάλαι οὐ Υ et Ε (Bus.).

manages to do so and finds what he was seeking. Here what happens is, that one initiates many processes before he arrives 10 at the stimulation of that one on which the object sought will ensue. Remembering depends upon the potential presence in consciousness of the causal process, and upon this, on the condition that, as mentioned, the transition be effected by one's own agency and by means of processes that one already possesses.

A starting point from which to begin must always be found. Hence commonplaces seem to be often the initial point in the act of recollection. The reason why these are 15 employed is that we pass quickly from one to another, *e.g.* from milk to white, from white to air, from this to wet, passing from which we call to mind the late autumn, which is the season we had in view.

It is true that in general the middle member also of a whole series of terms seems to be a starting point; if one does not recollect before, one will do so when he comes to it, or else there is no other point from which he can pass to the 20 recollection of the thing in question. Suppose for instance one has a series of thoughts A B C D E F G H ; if one has not remembered at H, one remembers at E, if he is seeking for G or F ; for from that point we can go in either direction both towards D and towards F. But if we are not seeking for one of these members of the series, *i.e.* G or F, by going to C we shall effect recollection ; if that is not so, by going to A we can. This is universally the process.

The reason why, though the same link is employed, 25 recollection sometimes is and sometimes is not successful, is that we can pass to a further distance at one time than at another from the same starting point, *e.g.* from C to F or to D. Hence, if the transition is mediated by some connecting link which has not lately been employed, one passes to the more familiar consequent, for the newly acquired habit has become exactly like a natural disposition. It is thus that we 30 explain why frequently we recollect quickly what we have been meditating upon. It is just in accordance with a natural tendency to follow one another in a particular order that things actually happen ; and it is frequent repetition that produces a natural tendency. But since in the realm of **452 b** Nature we meet with events contrary also to the order of Nature and due to chance, this is still more likely to occur in things due to custom, among which a natural order does

ὑπάρχει· ὥστε κινηθῆναι ἐνίοτε κἀκεῖ καὶ ἄλλως, ἄλλως
5 τε καὶ ὅταν ἀφέλκῃ ἐκεῖθεν αὑτόσε πῃ. διὰ τοῦτο καὶ
ὅταν δέῃ ὄνομα μνημονεῦσαι, παρόμοιον μέν, εἰς δ᾽ ἐκεῖνο
σολοικίζομεν. τὸ μὲν οὖν ἀναμιμνήσκεσθαι τοῦτον συμ-
8 βαίνει τὸν τρόπον.

8   τὸ δὲ μέγιστον, γνωρίζειν δεῖ τὸν χρόνον,
ἢ μέτρῳ ἢ ἀορίστως. ἔστω δέ τι ᾧ κρίνει τὸν πλείω καὶ
10 ἐλάττω· εὔλογον δ᾽ ὥσπερ τὰ μεγέθη· νοεῖ γὰρ τὰ
μεγάλα καὶ πόρρω οὐ τῷ ἀποτείνειν ἐκεῖ τὴν διάνοιαν,
ὥσπερ τὴν ὄψιν φασί τινες (καὶ γὰρ μὴ ὄντων ὁμοίως
νοήσει), ἀλλὰ τῇ ἀνάλογον κινήσει· ἔστι γὰρ ἐν αὐτῇ
τὰ ὅμοια σχήματα καὶ κινήσεις. τίνι οὖν διοίσει, ὅταν
15 τὰ μείζω νοῇ, ἢ ὅταν ἐκεῖνα νοῇ τὰ ἐλάττω; πάντα γὰρ
τὰ ἐντὸς ἐλάττω, καὶ ἀνάλογον καὶ τὰ ἐκτός. ἔστι δ᾽
ἴσως ὥσπερ καὶ τοῖς εἴδεσιν ἀνάλογον λαβεῖν ἄλλο ἐν
αὐτῷ, οὕτως καὶ τοῖς ἀποστήμασιν. ὥσπερ οὖν εἰ τὴν
ΑΒ ΒΕ κινεῖται, ποιεῖ τὴν ΓΔ· ἀνάλογον γὰρ ἡ ΑΓ
20 καὶ ἡ ΓΔ. τί οὖν μᾶλλον τὴν ΓΔ ἢ τὴν ΖΗ ποιεῖ;
ἢ ὡς ἡ ΑΓ πρὸς τὴν ΑΒ ἔχει, οὕτως ἡ [τὸ] Θ πρὸς
τὴν Ι ἔχει. ταύτας οὖν ἅμα κινεῖται. ἂν δὲ τὴν ΖΗ
βούληται νοῆσαι, τὴν μὲν ΒΕ ὁμοίως νοεῖ, ἀντὶ δὲ
τῶν ΘΙ τὰς ΚΛ νοεῖ· αὗται γὰρ ἔχουσιν ὡς ΖΑ
25 πρὸς ΒΑ.

ὅταν οὖν ἅμα ᾖ τε τοῦ πράγματος γίνηται κίνησις
καὶ ἡ τοῦ χρόνου, τότε τῇ μνήμῃ ἐνεργεῖ. ἂν δ᾽ οἴηται

452 b, 13 αὐτοῖς Ε Μ Υ, αὐτῇ etiam vet. tr. et Mich.   14 τίνι] τίνα Biehl, err.
typograph.   15 vulgo: νοῇ; ἢ ὅτι ἐκεῖνα νοεῖ, ἢ τὰ ἐλάττω; ἢ ante ὅτι om. Ε Μ Υ,
ἐκεῖνα νοῇ ἢ Μ, νοεῖν L S U, textum receptum de coniectura Freudenthalii scripsit
Biehl.   16 καὶ L M S U, ὥσπερ Biehl.   19 Γ Δ Biehl M Sylb., ΑΔ
reliqui codd. et edd., etiam vet. tr. et Mich., qui autem γ δ Aristoteli scribendum
fuisse annotat, ΓΔ recte coni. etiam Freudenth.   20 ἢ τὴν om. E.
21 ΑΓ] ΑΖ con. Freudth., codd. et edd. except. Biehl ΑΓ | τὸ] κ Υ, ν Ε, om. Μ.
22 τὴν Ι] τὸ μ L, τὴν ι Ε Μ Υ, τὴν Μ Biehl. | οὖν fort. γὰρ.   23. μὲν om. Ε |
Β] θ Μ, om. Υ.   24 Λ] α Ε Υ   25 πρὸς] ϛ Μ.

not prevail to the same degree. Hence in some cases we are impelled to pass both to one point and to another, especially when something diverts us from the one to the other. Hence 5 too, when we have to remember a name, we may recollect one like it and commit a verbal blunder as regards the proper one. This is the explanation of the way in which recollection occurs.

But there is a most important fact to be noticed—that we must have apprehension of time either determinate or indeterminate. Let us grant as real something by which we discriminate greater and less periods. It is reasonable that 10 we should do so in the same way as we discriminate extended magnitudes ; we know things that have great size and are at a distance, not by our thought reaching out to them there, as some say our sight does (for though they are non-existent they can equally be known), but by a psychic process analogous to them : there exist in the mind figures and changes similar to the external objects.

What then is the difference between knowing the objects of greater size (the objective) and knowing the other set (the 15 subjective) which are smaller ? All the inner are smaller and analogous to the outer, and probably, just as in the case of the knowable forms of things the subject has another corresponding one within him, so it is with distances. Thus, if AB, BE be the process, that produces AC, CD, for AC and CD are in the same ratio as AB and BE. Does not this then 20 give AF, FG quite as much as AC, CD? No, for AC is to AB as H is to I. These processes, then, occur together, but, if one wants to think FG, while he equally at the same time thinks BE, instead of the ratio of H to I he thinks that of K to L, for the latter lines are in the same proportion as FA stands in to BA.   25

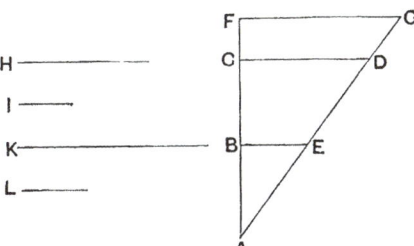

Hence when the process corresponding to the concrete object and that corresponding to the time are coincident we have an act of memory. If one thinks that they are coincident

μὴ ποιῶν, οἴεται μνημονεύειν· οὐθὲν γὰρ κωλύει δια-
ψευσθῆναί τινα καὶ δοκεῖν μνημονεύειν μὴ μνημονεύοντα.
30 ἐνεργοῦντα δὲ τῇ μνήμῃ μὴ οἴεσθαι ἀλλὰ λανθάνειν
μεμνημένον οὐκ ἔστιν· τοῦτο γὰρ ἦν αὐτὸ τὸ μεμνῆσθαι.
ἀλλ᾽ ἐὰν ἡ τοῦ πράγματος γένηται χωρὶς τῆς τοῦ χρόνου
ἢ αὕτη ἐκείνης, οὐ μέμνηται. ἡ δὲ τοῦ χρόνου διττή
453 a ἐστιν· ὁτὲ μὲν γὰρ μέτρῳ οὐ μέμνηται αὐτό, οἷον ὅτι
τρίτῃ ἡμέρᾳ ὁδήποτε ἐποίησεν, ὁτὲ δὲ καὶ μέτρῳ· ἀλλὰ
μέμνηται καὶ ἐὰν μὴ καὶ μέτρῳ. εἰώθασι δὲ λέγειν
ὅτι μέμνηνται μέν, πότε μέντοι οὐκ ἴσασιν, ὅταν μὴ
5 γνωρίζωσι τοῦ πότε τὸ ποσὸν μέτρῳ.

5 ὅτι μὲν οὖν οὐχ οἱ
αὐτοὶ μνημονικοὶ καὶ ἀναμνηστικοί, ἐν τοῖς πρότερον
εἴρηται. διαφέρει δὲ τοῦ μνημονεύειν τὸ ἀναμιμνήσκεσθαι οὐ μόνον κατὰ τὸν χρόνον, ἀλλ᾽ ὅτι τοῦ μὲν
μνημονεύειν καὶ τῶν ἄλλων ζῴων μετέχει πολλά, τοῦ
10 δ᾽ ἀναμιμνήσκεσθαι οὐδὲν ὡς εἰπεῖν τῶν γνωριζομένων
ζῴων, πλὴν ἄνθρωπος. αἴτιον δ᾽ ὅτι τὸ ἀναμιμνήσκεσθαί
ἐστιν οἷον συλλογισμός τις· ὅτι γὰρ πρότερον εἶδεν ἢ
ἤκουσεν ἤ τι τοιοῦτον ἔπαθε, συλλογίζεται ὁ ἀναμιμνησκόμενος, καὶ ἔστιν οἷον ζήτησίς τις. τοῦτο δ᾽ οἷς καὶ
15 τὸ βουλευτικὸν ὑπάρχει, φύσει μόνοις συμβέβηκεν· καὶ
16 γὰρ τὸ βουλεύεσθαι συλλογισμός τίς ἐστιν.

16 ὅτι δ᾽ ἐστὶ σω-
ματικὸν τὸ πάθος καὶ ἡ ἀνάμνησις ζήτησις ἐν τοιούτῳ
φαντάσματος, σημεῖον τὸ παρενοχλεῖν ἐνίους, ἐπειδὰν μὴ
δύνωνται ἀναμνησθῆναι καὶ πάνυ ἐπέχοντες τὴν διάνοιαν,
20 καὶ οὐκέτ᾽ ἐπιχειροῦντας ἀναμιμνήσκεσθαι οὐδὲν ἧττον,
καὶ μάλιστα τοὺς μελαγχολικούς· τούτους γὰρ φαντάσματα κινεῖ μάλιστα. αἴτιον δὲ τοῦ μὴ ἐπ᾽ αὐτοῖς εἶναι
τὸ ἀναμιμνήσκεσθαι, ὅτι καθάπερ τοῖς βάλλουσιν οὐκέτι

___

453 a, 19 ἐπέχοντες Christ, Biehl, ἐπέχοντας Bek. codd.

without securing that they really are so one thinks one
remembers, for there is nothing to prevent one's being deceived
and thinking one remembers when one does not. When,
however, one actually remembers, it is impossible not to 30
know it or to be unaware that that is so, for it is just in
being aware of this that memory consists. But if the object-
processes occur independently of that corresponding to the
time, or the latter take place without the former, there is no
memory.

The time-apprehending process is twofold; sometimes one
does not remember the interval with exact precision, as *e.g.* 453 a
that someone did something the day before yesterday, but
sometimes our sense of time is accurate. All the same one
remembers, though not aware of the exact interval; we are
wont to say we do remember though we don't know when the
thing happened, when we cannot tell what is the exact extent
of the interval.

We have already asserted that it is not the same people 5
who remember well and who recollect well. Recollection
differs from remembering not merely in the superiority of the
sense of time which it involves, but in the fact that, while
many of the other animals possess memory, we may say that 10
none of those now known, except man, share in recollection.
The reason is that recollection is like a syllogism. One who
recollects comes to the conclusion that he saw or heard or had
some such experience previously and the process resembles a
search and, owing to its nature, recollection accrues only to
those that have the power of deliberation, for deliberation is 15
a sort of syllogistic process.

Evidence that this experience is of a corporeal nature, and
that in recollecting we search for an image in a corporeal
organ, comes from the fact that it distresses some people
when they cannot recall a thing though applying their mind
hard in attempting to do so and, when they no longer try to 20
recollect, none the less the disturbance goes on. This happens
especially with liverish people, for they are the class most
easily moved by images. The reason why recollection is not
under their control is, that, just as when one has thrown a

ἐπ' αὐτοῖς τὸ στῆσαι, οὕτως καὶ ὁ ἀναμιμνησκόμενος καὶ
25 θηρεύων σωματικόν τι κινεῖ, ἐν ᾧ τὸ πάθος. μάλιστα δ'
ἐνοχλοῦνται οἷς ἂν ὑγρότης τύχῃ ὑπάρχουσα περὶ τὸν
αἰσθητικὸν τόπον· οὐ γὰρ ῥᾳδίως παύεται κινηθεῖσα, ἕως
ἂν ἐπανέλθῃ τὸ ζητούμενον καὶ εὐθυπορήσῃ ἡ κίνησις.
διὸ καὶ ὀργαὶ καὶ φόβοι, ὅταν τι κινήσωσιν, ἀντικινούν-
30 των πάλιν τούτων οὐ καθίστανται, ἀλλ' ἐπὶ τὸ αὐτὸ
ἀντικινοῦσιν. καὶ ἔοικε τὸ πάθος τοῖς ὀνόμασι καὶ
μέλεσι καὶ λόγοις, ὅταν διὰ στόματος γένηταί τι αὐτῶν
σφόδρα· παυσαμένοις γὰρ καὶ οὐ βουλομένοις ἐπέρχεται
πάλιν ᾄδειν ἢ λέγειν. εἰσὶ δὲ καὶ οἱ τὰ ἄνω μείζω
453 b ἔχοντες καὶ οἱ νανώδεις ἀμνημονέστεροι τῶν ἐναντίων
διὰ τὸ πολὺ βάρος ἔχειν ἐπὶ τῷ αἰσθητικῷ, καὶ μήτ'
ἐξ ἀρχῆς τὰς κινήσεις δύνασθαι ἐμμένειν ἀλλὰ διαλύ-
εσθαι μήτ' ἐν τῷ ἀναμιμνήσκεσθαι ῥᾳδίως εὐθυπορεῖν.
5 οἱ δὲ πάμπαν νέοι καὶ λίαν γέροντες ἀμνήμονες διὰ τὴν
κίνησιν· οἱ μὲν γὰρ ἐν φθίσει, οἱ δ' ἐν αὐξήσει πολλῇ
εἰσίν· ἔτι δὲ τά γε παιδία καὶ νανώδη ἐστὶ μέχρι πόρρω
τῆς ἡλικίας. περὶ μὲν οὖν μνήμης καὶ τοῦ μνημονεύειν,
τίς ἡ φύσις αὐτῶν καὶ τίνι τῶν τῆς ψυχῆς μνημονεύει τὰ
10 ζῷα, καὶ περὶ τοῦ ἀναμιμνήσκεσθαι, τί ἐστι καὶ πῶς
γίνεται καὶ διὰ τίνας αἰτίας, εἴρηται.

thing one can no longer check its course, so a man engaged in recollection and on the hunt for an idea stimulates into activity a bodily organ in which the experience is localised. 25 Those feel the vexation most who happen to have fluid in the region of the sensory organ, for once the fluid substance is set in motion it is not easily brought to rest until the object sought for returns to mind and the process resumes its direct course. Hence, when they have set something in agitation, emotions of anger and fear, owing to the reaction of these organs, do not come to rest; on the contrary they react once 30 more on them. The phenomenon resembles that which occurs when a name or a tune or a sentence has come to be much on one's lips; after one has stopped, and without one intending it, one is prompted again to sing or to speak.

Dwarfs and those who have a greater development in the upper parts of the body have poorer memories than those of 453 b the opposite type, because they have too great a weight pressing upon the organ of consciousness; the processes can neither persist in it from the time of the initial experience (on the contrary they are effaced), nor in the act of recollection can they easily take a direct course. The very young and 5 the exceedingly aged remember badly because of their transitional state: the former are growing, the latter decaying rapidly; and besides, children are dwarf-like in type up to a considerably advanced time in their life.

This is our account of memory and remembering, the nature thereof and the psychical organ employed by animals in remembering; likewise of recollection, its nature, mode of 10 occurrence, and causes.

COMMENTARY

DE SENSU

CHAPTER I.

436 a 1. περὶ αἰσθήσεως καὶ αἰσθητῶν. This is the common title of the treatise and that known to Alexander of Aphrodisias. As, however, the discussion is to be not about the soul *per se*, but in particular about its connection with the body, *i.e.* not merely psychological but especially physiological, Alexander suggests that περὶ αἰσθητηρίων τε καὶ αἰσθητῶν would be a more legitimate title. Sometimes αἴσθησις is used loosely instead of αἰσθητήριον, even by Aristotle himself. Simon Simonius adopts this amended title, translating it 'De Organis Sensuum et Sensilibus.'

This is evidently the investigation promised in *De An.* i. ch. 1, 402 b 15, where Aristotle asks if the objects of sensation may not be more profitably treated of before the function of sensation itself. In the whole passage 402 b 5 sqq. he points out that a definition of soul in the abstract is not sufficient for a comprehension of what soul is, ἀλλὰ καὶ ἀνάπαλιν τὰ συμβεβηκότα συμβάλλεται μέγα μέρος πρὸς τὸ εἰδέναι τὸ τί ἐστιν. Thus we must proceed beyond our abstract definition and give an account of the various μόρια—faculties of soul, but these again cannot be understood apart from their ἔργα—functions, and, once more, point to an account of their ἀντικείμενα—objects. Aristotle doubts if these subjects should not be treated in the reverse order; to do so would be to begin with things 'notiora nobis'; for, as later psychology also has pointed out, it is the things presented to our senses and not the psychical functions through which they are apprehended, which are in the order of time the primary objects of consciousness.

As a matter of fact, Aristotle does not adopt this reverse order in his exposition, thinking it sufficient to have pointed out the danger of resting content with a merely abstract treatment.

Thus we come finally to a discussion of αἰσθητά, the objects of sense and the bodily organs through which they are apprehended. It is not to be thought, however, that the separation of topics in Aristotle's psychological writings is observed with perfect logical rigidity. The general outlines of what is here laid down have already been anticipated in *De An.* II. chs. 7–11, and the detailed treatment of sound which is omitted from this treatise is to be found there in ch. 8.

What in particular distinguishes this treatise from the *De Anima* is the greater detail with which αἰσθητά are treated and the attention devoted to the bodily organ of each sense.

διώρισται, διορίζειν is a technical term with Aristotle, almost equivalent to 'to define' (ὅρος, ὁρισμός = definition).

καθ' αὑτὴν, another technical term; it is defined in *Anal. Post.* I. ch. 4, 73 a 34 sqq. Those characteristics of a thing without which it would be impossible for it to be that thing, belong to it καθ' αὑτό. They are stated in the definition. Cf. also *Metaph.* VII. ch. 5, 1030 b 23 sqq. It is assumed that a thing can preserve its individuality though stripped of certain qualities. These latter are συμβεβηκότα. When Aristotle says he has given a definition of the soul *per se*, he means that he has stated the ultimate attributes that everything psychical (or rather everything living, for plants have ψυχή) must have. This definition appears in *De An.* II. ch. 1, 412 b 5 : εἴη ἂν ἐντελέχεια ἡ πρώτη σώματος φυσικοῦ ὀργανικοῦ.

The question is, whether the soul *per se* is here contrasted with its faculties, or whether—as Alexander suggests is also possible—he is opposing soul considered alone to soul considered in its relation to the body. To this it may be objected that Aristotle never does consider soul apart from body. It is clear that Aristotle here means just what he says, after a discussion of soul in general and its faculties he is to go on to investigate their ἔργα or, as he here calls them, the πράξεις of the living creatures. This is a progress in the direction of greater detail, for one and the same δύναμις is capable of being determined in various ways when it passes into activity or ἐνέργεια. This will involve the more detailed treatment of the bodily organ of each ἐνέργεια also. Hence the predominantly physiological character of this treatise.

For the reason why a definition of soul in general is not sufficient, see *De An.* II. ch. 3, 414 b 20 sqq. Things ἐν τῷ ἐφεξῆς, like souls and figures, have no common nature which can exist apart from the particular type, *e.g.* triangle, quadrilateral, etc. Such things have a nature, ' media inter univocorum et equivocorum naturam.'

436 a 2. δυνάμεων, δύναμις is the regular word for potentiality translatable by 'faculty,' by which term we also render μόριον. This latter term Aristotle inherited from the Platonic psychology. The word itself and the way in which Plato employs it suggest rather a theory of the separable and independent nature of the various faculties, the point of view, in fact, of 'faculty psychology.' Aristotle's is, however, far removed from any such theory.

436 a 3. ἐπίσκεψιν ποιεῖσθαι is an equivalent for θεωρίαν ποιεῖσθαι: cf. *Metaph.* I. ch. 8, 989 b 24-27.

τῶν ζωὴν ἐχόντων. This brings in plants, which also have ψυχή, and to which some of the phenomena proposed for discussion belong (*e.g.* νεότης καὶ γῆρας, ζωὴ καὶ θάνατος).

436 a 4. ἴδιαι, ἴδιος is that which is the peculiar possession of any one species.

κοιναί, κοινός is the reverse of ἴδιος. Alexander points out that Aristotle desires not merely to classify the psychical functions of animals but to discuss the things classified.

Simon would make out that the distinction falls wholly within the functions of animals and that here ἴδιαι and κοιναί mean respectively 'belonging to them *quâ* animal and *quâ* living' because there is no discussion of the functions of plants in the *Parva Naturalia*. However, the missing treatise *De Plantis* (cf. *De Long. et Brev. Vit.* 467 b 4) seems to have been intended to carry on the discussion of the most universal of all the conditions of life. Simon seems to be right in denying that by κοιναί Aristotle is referring merely to the functions which plants share with animals. But neither is it evident that the distinction falls wholly within the functions of animals as he asserts. As a matter of fact the *Parva Naturalia* though dealing chiefly with the functions of animals contain reference too to the phenomena of plant life. Possibly, however, Aristotle had no strict and complete classification in his mind, but merely wished to suggest that some functions might be the peculiar attributes of a certain species and of certain wider groups, as ἀνάμνησις of man and ἀναπνοή and ἐκπνοή of animals with lungs. Simon's view, however, derives confirmation from a passage further on (cf. note to 436 a 7).

436 a 5. πράξεις, πρᾶξις is here employed in an unusual sense, as though it were a general term—action—used instead of the specific, ἐνέργεια, which is *par excellence* the name for the function or activity of anything possessing mind (κυρίως γὰρ πρᾶξις λογικὴ ἡ ἐνέργειά ἐστιν. Alex. p. 4, l. 5 [W.]). But πρᾶξις has generally a very restricted application, meaning as a rule distinctively human actions into which deliberation and thought enter. Cp. *passim* in the *Ethics*, especially I. ch. 1, 1094 a 1; VI. ch. 2, 1139 a 31 etc.

ὑποκείσθω. ὑποτίθεσθαι is to state as a ὑπόθεσις. This word has both a technical and a general meaning. It is used to refer (1) to certain of the undemonstrable but indubitable principles which lie at the basis of the several sciences; this is its most common technical meaning.

Again it may be used (2) to indicate a statement which is assumed as an ultimate principle without proof for the purposes of a particular discussion, but which is demonstrable and will be proved when it is convenient to do so (cf. Alex. 4, l. 23 [W.]).

Alexander is wrong in saying that the ὑπόθεσις which is an indemonstrable principle of science is an ἀξίωμα. Aristotle (*Anal. Post.* I. ch. 10) distinguishes three classes of first principles, (1) the κοινὰ ἀξιώματα of all science, *e.g.* the Law of non-contradiction, (2) definitions of the subject of demonstration (τὰ πρῶτα 76 a 32) and their properties (πάθη), (3) ὑποθέσεις, which affirm the existence of the subject to which the science is to attach predicates, *e.g.* lines and figures in geometry (76 b 5). These two latter classes of ἀναπό-δεικτα are ἴδια—appropriate to the science in question; they are both species of θέσις (*Anal. Post.* I. ch. 2, 72 a 15 sqq.). It is thus evident that, according to this technical use, a ὑπόθεσις is that which 'renders conclusions unconditional and categorical' (Poste, *Posterior Analytics*, Appendix B, p. 140). It corresponds to what Mill (*Logic*, Bk I. ch. 8, §§ 6 and 7) calls a 'postulate'—the assertion that, *e.g.* the figure in geometry, the triangle, exists, which renders our conclusions *unhypothetical*. Without this postulate which asserts the existence of the things defined there is no way of distinguishing a science from any self-consistent system of mythology. Upon definitions alone a science cannot be built.

There appears, however, to be another technical use of ὑπόθεσις which was common in Greek geometry. The ὑπόθεσις is the Q.E.F. of a problem or Q.E.D. of a theorem, the proposition set up for proof. This seems to be the sense in which it is employed in *Eth. Nic.* VII. ch. 9, 1151 a 17 (cf. Mr Burnet's note on the passage), though Poste (*op. cit.* p. 105 *note*) cites it as an instance of the former usage.

It is quite clear that here Aristotle uses ὑποκείσθω in the wider sense of ὑπόθεσις. The conclusions of the *De Anima* which can be proved are to be used as ἀρχαί in this treatise. These, therefore, though not indubitable first principles, are still certain; they are not 'hypotheses' in the modern sense, which are statements the certainty of which is still in doubt and which are assumed in a merely provisional way.

436 a 7. πρώτων. In *Posterior Analytics* I. ch. 4, 73 b 33 sqq. it is shown that what is a universal and peculiar attribute of a species belongs to it primarily, e.g. the equality of its angles to two right angles belongs to the species *triangle* primarily and not to figure, the genus (τὸ καθόλου δὲ ὑπάρχει τότε, ὅταν ἐπὶ τοῦ τυχόντος καὶ πρώτου δεικνύηται).

To be πρῶτος then is to be ἴδιος, and πρώτων will refer to the ἴδιαι mentioned above, l. 4. To proceed from ἴδια to κοινά is to follow the 'ordo doctrinae,' while from κοινά to ἴδια is the 'ordo naturae,' and this latter is the method which on the whole Aristotle follows in the *De Anima* in spite of his statement in *De An.* II. ch. 2, 413 a 11 sqq.

Here, however, he is to begin with the ἴδια which belong to animal *quâ* animal (if we interpret ἴδιαι as Simon will have it, cf. note to 436 a 4), e.g. Sense and Memory, and later he will go on to those functions which animals share with other living things.

The 'ordo doctrinae' is also employed by him when he treats of sight before touch in the *De Anima*, and in treating of animals before plants; it often proceeds from the γνωριμώτερα ἡμῖν to the γνωριμώτερα φύσει, cf. *Physics* I. ch. I. Perhaps, however, πρώτων refers to ζῴων as opposed to τῶν ζωὴν ἐχόντων merely. This, which is Ziaja's interpretation, makes the upshot of the whole matter that he is going to treat of animals and their functions first, as in fact he does. This interpretation relieves us from the necessity of limiting ἴδιαι definitely to one or other of the two alternatives—peculiar to animal *quâ* animal, and—peculiar to individual species.

436 a 8. κοινὰ τῆς ψυχῆς ὄντα. The most important both of the generic and specific functions of animals are functions both of the soul and the body, and hence (as Thomas says) the necessity of a separate treatise.

436 a 9. μνήμη. Memory does not belong to all animals, cf. *De Mem.* 450 a 16 and 453 a 9, also *Metaph.* I. ch. 1, 980 a 29 sqq.; hence he says only that these functions belong to *almost* all animals (σχεδόν, l. 11).

436 a 10. ὄρεξις or τὸ ὀρεκτικόν (cf. *Eth.* I. ch. 13, 1102 b 30) is the general name for the appetitive or conative element in the soul. It appears in three specific forms, ἐπιθυμία, θυμός, and βούλησις; the latter is a function of the rational soul. Cf. *De An.* III. ch. 9, 432 b 5: ἐν τῷ λογιστικῷ ἡ βούλησις γίνεται καὶ ἐν τῷ ἀλόγῳ ἡ ἐπιθυμία καὶ ὁ θυμός.

The Aristotelian distinction between θυμός and ἐπιθυμία is not the same as the Platonic (cf. *Repub.* III. and IV., especially 439 E sqq.), for Aristotle in *Ethics* I. ch. 13, 1102 b 13 sqq. assigns both θυμός and ἐπιθυμία to that irrational part of the soul which truly is not absolutely irrational (κυρίως ἄλογον) in so far as it partakes in a way (μετέχει πῶς) in reason, but yet is irrational in so far as it opposes reason (ἀντιτείνει τῷ λόγῳ). According to Plato ἐπιθυμία belongs to the wholly irrational part of the soul. Nevertheless though, according to Aristotle, ἐπιθυμία and θυμός belong to the same φύσις τῆς ψυχῆς, yet they are distinguished in a way analogous to the Platonic; cf. *Eth.* VII. ch. 7, 1149 a 25 sqq. Ἐπιθυμία is a mere desire for what is pleasant as such, θυμός is passion acting without reflection, but not mere craving for pleasure, cf. Zeller, *Arist. and Earlier Peripatetics* II. pp. 112–13. Anger is an inadequate rendering of θυμός, as the tenderer emotions are also ascribed to it by Aristotle, cf. *Polit.* VII. ch. 7, 1327 b 40. τὸ ὀρεκτικόν has been already treated in the *De Anima*. The accurate distinction of θυμός and ἐπιθυμία really falls into the background in Aristotle, since their demarcation was not of importance for his psychology.

436 a 12. τῶν μετεχόντων ζωῆς, *i.e.* plants as well as animals. In addition to the above class there is second a class of 'communissima' such as νεότης καὶ γῆρας, ζωὴ καὶ θάνατος, and a third class which are κοινὰ ζώων ἐνίοις, *e.g.* ἀναπνοὴ καὶ ἐκπνοή. If by ἴδιαι in l. 4 Aristotle means, as Simon maintains, peculiar to animal *quâ* animal, then the first list—αἴσθησις etc.—is the tale of the ἴδιαι, and the four συζυγίαι form the constituents of the two latter classes.

436 a 14. συζυγίαι. Simon says, 'Est enim horum quasi privatio alterius.' They are related as a positive quality, and its στέρησις, *i.e.* the contradictory, within the same genus.

436 a 16. τί τε ἕκαστον αὐτῶν. The τί ἐστιν of anything consists of the characteristics revealed in its definition—the scientific 'connotation' of the name, cf. *Anal. Post.* II. ch. 3.

436 a 17. αἰτίας. ἡ αἰτία or τὸ αἴτιον is cause,—that, the existence of which entails the existence of the thing of which it is said to be the cause. According to Aristotle's logical theories it is impossible to prove the τί ἐστιν of anything; only its existence, *i.e.* that it occurs (συμβαίνει), can be demonstrated; and this is done by giving its αἴτιον.

436 a 18. φυσικοῦ. In *De An.* I. ch. 1, 403 a 29 sqq. there is a discussion of the spheres of the φυσικός and the διαλεκτικός, and it is first suggested that the physicist pays attention to the matter, the other to the λόγος or εἶδος (in his illustration the final cause) in natural phenomena. But the conclusion is come to, that the real φυσικός pays attention to both. Cf. also *Metaph.* VII. ch. 11, 1037 a 16 sqq.

περὶ ὑγιείας καὶ νόσου. This tractate, which should have followed the περὶ ἀναπνοῆς (cf. 480 b 22), is not extant.

436 a 19. ἀρχάς, the premisses from which deduction is made.

436 a 20. ἐστερημένοις. This word is applied both to those that lack and those that have been deprived of a quality. Cf. *Metaph.* V. ch. 22, 1022 b 22 sqq.

436 a 22. ἰατρικῆς. Aristotle cites a case in which we can explain a phenomenon in medicine by geometrical principles,—that circular wounds are slowest to heal (cf. *Anal. Post.* I. ch. 13, 79 a 15).

436 b 2. ἄρχονται, a reference to ἀρχαί (cf. l. 19 above).

436 b 4. μετ' αἰσθήσεως. That sensation cannot exist apart from the bodily life is affirmed in *De An.* II. ch. 2, 413 b 27. Ἡδονή, λύπη, θυμός, ἐπιθυμία, and ὄρεξις generally, occur *along with* sensation; it enters into their being: cf. *loc. cit.* 413 b 22–24.

436 b 5. δι' αἰσθήσεως. μνήμη is due to αἴσθησις: it is a ἕξις φαντάσματος (cf. *de Mem.* 451 a 17) and a φάντασμα is a κίνησις ὑπὸ τοῦ αἰσθέσθαι, *i.e.* a psychical affection originating with, and being a persistence of, a sense stimulation; it is the μονὴ τοῦ αἰσθήματος talked of in *Anal. Post.* II. ch. 19, 99 b 36 and *De An.* I. ch. 4, 408 b 18. Again the φάντασμα is called a ὑπόλειμμα τοῦ αἰσθήματος. Cf. *De Mem.* ch. 1, 451 a 4 and *De Insom.* 461 b 21, and also *An. Post.* II. ch. 19, 100 a 3, ἐκ μὲν οὖν αἰσθήσεως γίνεται μνήμη.

πάθη. A πάθος is (1) in its most general signification, any attribute of a thing whatsoever as opposed to the concrete reality itself (cf. *De Gen. et Corr.* I. ch. 4, 319 b 8 etc.). In accordance with the etymology of the word there is, however, generally the side implication of the πάθος, being a determination produced in a thing which is passive and suffers modification (πάσχει) by something else. Hence (2) πάθος, though often used indiscriminately, tends to be demarcated from a permanent quality and to refer to a more temporary attribute: cf. *Categ.* ch. 8, 9 b 28. It is often indistinguishable from συμβεβηκός.

If the subject—the thing which has the πάθος—is mind or one of its faculties, then the πάθος is some modification of consciousness. We must, however, distinguish as a special meaning that sense of πάθος (found in *De Mem.* ch. 1, 450 b 1), where it means mental perturbation.

For the use of πάθος cf. Burnet, *Eth. Nic.* p. 88. Here, according to Alexander, ὕπνος καὶ ἐγρήγορσις come under the designation of πάθη τῆς αἰσθήσεως: cf. *Comment. in De Sensu*, p. 7 (Wendland), l. 25: ταύτης γάρ τι πασχούσης ὁ ὕπνος. The explanation is that exhalations from food proceed upwards to the brain, condense and, descending once more, press upon the seat of consciousness (the heart), and so produce sleep. Cf. also *De Somn.* 454 a 22: ἄμφω γάρ ἐστι τὰ πάθη ταῦτα περὶ αἴσθησιν τοῦ πρώτου αἰσθητικοῦ.

436 b 6. ἕξις. A ἕξις is a fixed and determinate disposition (mere temporary disposition is διάθεσις). Cf. *Categ.* ch. 8, 8 b 27. Aristotle seems here to be describing the character of the four συζυγίαι mentioned above in 436 a 14 sq. Hence by ἕξεις he can hardly be referring to memory, which indeed is a ἕξις of the image left by sensation, not directly of sensation itself. Alexander thinks that by ἕξεις sensation itself is referred to. But, if we hold that one of the pairs of correlatives is indicated, perhaps νεότης καὶ γῆρας may be intended, though in what sense these are ἕξεις of αἴσθησις is not clear; they belong rather to τὸ θρεπτικόν—the 'nutritive soul.'

436 b 7. σωτηρίαι. ἀναπνοή preserves the life because it cools the heart—the ultimate organ of sensation, and prevents it from destroying itself by means of its own heat. Cf. *De Juvent.* ch. 3, 469 a 5 sqq. and *De Resp.* chapters 1, 8 and 16.

στερήσεις. νόσος and θάνατος are φθοραί and στερήσεις of life. στέρησις is used here in the sense of *de*privation (cf. note to 436 a 20).

436 b 8. διὰ τοῦ λόγου here is equivalent to 'deductively' as opposed to 'inductively'—δι' ἐπαγωγῆς (cf. *Phys.* III. ch. 3, 210 b 8 sqq.). No reference to *à priori* in the Kantian sense is intended.

436 b 9. αἰσθήσεως. The distinction between noun and verb seems here to correspond to that between faculty and function. Cf. μνήμη and μνημονεύειν *De Mem. passim*. In the famous passage in *Anal. Post.* II. ch. 19, 100 a 17 it is generally understood to be that between content and function—καὶ αἰσθάνεται μὲν τὸ καθ' ἕκαστον, ἡ δὲ αἴσθησις τοῦ καθόλου ἐστιν.

436 b 11–12. περὶ ψυχῆς. The reference is to *De An.* II. chapters 2, 3, 5 etc. Cf. 413 b 1 sqq.

436 b 14. ἰδίᾳ. This supports Simon's interpretation of ἴδιαι in 436 a 4 above.. If touch belongs peculiarly to each and every species, that must mean that it is a peculiar property of that nature which they all have in common. It is something which they have *quâ* animal. The usual meaning of ἴδιος is 'belonging to a species exclusively,' but as *each* species is here said to have the properties in question, the usual sense is out of the question.

436 b 15. Cf. *De An.* II. ch. 3, 414 b 2 sqq. By touch we discriminate dry and moist, hot and cold—the ultimate properties of things material and also important characteristics of τροφή (ἡ γὰρ ἀφὴ τῆς τροφῆς αἴσθησις). Compare also III. ch. 12, 434 b 9 sqq. Touch is necessary for the animal's preservation.

In the former passage (II. ch. 3) we find that γεῦσις also discriminates characteristics of τροφή and cf. below ch. 4. Taste discriminates flavour, but χυμός is simply a ἥδυσμα of the fundamental characteristics of τροφή—the tangible ones, and hence γεῦσις is a species of touch (441 a 3 below).

436 b 19. τοῦ θρεπτικοῦ. The omission of μορίου (which is read by L S U P and Bek.) after θρεπτικοῦ makes this passage intelligible. Aristotle here refers to that which nourishes, not to the 'nutritive faculty' of the soul. (1) In the first place, it is not χυμός but γεῦσις which should be a πάθος of any of the faculties of the soul, and (2) that would be a πάθος, not τῆς θρεπτικῆς δυνάμεως, but τοῦ αἰσθητικοῦ.

The first of the above reasons makes us reject Alexander's interpretation of τοῦ θρεπτικοῦ μορίου as τοῦ γευστικοῦ, which wants explanation and besides makes this statement a tautology.

Alexander himself suggests that the meaning is τὸ μόριον τρέφειν δυνάμενον, *i.e.* the nutritive object. But μόριον is strange and is better omitted as in E M Y.

Hammond does not notice the importance of the alteration in Biehl's text, and translates: 'flavour is an affection of the nutritive soul,' and explains that 'flavour as a property of food affects the processes of growth or the nutritive soul.'

But τὸ θρεπτικόν here = τροφή.

436 b 20. Aristotle is clearly demarcating animals in general

R. 9

from the smaller number that possess local movement, by a distinction in their sensational consciousness also. In all animals we have touch and taste, but in those that have κίνησις κατὰ τόπον we have also the senses which are stimulated by a medium external to the body (διὰ τῶν ἔξωθεν). The *objects* of touch and taste are external as well as those of the other senses, and hence it is no *differentia* of the senses of sight, hearing, and smell to be 'excited by external objects' as Hammond translates : cf. *De An.* III. 12, 434 b 14 : αἱ γὰρ ἄλλαι αἰσθήσεις δι' ἑτέρων αἰσθάνονται, οἷον ὄσφρησις ὄψις ἀκοή.

For a discussion of the media (air, water and τὸ διαφανές) cf. ch. 3–5, the discussion of the special senses, and Bäumker, *Des Aristoteles Lehre von den Äussern und Innern Sinnesvermögen*, pp. 38 sqq.

436 b 22. σωτηρίας ἕνεκεν. For the question of Aristotle's teleological interpretation of nature cf. Zeller, *Arist.* I. pp. 359 sqq.

προαισθανόμενα, *i.e.* perceiving their food before they are in actual contact with it.

437 a 1. φρονήσεως. φρόνησις is here used in a wide and general sense as equivalent to διάνοια—the faculty which gives us universals ; but used more accurately, as in *Eth. Nic.* VI., it is περὶ ὧν ἔστι βουλεύσασθαι (1141 b 9), *i.e.* knowledge of τὰ πρακτά. Cf. 1140 b 4 : λείπεται ἄρα αὐτὴν (sc. φρόνησιν) εἶναι ἕξιν ἀληθῆ μετὰ λόγου πρακτικὴν περὶ τὰ ἀνθρώπῳ ἀγαθὰ καὶ κακά.

The φρόνιμος is able to determine what is good and profitable πρὸς τὸ εὖ ζῆν ὅλως, *i.e.* for his general welfare. φρόνησις is one of the 'intellectual virtues.' Some of the animals seem to have φρόνησις : cf. *Metaph.* I. ch. 1, 980 b 22, where some are said to be φρονιμώτερα than others.

437 a 3. νοητῶν. νοητά are the objective counterpart of νοήματα, which are concepts generally, the contents of νόησις or νοῦς, *i.e.* intellect. Cf. *De An.* I. ch. 3, 407 a 7 : ἡ νόησις τὰ νοήματα, and *Metaph.* XII. ch. 7, 1072 b 22 : τὸ γὰρ δεκτικὸν τοῦ νοητοῦ...νοῦς. φρόνησις τῶν νοητῶν is equivalent to θεωρία or ἐπιστήμη, which are regularly opposed to πρᾶξις as well as to a knowledge of τὰ πρακτά. Cf. *Eth.* VI. ch. 5, 1140 b 1 : οὐκ ἂν εἴη ἡ φρόνησις ἐπιστήμη, and cf. ch. 3, 1139 b 17 sqq. ἐπιστήμη concerns τὰ ἐξ ἀνάγκης, φρόνησις those things which ἐνδέχεται ἄλλως ἔχειν. Hence, in the strict sense of the terms, the expression φρόνησις τῶν νοητῶν contains a contradiction.

437 a 5. καθ' αὐτήν, *i.e.* sight in its own sphere, in the objects directly presented to it. To the sphere of sight belong colour and the mathematical qualities of objects perceived by sight—τὰ κοινὰ αἰσθητά (cf. ll. 9–10 below). Compare *De An.* II. ch. 6, 418 a 9, where the κοινὰ αἰσθητά are said to be perceived καθ᾽ αὑτά. Besides those things which are thus perceived there are others that are perceived κατὰ συμβεβηκός, *e.g.* we perceive by sight qualities referring to another sense, which are 'complicated' with the visual one in the same object, and again we can perceive all sorts of other determinations of the visible object, *e.g.* that such and such a white object is 'the son of Diares' (418 a 21). Here some modification of the visual quality must pass as a symbol for or mean the other characteristics which we infer from it. But it is in the perception of these associated elements that hearing contributes more to intellectual life, for to the audible sounds we have by convention (κατὰ συνθήκην) attached the concepts by which we think the whole of reality so far as it is known to us.

πρὸς δὲ νοῦν. νοῦς seems to be best described as the faculty of conceptual thought. Though sometimes defined so widely as to take in all mental activities superior to αἴσθησις (cf. *De An.* III. ch. 4, 429 a 23 : λέγω δὲ νοῦν ᾧ διανοεῖται καὶ ὑπολαμβάνει ἡ ψυχή: cf. also *De An.* III. ch. 3, 427 b 27–29), in its most characteristic application it refers to the highest faculty of all. That seems to be the apprehension of concepts in abstraction from the imagery, the sensuous setting or ὕλη by which they seem generally to be attended. Cf. *De An.* III. ch. 4, 429 b 21 and Rodier's notes to the preceding passage, also ch. 6, 430 b 30. Such simple concepts seem to form the starting point of all scientific knowledge, and in *Eth.* VI. ch. 6, 1141 a 7 νοῦς is said to be the faculty for apprehending them, not a faculty of discursive thought. Cf. also *Anal. Post.* II. ch. 19, 100 b 12.

κατὰ συμβεβηκός. Cf. above, note to καθ᾽ αὑτήν. Aristotle does not mean to equate κατὰ συμβεβηκός and πρὸς νοῦν; as we saw, by sight we may perceive objects κατὰ συμβεβηκός. But it is audible sound alone which is elaborated into a system corresponding to the scheme of ideas and in each item suggestive of them.

437 a 8. τὰ κοινά. Cf. *De An.* II. ch. 6, 418 a 17, III. ch. 1, 425 a 14, III. ch. 3, 428 b 22, and also below ch. 4, 442 b 2 sqq. ἠρεμία is here omitted from the list, though codex L reads στάσις.

437 a 11. φωνῆς. Cf. *De An.* II. ch. 8, 420 b 5 sqq. The general description of φωνή is ψόφος τίς ἐστιν ἐμψύχου. The narrower usage appears in 420 b 32 : σημαντικὸς γὰρ δή τις ψόφος

9—2

ἐστὶν ἡ φωνή. It is sound which conveys a meaning. In 420 b 22 we find that it is φωνή which permits of the realisation of τὸ εὖ: cf. above 437 a 1. The ἀναγκαῖα (cf. 420 b 19, where γεῦσις is said to be ἀναγκαῖον) are the things chosen σωτηρίας ἕνεκεν. Aristotle means quite clearly that intelligence and the higher life generally depend upon ἀκοή and its special object φωνή. For the special reasons why sounds are best fitted to represent concepts, cf. Stout, *Manual of Psychology*, pp. 464 sqq.

437 a 15. σύμβολόν. A σύμβολον is the token given by any of the parties to a compact (συνθήκη). Hence the apprehension of the meaning of a word is conventional and κατὰ συμβεβηκός, for φύσει τῶν ὀνομάτων οὐδέν ἐστιν (*de Interp.* 16 a 27). The opposite doctrine had been maintained in the *Cratylus* (ch. ix. sqq.). Cf. also 16 a 19. No sound is a word unless it become a conventional sign.

CHAPTER II.

437 a 19. δυνάμεως. δύναμις is the characteristic word for faculty or potentiality, not *function* (as Hammond has it), the appropriate word for which is ἔργον.

437 a 20. πρότερον. In *De An.* II. *loc. cit.*

437 a 22. στοιχεῖα. The four physical elements—the primary differentiations of πρώτη ὕλη—are fire (πῦρ), water (ὕδωρ), earth (γῆ), and air (ἀήρ). Each has a pair of ultimate qualities one of which it shares with another of the elements and the other with another. Thus there are four ultimate qualities and those elements are most opposed to each other which have no qualities in common. Thus fire is hot and dry (θερμὸν καὶ ξηρόν); water is cold and moist (ψυχρὸν καὶ ὑγρόν). These are contraries of each other. But fire and water share their heat and moisture respectively with air, their dryness and coldness with earth. Thus these latter two elements are relatively to each other contrarily opposed. Thus

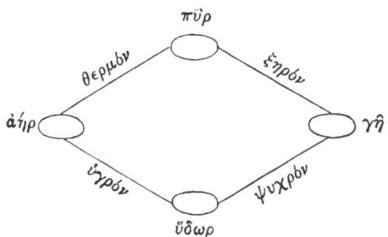

Cf. Zeller, *Arist.* I. pp. 480 sqq.

437 a 23. τέτταρα. The traditional four elements were first distinguished by Empedocles. Cf. Burnet, *Early Greek Phil.* p. 59, also pp. 240 sqq. Empedocles referred smell to air also. Theophrastus, *De Sensu*, 7 (*R. P.* 177 b, 8th ed.), says he did not assign any particular element as connected with touch and taste. Aristotle's statement here need not mean more than that there was a general tendency to correlate each sense with a particular element, and that the disparity of the number of the senses and the elements respectively caused a difficulty when it was attempted to carry out the correlation completely.

437 a 24. πέμπτης. Hearing and smell on the Empedoclean theory, touch and taste on the Aristotelian are grouped together.

437 a 25. θλιβομένου. Apparently the sensation caused by concussion of the optic nerve owing to a blow in the region of the eye. The words used however do not convey a very graphic description of this experience. Perhaps Aristotle is here generalising so as to include such light sensations as are caused by chemical changes in the eye itself. The theory is to be referred to Alcmaeon of Kroton. Cf. Theophrastus, *De Sensu*, 26 : ὅτι δ' ἔχει πῦρ (ὁ ὀφθαλμός)...δῆλον εἶναι· πληγέντος γὰρ ἐκλάμπειν.

437 a 31. ἑαυτὸν. Because in the dark no other object is visible, the eye, being of the nature of fire, will be visible. It should thus be visible at any time in the dark. As this is not the case, the theory is rejected.

Aristotle next goes on to give his own account of the phenomenon, which professes to explain why this sensation of light experienced in the dark occurs only when the eye moves rapidly.

437 a 34. λεῖα. Cf. 437 b 7, where he adds confirmatory instances. From *Meteor.* iii. ch. 4, 373 a 35 : ἀνακλωμένη μὲν οὖν ἡ ὄψις ἀπὸ πάντων φαίνεται τῶν λείων, and 372 a 31 we should infer that this was really a case of reflection. Though, however, smoothness is assigned as the source both of luminousness in the dark and of reflection generally, the two phenomena are never identified. Cf. *De An.* ii. ch. 7, 419 a 2 sqq., where fungi, horn and scales are enumerated along with the eye and the heads of fishes, as a class of ἀνώνυμα which are πυρώδη φαινόμενα καὶ λάμποντα. Note πυρώδη φαινόμενα is all he says. He would not allow that they were really πυρώδη, for in that case they would really produce light. Thus according to Aristotle these substances were not in the strict sense phosphorescent (Bäumker, p. 26).

φῶς is the ἐνέργεια or ἐντελέχεια τοῦ διαφανοῦς (cf. *De An.* ii. ch. 7, 418 b 9, 419 a 11)—the proper function of the transparent medium.

Again, in ch. 3, 439 a 21 below, it is said to be the presence of something of the nature of fire in the transparent medium. Since, then, it requires something of the nature of fire to produce light and the eye does not consist of fire, it cannot be said to produce light. Hence it would be suggested that the phenomenon is one of reflection, though where the light is to come from when the eyes are closed is not apparent.

437 b 2. φαίνεται (2). There are many instances of φαίνεται taking this sense (cf. 3, 440 a 8 etc.). But most interpreters take φαίνεται δὲ τοῦτο to mean 'This is evident,' *i.e.* what was said before about the eye not producing light is evident because of what follows. But that is not the sense required. The 'one becoming two' is not the reason why the eye does not emit light. But the eye is seen because, though really one, it appears when quickly moved to be two.

437 b 3. δύο γίγνεσθαι τὸ ἕν. This is very difficult to understand. Simon prefers to take Alexander's second interpretation, that one part of the eye sees the other—that which is 'in loco naturali' sees that which is not. But the interpretation does not explain why *swiftness* of motion is essential to the phenomenon. Probably Aristotle was thinking of common instances of a single object appearing to be made double by rapid motion (as *e.g.* a vibrating string) and applied this in a confused way to the present case. He apparently thought that the eye, when at the one position, could see itself at the other if the oscillation between the two was so rapid that it appeared to be at both points at the same time. It will not do to say, as Ziaja does, that the eye regains its former position before the light from it, when at the place from which it has moved, arrives. According to Aristotle the propagation of light is instantaneous and one must not read into his words a theory of light vibrations.

437 b 5. τὸ ὁρώμενον. The eye at the position to which it moves.

437 b 7. Cf. 437 a 34 above.

437 b 12. ἀνακλάσει. Aristotle does not mean to identify the present phenomenon with reflection but merely to adduce another instance illustrating the apparent duality of the eye by the apparent duality of seer and seen caused by reflection in a mirror.

Ἐμπεδοκλῆς. Cf. Burnet, *Early Greek Philosophy*, pp. 264 sqq., *Meno* 76 c, and *De Gen. Animal.* v. ch. 1, 779 b 15.

437 b 13. Τιμαίῳ. For the Platonic theory of sight-perception compare *Timaeus* ch. VII. 31 B and ch. XXX. 67 C sqq., and especially ch. XVI. 45 B sqq.

437 b 16. ὁ Τίμαιος. Cf. *Timaeus*, 45 D.

437 b 17. κενόν. κενός and its adverb κενῶς are constantly used in the sense of 'irrelevant': cf. *De An.* I. ch. 1, 403 a 2 of definitions that are mere vague generalities.

Cf. also *Eth. Nic.* II. ch. 7, 1107 a 30 etc. : but it may mean as well 'unfounded,' as in *An. Post.* I. ch. 3, 73 a 18. Here probably both implications are to be assigned to the word. The thought is, that it is absurd to talk of the ἀπόσβεσις of sight, because the notion of 'quenching' has nothing to do with the nature of light. Hence the theory is groundless because of the irrelevancy of the ideas to the phenomena in question. In addition, even if they were relevant, the theory would conflict with facts. The argument of the whole passage is that ἀπόσβεσις can be predicated only of τὸ πῦρ and ἡ φλόξ, not of light, for, as we saw before (cf. note to 437 a 34), light is not fire though it requires the presence of πυρῶδές τι. Plato and Empedocles, however, when alleging that the light which issues from the eye is quenched in darkness, imply that it is of the nature of fire which is θερμὸν καὶ ξηρόν and is quenched by either moisture or cold, the contrary qualities. (The Aristotelian theory is that things are neutralised by and pass into their opposites.) Now φῶς is not of the nature of πῦρ and hence to talk of its ἀπόσβεσις is absurd.

Secondly, even if there were something of the nature of fire in light though imperceptible, it would be extinguished by wet and cold weather; which is not true.

For the distinction of πῦρ and φῶς cf. also *Top.* v. ch. 5, 134b 28.

437 b 20. τῷ φωτί. The mere bringing forward of the fact that light is not quenched by wet shows that Aristotle really means to deny that it is of the nature of fire.

Alexander, however, evidently troubled by the fact that light is warm and hence perhaps should be identified with fire, suggests an emendation or rather a reconstruction of the passage which would make out that Aristotle, while conceding that fire is 'dry' and 'warm,' points out that darkness which is supposed to extinguish it has neither of the opposed qualities and hence cannot do so. On this interpretation the rest of the passage would run—'but if darkness is really, though imperceptibly, cold and wet, we should expect the marked presence of those characteristics to make a difference to sight by daylight. But this is not found to hold good.'

437 b 22. ὕδατι. It would not be correct to say that light is not diminished when it penetrates water; ὕδωρ frequently signifies rain or rainy weather.

Similarly πάγος must be here frosty weather, not ice.

437 b 25. τοιοῦτον, *i.e.* the behaviour of light in cold or damp weather.

437 b 27. οὕτως. Cf. *R. P.* 177 b. Burnet, *Early Greek Philosophy*, pp. 231–2. They are vv. (Stein) 316–23, Fr. 84 (Diels, *Die Fragmente der Vorsokratiker*).

438 a 1. λοχάζετο. ἐχεύατο—suffused, is another reading which would make the construction easier.

438 a 3. διαθρῶσκον. διίεσκον, suggested by Blass, *N. Jahrb. f. Phil. u. Päd.* 1883, p. 19, would improve the grammar of the passage. Translate 'but they (αἱ δ') let the fire through.'

438 a 4. ἀπορροίαις. Cf. Empedocles and Plato *loc. cit.* in note to 437 b 13. Aristotle's words imply that Empedocles had no consistent theory but had recourse alternately to the doctrine that fire issued from the eyes and illuminated objects, and to that according to which effluences from bodies entered into the pores of the eye and so created perception.

The fact seems to be that Empedocles intended to account for vision by postulating that both those operations took place, but had great difficulty in reconciling them, and that thus at one time we hear more about the one than about the other.

The difficulties attending the acceptance of either one or both theories are pointed out below by Aristotle in 438 a 26 sqq.

We may conjecture as Hammond does, *Aristotle's Psychology*, p. 152 note, that he imagined that the images of things entering by means of the pores through the outer covering of the eye are illuminated by the fire issuing from the pupil. But it is not clear that he said anything so definite unless Aristotle means (in ll. 29–30 below) that τὸ ἐν ἀρχῇ συμφύεσθαι τοῦ ὄμματος was one of the positions held by Empedocles. It is manifest from what Theophrastus says (*R. P.* 177 b) that, according to the Empedoclean theory, fire existed both in the external world and in the eye, and that the effluences from things which produced the perception of visible objects consisted of fire. Fire was the finest of all substances and could thus penetrate the finest of the pores. Through the passages of the water we perceived dark objects.

This must surely mean that objects throw off effluences composed both of fire and water and that the fire penetrating through the fine pores is perceived by its 'like' fire, and the water, a crasser substance, can enter only by the wider pores and is recognised by its 'like' the water in the eye; cf. *R. P.* 177 b. Of course it is *quâ* light that objects are visible (dark being but a privation of light), and hence the really important part in vision is that played by the fire. Thus Aristotle is justified in regarding the Empedoclean theory as one which referred vision to fire.

438 a 5. Δημόκριτος. Cf. Zeller, *Presocratic Philosophy*, II. pp. 266 sqq., cf. p. 268. This doctrine was also shared by Leucippus and Epicurus.

The theory of Democritus was also one of ἀπόρροιαι. Things threw off εἴδωλα which affected the sense organs. But in the case of sight it seems to have been not actually the εἴδωλον thrown off from the object but the impression caused by this in the air which was reflected in the eye. (Cf. Theophrastus, *de Sensu*, 50, Zeller, *op. cit.* II. p. 219.) This was connected with his doctrine that we did not perceive things as they were in themselves but only as they affected the senses. Nevertheless he seems to hold that the medium is at the same time affected by an effluence from the seeing eye, but how it is possible to reconcile this with any intelligible theory of reflection it is difficult to see.

It is noteworthy that Plato too had some such theory of interaction between the effluence from the eye and from the external object; cf. *Timaeus*, 45 c.

The effluences are, however, according to him, fire (cf. the comparison of the eye to the sun in *Rep.* VI. 508). But he also agrees with Democritus in holding that by like we perceive like and that perception takes place with the whole soul.

438 a 6. ἔμφασιν. Cf. notes to 437 a 34 sqq. ἔμφασις means the appearing or being visible of one body in another: cf. *Meteor.* III. ch. 4.

438 a 8. ἐκείνῳ. The visibility or being seen of the reflected object exists not in the eye in which the reflection takes place but in the eye of the spectator who sees the reflection.

I have here followed Ziaja and Bender in opposition to Alexander, Simon, Thomas, St Hilaire and Hammond. Hammond appears to make τοῦτο refer to τὴν ἔμφασιν and then to supply a new subject— τὸ ὁρᾶν—as the subject of ἔστιν. This is surely in defiance of grammar.

If one took τοῦτο to mean τὸ τὴν ἔμφασιν ὁρᾶν the sense would be plain enough and would be exactly what we require. This is however to give a very liberal interpretation to τοῦτο which should mean τὸ ἐμφαίνεσθαι, which is the appearance of an εἴδωλον in a smooth surface. Now, though Aristotle could not say that the εἴδωλον (a special term used by Democritus) was not ἐν ἐκείνῳ (the reflecting eye), he can quite well maintain that the appearing of the εἴδωλον in the reflecting surface is not itself in the surface. Alexander also takes τὸ ὁρᾶν as the subject of ἔστιν and interprets ἐν ἐκείνῳ as ἐν τῇ ἐμφάσει. Simon and St Hilaire differ from him only in taking ἐν ἐκείνῳ to mean ὅτι τὸ ὄμμα λεῖον.

If, therefore, we were to follow Alexander we should render— 'For reflection occurs because the eye is smooth; but vision does not lie in the reflection or take place by means of it, but occurs in the seer, i.e. is an affection of one who has the power of sight.' According to Simon and St Hilaire we should turn the latter part of the sentence thus 'but vision does not lie in this property of the eye, etc.'

In addition to the syntactical objections to these interpretations, they have the demerit of making Aristotle reason in a circle. In arguing against the theory that vision is reflection, to state as one's reason that vision does not lie in the reflection of things in the eye and in its property as a reflecting structure, is merely to reiterate one's objection without proving it. ἐκείνῳ must refer to τὸ ὄμμα and the argument is to the effect that reflection must presuppose vision, because the mirroring of anything is a fact not for the subject in whose eye it takes place but for a second person who sees it.

438 a 13. ὄψιν. Note that ὄψιν, the word for the sense-faculty, is used as though it referred to the sensorium. Cf. Neuhäuser, *Aristoteles Lehre von den sinnlichen Erkenntnissvermögen und seinen Organen*, p. 79, and cf. note to 438 b 22 below.

438 a 14. διαφανές. The whole nature of τὸ διαφανές will be treated below in ch. 3.

438 a 16. εὐπιλητότερον. εὐυπολημπτότερον is the variant reading (L S U Alex.) which, if possible, only repeats the idea of εὐφυλακτότερον. With εὐπιλητότερον the καὶ becomes epexegetic.

Aristotle is here referring to what are now called the aqueous and vitreous humours.

438 a 21. τοῖς ἔχουσιν αἷμα. The sanguineous and non-sanguineous animals were two main divisions in Aristotle's *Zoology*. Cf. *De Part. Anim.* IV. ch. 5, 678 a 33. Insects and Crustaceans were placed in the latter class as the fluids in their bodies, not being red, were not thought to be blood.

438 a 26. ἄλογον. Aristotle here returns to his criticism of the
Empedoclean and Platonic theory. Cf. above 437 a 24—438 a 5.

The transition to this topic once more is probably to be explained
by the fact that Democritus, too, held a theory according to which
something emanates from the eye. Hence Aristotle first mentions
the doctrine in its most general form (ὅλως τὸ ἐξιόντι τινὶ...ὁρᾶν) and
then glides on to discuss the specially Empedoclean and Platonic
theories.

438 a 28. συμφύεσθαι. The fire from the eye unites with that
which is the effluence from external bodies.

438 a 29. τινες. Probably the more scientific Platonists or
interpreters of Empedocles.

ἐν ἀρχῇ. Alexander and Simon interpret as I have translated.
Aristotle proposes to simplify the phenomenon by supposing that
the union of fire with fire takes place in the eye itself *before* the
internal fire issues out, *i.e.* in the starting place of the internal fire
according to the more complex theory. It will be easier, he thinks,
to support the theory if one omits that part which makes the union
of fire with fire take place outside the eye.

One must not translate with Hammond 'It would be better to
assume that the combination of the eye with its object were in the
eye's original nature.'

In the first place, this makes Aristotle propose to supersede the
older theory by an explanation which merely shelves the difficulty
and refers it to a 'faculty.' Secondly, Aristotle is talking not of a
combination of eye with object but of fire with fire; as is apparent
from the next sentence, apart from which this one cannot be understood.

Simon quotes *De Part. Animal.* III. ch. 4, 665 b 14 (ὅπου γὰρ ἐνδέχεται μίαν βέλτιον ἢ πολλάς) as an illustration of the principle of
parsimony in Aristotle.

438 a 31. φωτὶ πρὸς φῶς. Alexander affiliates this and the
following statement—οὐ γὰρ τῷ τυχόντι κ.τ.λ.—to the doctrine expounded in *De Gen. et Corr.* I. ch. 10, where we find, 327 b 20: οὐ
γὰρ ἅπαν ἅπαντι μικτὸν ἀλλ᾽ ὑπάρχειν δεῖ χωριστὸν ἑκάτερον τῶν μιχ-
θέντων, *i.e.* only concrete objects (χωριστά), *i.e.* σώματα, can be mixed;
now light is a πάθος of the definite type ἕξις (cf. *De An.* III. ch. 5,
430 a 15) and hence cannot experience μίξις. This explanation
assumes that the σύμφυσις here talked about is a case of μίξις, which
is not quite evident. Neither is it evident that the union of light

with light (συμπαγὲς γενόμενον) mentioned in Plato, *Tim.* 45 C, against which this argument is directed, is properly a case of μίξις. Plato uses the term συμφυές below in 45 D probably hardly in the exact sense in which συμφύεσθαι is here employed. It need mean no more than 'kindred.'

συμφύεσθαι means no more than to grow together or unite, and not the union of two different substances which results in the production of a third distinct one, which is the sense in which Aristotle employs μίξις. Hence Alexander's discussion of the blending of lights (he denies that they can be united) seems to be irrelevant, and whether σύμφυσις can be brought under the category of μίξις is not clear.

Besides, if Alexander's were the correct interpretation, a Platonist might still reply that according to his theory light is nothing ἀσώματον, and hence (according to Aristotelian principles) *could* combine with other light. Cf. *Timaeus*, 45 C: ἓν σῶμα οἰκειωθὲν συνέστη by the union of the internal and the external light.

Perhaps Aristotle need mean no more than that the union of light with light is on the Platonic theory quite unexplained. Compare next note.

438 b 1. τὸ τυχόν. The commonest interpretation and that in consonance with Alexander's explanation (cf. above) is 'Not everything will unite with anything else' and that is referred to the doctrine οὐ γὰρ ἅπαν ἅπαντι μικτόν in *De Gen. et Corr.* I. ch. 10.

According to the translation I suggest the argument would run, 'How will this unexplained "union" of the Platonists produce sight? When we see, we see something definite, *i.e.* it is not with τὸ τυχόν that the union is effected. The theory is not capable of explaining in detail how we see.'

438 b 3. ἐν ἄλλοις. *De An.* II. ch. 7, 418 b 1, 419 a 9, III. ch. 5, 430 a 16.

438 b 5. This seems to contradict what is said below in ch. 6, 446 b 31: ἀλλ᾽ οὐ κίνησις (τὸ φῶς). It is true that κίνησις is frequently used for all the four varieties of change and as equivalent to μεταβολή—change in general, not merely to φορά—local motion, which is its most characteristic sense. The four species of change are 1. (κατ᾽ οὐσίαν) γένεσις καὶ φθορά: 2. (κατὰ τὸ ποσόν) αὔξησις καὶ φθίσις: 3. (κατὰ τὸ ποῦ) φορά: 4. (κατὰ τὸ ποιόν) ἀλλοίωσις. Hence, if light is an ἀλλοίωσις (qualitative change) and κίνησις is here used vaguely as including it, there is no contradiction between the two statements. We shall, however, maintain when we come to chapter 6, that in the Aristotelian theory the propagation of light is not even to be described as ἀλλοίωσις.

438 b 10. ἡ ψυχή is wider than consciousness, but Aristotle, though of course meaning merely consciousness here, is forced to use the wider term for want of a special word to designate conscious life in general without suggesting any one special faculty. We shall be forced to translate ψυχή thus more than once.

438 b 11. ἐντός. This surely must mean ἐντὸς τοῦ ὄμματος. The faculty or δύναμις of the special sense of sight resides within the eye. If this statement is capable of being generalised at all, it can be extended only so far as to include the organs of the other two mediated senses (hearing and smell). This cannot be taken as a reference, as Alexander (p. 36) and Neuhäuser (pp. 65 and 127) seem to think, to the central sense, which resides further within the body (in the heart). It is not the function of this central faculty to discriminate the objects of the special senses. It is the seat rather of that self-consciousness which also discriminates the various special senses (cf. *De An.* III. ch. 2), and is generally the organ of κοινὴ αἴσθησις and φαντασία.

If the faculty of vision resided in the central organ then surely according to Aristotle's argument there would need to be a transparent medium extending through the body right up to it, and it itself would need to have the same property. Neuhäuser indeed maintains that something like this is, according to the Aristotelian theory, the case. But a much simpler explanation is possible.

Something internal is the organ, Aristotle says, and hence it must be transparent. The interior of the eye is that which fulfils the conditions. Why the organ should be transparent is due to his general theory that it should be capable of receiving the same determinations as those existing in the world outside, *i.e.* should be δεκτικὸν τοῦ εἴδους of the external bodies (*De An.* II. ch. 12, 424 a 18). Cf. Introduction, sec. IV. pp. 7 sqq.

The statement that the sense faculty resides within is not a deduction from what is said in the *De Anima* about the internal or central sense; it is a truth said to be given by observation (δῆλον) and Aristotle at once proceeds to adduce a confirmatory instance.

If we hold with Neuhäuser that the seat of perception is really always a central organ—even in the case of the special senses—and that Aristotle held a theory according to which substance of the same kind as that composing the peripheral organ extended along the πόροι up to the central chamber of the heart, then perhaps ἐντός might mean 'in the central region.' Perhaps Alexander, when he says πόρους ἐν οἷς τὸ διαφανές, may also be referring to a similar theory. It seems an extraordinary hypothesis (cf. Introduction, sec. VI.) and it is not at all clear whether Neuhäuser has succeeded in substantiating it or merely in disproving the rival theory, viz. that the blood is, in Aristotle's eyes, the medium of communication between the end organ and the central one. Cf. note to 439 a 2 : Neuhäuser, *Aristoteles Lehre von den sinnlichen Erkenntnissvermögen und seinen Organen*, pp. 111–129.

438 b 14. τοὺς πόρους. Those who (*e.g.* Thomas, etc.) think that the reference is here to the central sense must hold that the πόροι are the optic nerves, which Aristotle imagined to be ducts leading to the brain and ultimately to the heart. Cf. *Hist. Animal.* IV. ch. 8, 533 a 13, *De Part. Animal.* II. ch. 10, 656 b 17. Alexander, however, seems to understand them to be the πόροι of the older philosophers—the passages through which (according to their view) the eye's internal fire issued. Cf. Theoph. *De Sensu*, 7 (*R. P.* 176 b) and Arist. *De Gen. et Corr.* I. ch. 8, 324 b 26.

Alexander says τοὺς πόρους ἐν οἷς τὸ διαφανές ἐστι and since the nerves are not (except on Neuhäuser's theory) transparent we can assume only that he means the passages supposed to exist in the eye itself. Blindness ensuing on the cutting of the optic nerve would show rather that the sense was not localised in the eye, but we have seen reason (see previous note) for maintaining that this is not the Aristotelian view. Hence Aristotle is not here referring to such a serious wound as one which would sever the optic nerve but to a more superficial injury to the eye. This is also borne out by the simile which follows. You cut the wick and the flame goes out; and so you destroy the channel communicating the external light to the pupil and sight is destroyed. This interpretation also gives παρά its characteristic sense. On the other hand we must remember that παρά need mean no more than 'on.' To read ὥστε τμηθῆναι in this line along with Mr Bywater (*Journal of Philol.* XXVIII. p. 243) would probably be better.

438 b 19. τοῦτον τὸν τρόπον. Cf. above 437 a 21. Aristotle does not commit himself to the proposed reduction.

438 b 22. ψόφων. Cf. *De An.* III. ch. 1, 425 a 4 : ἡ δ' ἀκοὴ ἀέρος. πυρὸς δὲ τὴν ὄσφρησιν. This statement seems to contradict what is said in *De An.* III. ch. 1, 425 a 5 : ἡ δ' ὄσφρησις θατέρου τούτων (sc. ὕδατος καὶ ἀέρος)...τὸ δὲ πῦρ ἢ οὐθενὸς ἢ κοινὸν πάντων. If then we take ὄσφρησις to be the sense organ here (a very common use; cf. above 438 a 13, Bonitz, *Ind.* p. 538 a 30), the two passages are in disagreement. Again the statement in ll. 25–26 beneath ἡ δ' ὀσμὴ καπνώδης ἀναθυμίασίς ἐστιν is in contradiction with ch. 4, 443 a 23 sqq., where it is denied that ὀσμή is of the nature of ἀναθυμίασις.

These considerations have led Alexander and most interpreters to maintain that here Aristotle is not putting forward his own theory (οὐ γὰρ δὴ ἀρέσκοντα αὐτῷ λέγει, Alex. 38, l. 14 [W.]), but merely discussing the consequences and the detailed working out of the doctrine suggested by the earlier philosophers—namely the ascription of each sense organ to a separate element.

On this interpretation the reading of the majority of the codices ὡς εἰ δεῖ in ll. 18–19 above, which Biehl adopts and Bäumker, p. 48, prefers, is particularly welcome. E M and Y read merely φανερὸν ὡς δεῖ and Bekker follows.

Thus it is contended that Aristotle's adoption of the correspondence of each sense organ to a separate element is merely hypothetical. Nevertheless it is strange that if this is so, Aristotle should go on to work out the connection between smell and fire by the aid of his own technical terms and connect it with his own theory of the excessive coldness of the brain. It almost looks as though the doctrine were one which had attractions for Aristotle and which was left as an unexpunged suggestion even after the possibility of reconciling it with the rest of his philosophy had been removed.

But, as it is stated, there are great difficulties to be overcome. The proof in ll. 22–25, as Alexander recognises, merely shows that the organ of smell is *potentially* (δυνάμει) of the nature of fire and is *actually* cold. It is not on all fours with the former two sense organs which are *actually* (ἐνεργείᾳ) water and air respectively.

Hence Hayduck (*Prog. Kön. Gym. zu Meldorf*, 1876–7) proposes not to take those lines (ὁ γὰρ ἐνεργείᾳ κ.τ.λ.) as a proof of the previous statement and to read ὁ δὲ ἐνεργείᾳ κ.τ.λ. He also proposes to omit l. 25 ἡ δ' ὀσμὴ...l. 27 πυρός as being in hopeless disagreement with the other passage at 443 a 23 sqq. His explanation is that Aristotle, beginning with a discussion of the organs corresponding to each sensuous function, naturally mentions the act of smelling and so proceeds to discuss its peculiar organ, which, though not parallel to the organs of sight and hearing in that it does not consist of any single element, he yet takes the opportunity of discussing. It seems however that Aristotle is really attempting to make the sense of smell in some way parallel to the other two and that ll. 22 sqq. are intended to prove this. Hence the elaborate doctrine about the coldness of the region in which the sense organ is situated and which is potentially warm ; and we hear elsewhere that ἡ τῆς ὀσμῆς δύναμις θερμὴ τὴν φύσιν ἐστίν (444 a 27). So that, in spite of the fact that he has not proved the sense organ to consist of actual fire, Aristotle evidently wishes to establish some connection between fire and odour. Hence Ziaja (*De Sensu*, p. 11) maintains that he does not intend here to discuss the nature of the sense organ of smell and that there is no conflict between this passage and any other. He points out how, when the brain is said to be ὑγρότατος καὶ ψυχρότατος τῶν ἐν τῷ σώματι μορίων, that agrees with the passage in *De An.* 425 a 3 sqq. where it is held that the sense organs are composed only of air and water. This latter statement however, it must be observed, is not perfectly unqualified, for Aristotle goes on to say that fire, though not a special ingredient of any one, may be said to exist in all (οὐθὲν γὰρ ἄνευ θερμότητος αἰσθητικόν) and that earth is either in none or is specially incorporated in the organ of touch (cf. below ll. 32 sq. : τὸ δὲ ἁπτικὸν γῆς). This passage (*q.v.*) shows the difficulty which there is in extracting a consistent statement from Aristotle as to the nature of the sense organs, and the fact that his theories on this subject seem to fluctuate makes it difficult to avoid thinking that here he at least starts with an attempt to work a parallel between the organs of sight and hearing on the one hand and that of smell on the other. It is quite evident, as Rodier, *De An.* II. p. 349, points out, that τὴν ὄσφρησιν must here mean τὸ τῆς ὀσφρήσεως αἰσθητήριον, otherwise it could not support the statement φανερὸν ὡς εἰ δεῖ κ.τ.λ.; besides Aristotle plainly means the sense organs in the other cases—τὸ ὁρατικόν, τὸ τῶν ψόφων αἰσθητικόν, τὸ ἁπτικόν.

Hence, unless we adopt Hayduck's bold emendations, we must conclude (1) that the doctrine here is a tentative construction of a parallel between the organs of smell, touch and taste and those of sight and hearing ; (2) that the parallel consists in assigning each to a special element (touch and taste, being generically the same, share one between them) ; (3) that though Aristotle cannot work out the parallel in the case of smell and the attempt to do so endangers conflict with the rest of his teaching, the theory has attractions for him owing to its symmetry and the fact that in so far as it can be

R.   10

worked out it connects with his account of the nature of the brain ; and hence it was not deleted, but became incorporated with the remainder of his preserved writings.

γάρ. On Hayduck's suggestion this is changed to δέ, and the following statement is not a reason for the preceding one but a new premise from which, in combination with the preceding one, διὸ καὶ κ.τ.λ., ll. 27 sqq., is deduced.

438 b 23. δυνάμει. Cf. *De An.* II. ch. 5, 418 a 3 : τὸ δ' αἰσθητικὸν δυνάμει ἐστὶν οἷον τὸ αἰσθητὸν ἤδη ἐντελεχείᾳ. Cf. also II. ch. 12, 424 a 17–20 : ἡ μὲν αἴσθησίς ἐστι τὸ δεκτικὸν τῶν αἰσθητῶν εἰδῶν ἄνευ τῆς ὕλης and III. ch. 2, 425 b 23 : τὸ γὰρ αἰσθητήριον δεκτικὸν τοῦ αἰσθητοῦ ἄνευ τῆς ὕλης ἕκαστον, etc.

The theory is, that the sense organ is potentially capable of receiving the 'form' *i.e.* the perceptible properties of the object of sense. In the act of perception object and sense are one, but, when the sense organ is not stimulated, it is only potentially percipient, the object only potentially perceived. Cf. 425 b 26 : ἡ τοῦ αἰσθητοῦ ἐνέργεια καὶ τῆς αἰσθήσεως ἡ αὐτή ἐστι καὶ μία. In the act of perception the organ becomes like its object ; previously to perception it is unlike ; cf. 418 a 5, 6 : πάσχει μὲν οὐχ ὅμοιον ὄν, πεπονθὸς δ' ὡμοίωται καὶ ἔστιν οἷον ἐκεῖνο.

Note that Aristotle has no need to assume that the sense organs consist of the elements because like is perceived by like. The organ was not like its object in consisting of the same material but in receiving its εἶδος or λόγος—the pattern according to which it was constructed. Cf. Introduction, sec. IV.

438 b 24. ποιεῖ. The external object is the agent in perception ; the sense organ is passive. Cf. *De An.* II. ch. 5, 417 b 20 : τὰ ποιητικὰ τῆς ἐνεργείας ἔξωθεν, τὸ ὁρατὸν καὶ τὸ ἀκουστόν, ὁμοίως δὲ καὶ τὰ λοιπὰ τῶν αἰσθητῶν.

If we read ὃ in l. 25 below we cannot translate 'the latter (sc. the sensation) must have an antecedent potential existence,' as Hammond does, but 'the sensation is what it previously had the potentiality of becoming.'

438 b 27. τὸν ἐγκέφαλον. The brain was not the organ of sensation according to Aristotle but played a subsidiary part in the bodily economy as neutralising the heat of the heart. On the other hand excessive cold in the brain was tempered (at least in man) by the dry warmth of odours which were healthful and hence delightful. Cf. below ch. 5, 444 a 9 sqq.

438 b 29. This is an application of the general Aristotelian doctrine that opposites pass into each other. Things are only opposite in so far as they have the same ὕλη and it is through having the same ὕλη that they can pass into each other. Hence the ὕλη is potentially capable of being either. Cf. *Phys.* I. ch. 9, 192 a 21: φθαρτικὰ γὰρ ἀλλήλων τὰ ἐναντία, and IV. ch. 9, 217 a 22: ἐστὶν ὕλη μία τῶν ἐναντίων, θερμοῦ καὶ ψυχροῦ καὶ τῶν ἄλλων τῶν φυσικῶν ἐναντιώσεων, etc.

τοῦ ὄμματος. Cf. *De Gen. Animal.* II. ch. 6, 743 b 28 sqq., 744.

438 b 33. γῆς. Cf. *De An.* III. ch. 1, 425 a 7: cf. above note to 438 b 22.

τὸ δὲ γευστικὸν κ.τ.λ. Cf. 441 a 3 sq. : ἡ γεῦσις ἁφή τις ἐστίν and *De An.* III. ch. 12, 434 b 18. Comment on this doctrine will be postponed until we come to chapter 4, where taste is discussed at length.

439 a 2. πρὸς τῇ καρδίᾳ. It is true that the organs of taste and touch transmit κινήσεις—sense affections—to the heart, but we cannot translate πρὸς τῇ καρδίᾳ by 'conduct to the heart,' as Hammond does, because, according to Aristotle's general theory, *all* sense organs should do so, and besides Aristotle is here not discussing the question of the communication of the exterior sense organs with the inner πρῶτον αἰσθητήριον, but the nature of the composition of those sensoria. It is true that Aristotle does not make clear how the κινήσεις from the special senses are conveyed to the heart (cf. Zeller, *Aristotle* II. pp. 67–70, English Trans.). Alexander says that there are three πόροι extending from the heart to the brain and then to the three sense organs of sight, hearing and smell respectively, but in the case of taste and touch the πόροι communicate directly with the end organs; by these the κινήσεις are transmitted. For confirmation of this cf. *De Juvent.* ch. 3, 469 a 12 sqq. ; *De Insom.* ch. 3, 461 a 1 sqq. The blood seems to some to be the medium of transmission but we cannot certainly say so. According to Neuhäuser it certainly is not. The medium is a substance of the same nature as the end organ extending (in the case of the three senses of which the organs are localised in the head) along πόροι first to the brain and ultimately to the heart. Cf. Introduction, sec. VI. and Neuhäuser, pp. 110 sqq. It is true also that the heart, which is the organ of the common sense (cf. *De Juvent.*, *De Insom. loc. cit.* above and *De Somno* ch. 2, 455 a 21 : τὸ κύριον αἰσθητήριον), seems to be also the special organ of touch (cf. 455 a 23 : τοῦτο (τὸ κύριον αἰσθητήριον) τῷ ἀπτικῷ μάλισθ᾽ ὑπάρχει), between which and its object the flesh seems to be the medium (cf. *De An.* II. ch. 11, 423 b 26 : τὸ μεταξὺ τοῦ ἀπτικοῦ ἡ σάρξ, and III. ch. 2, 426 b 15 : ἡ σὰρξ οὐκ ἔστι τὸ ἔσχατον αἰσθητήριον). But however that may be—and if the latter point is to be insisted upon we had better translate 'their organ is situated in the region of the heart'—the question is here not one of communication, but of the origin of the organs in question. If the organ of smell is actually cold and potentially warm and apprehends what is in actuality warm (ὀσμή), so conversely the organ of taste and touch should be actually warm but potentially cold if it apprehends what is actually cold, viz. γῆ.

Alexander, however, will not allow that γῆ is the proper object of touch. Certainly it is the Aristotelian theory that touch perceives not merely the qualities of γῆ, *i.e.* τὸ ψυχρόν and τὸ ξηρόν, but all the four ultimate (and primary in that sense) qualities of objects (cf. above note to 437 a 22) and others as well (cf. *De Gen. et Corr.* II. ch. 2, 329 b 17 sqq.). Hence once more we have evidence that the above argument is at best only tentative.

If we take it that the organ of touch is actually of the nature of earth and has the characteristic qualities of earth, then it is impossible to see how it is connected with the heart, which is the seat of warmth. If it is potentially of the nature of γῆ then it will, like the heart, have actually the opposite qualities. But in that case we shall have failed to account for the perception of τὸ θερμόν, as well as other qualities, by it, in the sense of reconciling that to the general Aristotelian doctrine that the organ is unlike the object before sensation but in the act of perception becomes qualitatively identical with it, as is stated in *De An.* II. ch. 5, 417 a 20.

Cf. also *De Part. Animal.* II. ch. 10, 656 a 29 : καὶ διότι αἱ μὲν δύο φανερῶς ἠρτημέναι πρὸς τὴν καρδίαν εἰσίν, ἥ τε τῶν ἁπτῶν καὶ ἡ τῶν χυμῶν.

αἰσθητήριον. One more proof that the whole passage is a discussion of sensoria.

CHAPTER III.

(This chapter begins the treatment of the objects of the special senses. It treats of colour.)

439 a 9. ἐν τοῖς περὶ ψυχῆς. Cf. *De An.* II. ch. 7–12.

439 a 10. ἔργον. In *De An.* I. ch. 1, 402 b 12 Aristotle talks about the function (ἔργον) of the sense. The function of the sense is to perceive, that of the object to cause perception; but as we shall see (cf. note to 439 a 17–18), when functioning, sense and its object are qualitatively identical.

ἐνεργεῖν. This practically repeats the sense of ἔργον. ἐνέργεια contains more explicitly the notion of the realisation of an end than ἔργον, but the two are often almost identical and tend to replace each other in our texts, *e.g.* in *De Mem.* ch. 1, 449 b 20.

439 a 11. τὸ τί ἐστιν is the essential nature of a thing as revealed in its definition (without going on to state its additional properties). Aristotle is now to discuss what each object of sense is in its own objective nature apart from its action on the sense organs.

439 a 17–18. ἐν τοῖς περὶ ψυχῆς. Cf. *De An.* III. ch. 2, 425 b 26: ἡ δὲ τοῦ αἰσθητοῦ ἐνέργεια καὶ τῆς αἰσθήσεως ἡ αὐτὴ μέν ἐστι καὶ μία, τὸ δὲ εἶναι οὐ τὸ αὐτὸ αὐταῖς.

Similarly in *De An.* II. ch. 5, 417 a 20, we learn that, in the act of sensation, object and sensorium are alike. Whatever is said in this connection of the sensorium holds of the sense faculty and, as we have seen, Aristotle often uses the name of the faculty inter-changeably for that belonging to the organ. His theory shows in this respect what we might call a thorough-going psycho-physical parallelism.

It is by his distinction between the actual and the potential object of sense that Aristotle attempts to explain the problem about the independent existence of external objects of sense. Considered κατὰ δύναμιν or as ὑποκείμενα (cf. *Metaph.* IV. ch. 5, 1010 b 30 sqq.) they have an independent existence, κατ᾽ ἐνέργειαν not. Apart from

actual perception the sense also is a δύναμις merely and, as potentialities, sense and its object are different and have different names—
χυμός and γεῦσις, ψόφος and ἀκοή, χρῶμα and ὄψις etc. But the
ἐνέργεια of each is one and the same, *e.g.* ψόφησις and ἄκουσις are
one and the same.

It is, however, impossible for Aristotle to maintain this attitude
towards external reality consistently. If the sense is that which is receptive of the εἶδος of things, how can it be said to receive that which
prior to this reception had no existence? It is not sufficient to say
that its ὑποκείμενον existed; if we strip the external world of all εἶδος,
nothing is left but the πρώτη ὕλη, and this, being perfectly undifferentiated, cannot account for the difference of the εἶδος which we
apprehend at different times. Aristotle is forced to think of the
εἶδος as existing antecedently to the perception of it, and consequently we find in *De An.* II. ch. 5, 418 a 3: τὸ δὲ αἰσθητικὸν
δυνάμει ἐστὶν οἷον τὸ αἰσθητὸν ἤδη ἐντελεχείᾳ. Thus the object apart
from perception, which is said (in *Metaph.*, *loc. cit.*) to cause the
perception and is yet called a ὑποκείμενον, cannot be regarded as
a mere ὑποκείμενον, for to exist ἐντελεχείᾳ is to have εἶδος (cf.
Metaph. IX. ch. 8, 1050 b 2 and Bonitz ad 1043 a 18, cf. also
Ind. p. 219 a 25). According both to ancient and modern
physical atomism this ὑποκείμενον, which is yet something actual
and not mere ὕλη, would be described in terms of spatial configuration, mass and motion—the primary qualities from the atomistic
point of view. This solution however could not be entertained by
Aristotle, for whom the qualities relative to the special senses
were as primary determinations of physical reality as motion, figure
and mass (cf. notes to ch. 6, 445 b 6 sqq.). The atomistic solution
is only a makeshift; but we are left with a bad contradiction in the
Aristotelian theory.

439 a 20. περὶ φωτός. Cf. *De An.* II. ch. 7, 418 b 11 : τὸ δὲ φῶς
οἷον χρῶμά ἐστι τοῦ διαφανοῦς, ὅταν ᾖ ἐντελεχείᾳ διαφανὲς ὑπὸ πυρὸς ἢ
τοιούτου οἷον τὸ ἄνω σῶμα (τὸ ἄνω σῶμα is the upper fire, the celestial
ether).

τοῦ διαφανοῦς. For Aristotle's theory of τὸ διαφανές cf. Introduction pp. 20 sqq. At first sight it seems strange to define light as
the colour of the transparent medium, especially as he goes on (in 439 b
11 below) to define colour as the limit of the transparent element in
bodies. But that which renders bodies visible is colour and, though
an object must have a definite boundary or surface for this colour to

be detected, still we are bound to assume that throughout, so far as it is a coloured thing, its nature is the same (439 a 35 below). This quality on which its colour depends and which transpierces it through and through is light (φῶς), which is, however, but the activity or the proper function of that property—τὸ διαφανές—which permeates all bodies to a greater or less degree. Cf. *De An.* II. ch. 7, 418 b 9: φῶς δέ ἐστιν ἡ τούτου ἐνέργεια, τοῦ διαφανοῦς ᾗ διαφανές, and 419 a 11: ἡ δ' ἐντελέχεια τοῦ διαφανοῦς φῶς ἐστίν.

Thus though φῶς is not χρῶμα in the sense in which that is the πέρας of the transparent element in bodies, still it is the colour principle which transfuses all substances.

439 a 21. By κατὰ συμβεβηκός Aristotle means, not 'casually,' but 'indirectly' *i.e.* subject to some condition being fulfilled, not in its own nature without further determination. Relatively to the thing which has a certain attribute only upon the supervention of some condition, that attribute is contingent, and it seems to be with this in mind that Kant identifies the contingent and the conditioned in the proof of the antithesis in the fourth antinomy. But, from another point of view, when we take into account the dependence of this attribute upon its conditions it is seen to be necessary. κατὰ συμβεβηκός in Aristotle is by no means equivalent merely to 'due to chance' but in its general sense is used simply as opposed to καθ' αὑτό, due not to the essence of the thing to which it belongs but to some external condition.

πυρῶδες. Cf. *De An.* II. ch. 7, 418 b 12 quoted above in note to 439 a 20 and again 419 a 24: τὸ γὰρ διαφανὲς ὑπὸ τούτου (sc. πυρὸς) γίνεται διαφανές. It is fire, then, or anything of the nature of fire, the sun or the celestial ether (τὸ ἄνω σῶμα), which raises the transparent medium from a state of mere potentiality in which it is ἄχρουν—colourless and invisible (418 b 28)—to a state in which colour is actually visible. The fire evidently makes it actually transparent, and this state of actual transparency, this ἐνέργεια, is light. We cannot say with Hammond that 'light is that which converts the potentially diaphanous into the actually diaphanous.' It is fire which performs this function.

439 a 22. παρουσία (cf. *De An.* 418 b 16 and 20) seems here to be reminiscent of its technical Platonic signification—immanence, and thus we could define light as 'the immanence of fire in the transparent medium.'

But there are two points of view from which light can be

regarded, (1) as a state of illumination, cf. *De An.* III. ch. 5, 430 a 15, and (2) as though it were the stimulation proceeding from the coloured object to the eye (cf. *De An.* II. ch. 7, 418 a 31: πᾶν δὲ χρῶμα κινητικόν ἐστιν τοῦ κατ' ἐνέργειαν διαφανοῦς).

Yet according to this passage in the *De An.* it is implied that the state of illumination must be already realised for the stimulation which causes vision to take effect. Aristotle, though frequently asserting that there is a stimulation proceeding from object to eye and talking as though this were light, yet in chapter 6 below turns round and says that light is not a stimulation at all. According to the interpretation of that chapter which I adopt, it is not a stimulation of the type ἀλλοίωσις even (*i.e.* qualitative change). Yet light is still said to cause us to see (447 a 12), and if it is not the stimulus through the medium, what *is* that stimulus? It appears as though Aristotle, influenced by the apparent instantaneousness of light transference, were trying to combine into one the notion of it (1) as a ἕξις, the state of illumination, and (2) as an action passing from the object to the eye, two notions which will not unite.

Compare chapter 6, 446 a 22—447 a 12, and Introduction, sec. VII.

439 a 23. τὸ διαφανές is no *proprium* of air or any one transparent substance.

439 a 25. φύσις καὶ δύναμις. Cf. *De An.* II. ch. 7, 418 b 8: ἐστὶ φύσις ὑπάρχουσα ἡ αὐτὴ ἐν αὐτοῖς ἀμφοτέροις (sc. ὕδατι καὶ ἀέρι) καὶ ἐν τῷ ἄνω σώματι.

χωριστή. Light is not a substance. χωριστά is a common designation for substances. Cf. *De Gen. et Corr.* I. ch. 10, 327 b 21.

439 a 26. Cf. below 439 b 10. τὸ διαφανές is found in all, not merely in certain bodies.

439 a 29. ἀορίστῳ. φῶς as the general colour principle permeates bodies through and through in so far as they share in the material condition of colour phenomena.

439 a 31-32. ἐκ τῶν συμβαινόντων. Cf. 438 b 12-13 and note ἐπὶ τῶν συμβαινόντων δῆλον.

439 a 33. Πυθαγόρειοι. Cf. Plut. *Epit. Mem.* I. 15; Stobaei *Eclog.* I. 15 quoted by Diels, *Dox. Gr.* p. 313.

439 a 34-35. The point is that colour is not the boundary or surface of the *body* but, as appears in 439 b 12 below, of the transparent element in the body.

439 b 2. We may supply εἶναι after ἐντός, not necessarily χρωματίζεσθαι. Aristotle does not actually say that colour, in the sense of definite tint, pervades the body through and through. That resides in the surfaces. But the colour principle, which is made definite only when the body has a definite surface, must pervade the body in every part in so far as it is διαφανές. This colour principle can be nothing else than φῶς, and its opposite is σκότος.

Most of the commentators, however, will have it that here Aristotle is distinguishing bodies which are coloured 'externally' *e.g.* air and water, which have no proper colour of their own, and those coloured 'internally' *i.e.* with a proper colour of their own, opaque bodies, and that he here declares that it is an identical principle in each class that makes them receptive of colour. The difference between the two classes of objects is that the former set, having no definite surface, have no definite limit of the διαφανές in them and it is a definite boundary that gives definite colour. But it is solely the want of definiteness in their limits which causes the indefiniteness of the colour. Since they show colour of some kind, they must have the constitution which renders colour possible. This is their transparency, which we must hence ascribe to opaque bodies also.

If we accept this theory the translation will run as follows : 'We must, however, believe that the type of construction which internally and of its own nature takes on colour is the same as that which receives its colour from without. Now air and water show colour, for the gleam they have betrays tint.'

The advantage of this interpretation is that it does not make Aristotle say that the colour pervades the whole of an opaque object, for this, unless we explain the distinction between definite and indefinite colour as above, seems to conflict with his statement that colour resides on the surface. Cf. also *Top.* v. ch. 8, 138 a 15.

φαίνεται. Simon would translate 'appear to be coloured,' as though they really were not. But, though colour were held to pervade pellucid substances which have no definite surface, that would not entail as a consequence that it permeated opaque bodies as well—which is the conclusion against which Simon wishes to argue.

439 b 3. αὐγή. Thomas and Simon translate this by 'aurora,' on what grounds it is difficult to discover. Perhaps it means the *ray* *e.g.* of the sun falling upon these bodies.

439 b 6. σώμασιν. Alexander says that Aristotle here means to indicate στερεά—solids, as though they were more properly σώματα

than air and water. But the distinction should properly be between pellucid and opaque bodies as in ll. 13–15 below. Aristotle had already, in *De An.* II. ch. 7, 418 b 7, noticed that many στερεά were transparent. Probably here he leaves this latter class out of account. (Cf. ch. 5, 445 a 17 sqq. and notes on σῶμα and σωματοῦσθαι: cf. beneath 439 b 18.) The argument certainly requires σώμασιν here to mean definitely bounded or solid bodies. The omission of the class of transparent solids from consideration is simply a sign of the inadequacy of the theory.

439 b 10. ποιεῖ. τὸ διαφανές is the 'material' cause of colour, *i.e.* it accounts for its possibility.

439 b 12. χρῶμα κ.τ.λ. This is the definition, the τί ἐστιν of χρῶμα *per se*, and, in stating this, the *De Sensu* makes an advance on the *De Anima* which defined it merely in reference to the organ of sight as κινητικὸν τοῦ κατ' ἐνέργειαν διαφανοῦς.

439 b 14. ὅσοις κ.τ.λ. These are the 'corpora terminata' or στερεά of the commentators, which have a colour of their own and ἐντὸς χρωματίζεται. Many interpreters, however, disjoining κατὰ τὸ ἔσχατον from ὑπάρχειν and uniting it with ὁμοίως, find themselves in a difficulty and *identify* those referred to by καὶ ὅσοις with αὐτῶν τῶν διαφανῶν!

439 b 20. διελομένους. διαιρεῖσθαι constantly means to break up a genus into species or to discriminate species from each other. But, as Aristotle has not yet given any classification of the 'intermediate' colours, *i.e.* those over and above black and white, we must interpret ἤδη διελομένους (the reading of all mss. and edd.) as meaning merely 'after recognising the distinction' between the other colours and black and white. This is to take διελομένους in its vaguest sense. It is thus much better to read εἴδη instead of ἤδη. The phrase then becomes a common one and gives διελομένους its wonted sense. Cf. *Politics* IV. ch. 10, 1295 a 8 : τυραννίδος δ' εἴδη δύο μὲν διείλομεν etc. It is true that, owing to the aorist διελομένους, we seem still to be committed to the promise of a preliminary classification of the species of colour which is not fulfilled. The full list of the colours appears only in ch. 4, 442 a 22 sqq. Thus a minor inaccuracy is left in any case, and it may be argued that ἤδη διελομένους need give no more than this sense. But εἴδη is a rather tempting emendation.

Aristotle's theory is that the chromatic tones are obtained by a mixture of substances which already have the basal tones of white and black. The chromatic tones are intermediate between black and white, which appear to be regarded as lying at the two extremities of a *continuum* in the centre of which the other tints are found. Aristotle does not however attempt to assign its exact place in the scale to any one colour or state its affinity to either of the extremes. Each distinct colour depends upon the proportion in which the black and white, out of which it is formed, are mingled. But he does not venture to state the proportion which obtains in any one case. Cf. also *Metaph.* x. ch. 2, 1053 b 30.

439 b 26. μικτόν. The doctrine of composition or mixture is referred to again directly: cf. especially 440 b 14 sqq.

439 b 29. A λόγος appears to be the relation which prevails between two numbers when a division of the greater by the less yields a rational quotient. Numbers that are not so related are said to be οὐκ ἐν λόγῳ (cf. 440 a 16). λόγος then is not ratio in general but commensurate ratio. The incommensurate is the irrational —ἄλογον. Thus we cannot translate οὐκ ἐν λόγῳ, μὴ ἐν ἀριθμοῖς etc. by 'disproportionate,' for that applies to a ratio when one of the terms is excessive, not to one where the quantities are incommensurate.

439 b 34. εὐλογίστοις—easily reckoned, from λογίζεσθαι to reckon. Cf. *Metaph.* xiv. ch. 6, 1092 b 27.

440 a 2. The reason is that the εὐλόγιστοι ἀριθμοί, *i.e.* proportions where the division of one term by the other takes very little trouble, are few in number. The author of the *Problems* in 920 a 27 avers that the most agreeable harmony is that of the octave, and the reason for this is that the terms are whole numbers 2 and 1, or 4 and 2, and the division yields no remainder. The next harmony in order of pleasantness is that of the fifth, where the two notes are related as 1 to 1½, and so on.

440 a 5. τεταγμένας. The proportion of elements may be uniform in every part, *i.e.* the combination is according to a regularly recurring pattern, *e.g.* 3 : 1, 3 : 1, 3 : 1 etc., not 2 : 1, 4 : 1, 3 : 1 etc.

440 a 6. μὴ καθαραί. Some commentators (*e.g.* Simon, Hammond) identify the ἄτακτοι χρόαι with the μὴ καθαραί, but, unless we read τοῖς αὐτοῖς before ἀριθμοῖς in l. 6 as Biehl suggests, this is impossible, for Aristotle has immediately before said that both the τεταγμέναι and the ἄτακτοι are ἐν ἀριθμοῖς.

The impurity referred to must be want of saturation, *i.e.* want of colour, if it is caused by absence of proportion between the elements, and all chromatic colour involves a proportion between its components. But one may ask, why does impurity seem to occur only in the second class of colours—those due to an irregular structure? The reason I would suggest is this—Aristotle identifies the most pleasing colours with those which depend upon a regularly recurring structure in the combination of their elements. Relatively to these, other colours are not so pleasing and hence not regarded as so pure, καθαραί, if purity is a mark of excellence (as frequently in Plato, cf. *Philebus* 57 A *et passim*); but the colours of this second class contain in themselves differences in purity. Their impurity we may assign to a total want of commensurate proportion in their composition. Unless some such explanation as this is adopted we shall have to make αὐτὰς ταύτας refer to both classes of colours; but this is to strain the Greek.

440 a 8. τὸ φαίνεσθαι κ.τ.λ. Literally 'the shining of one colour through another.'

This second theory is, like the first, also rejected by Aristotle.

440 a 12. διὰ δ' ἀχλύος. The reason for this is discussed in *Meteorology* III.

440 a 16–21. It is difficult to see what connection this paragraph has either with what precedes or what follows. Thurot and Susemihl (*Philol.* 1885) think that it is misplaced in the text. It refers back to the theories of Empedocles and Democritus mentioned in chapter 2.

440 a 17. ἀπορροίας. Cf. 438 a 4.

440 a 19. εὐθὺς—directly, without the intervention of any intermediate steps in the argument.

440 a 21. ἀφῇ. Why was it necessary for the atomists to identify all sensation with touch? Surely because differences in sensation corresponded to differences in the tangible properties of things. Cf. chapter 4, 442 b 1 and 11: οἱ δὲ τὰ ἴδια εἰς ταῦτα ἀνάγουσιν κ.τ.λ. The argument runs—if sensation is to be effected by contact, contact with a medium which is sensitive to stimulation will explain perception better than a theory according to which the actual particles of the distant objects impinge upon the sense organs. On the other reading (L S U Alex. vet. tr.) ἢ ἀφῇ καὶ ταῖς ἀπορροίαις there is no argument.

Thomas and Alexander try to connect this with what follows; but Aristotle goes on to talk of κινήσεις impinging on the sense organ, not effluxes.

440 a 23. μέγεθος is almost always a spatial quantum, but cf. μέγεθος χρόνου ch. 7, 448 b 4.

The discussion on the possibility of the existence of imperceptible quanta is contained in chapter 6, 445 b 3 sqq.

χρόνον ἀναίσθητον. Aristotle argues at length against there being any such thing as an imperceptible time in ch. 7 below 448 a 21 sqq. The two moments of time in which the two sensations arrive would, on this hypothesis, be indistinguishable as two distinct moments, but would appear as one single moment which had no parts. Now, as time is a *continuum*, each part of it must be capable of resolution into other parts. Hence the supposition of an atomic time is absurd, no part is imperceptible. Cf. notes to chapter 7, and Introduction, sec. VIII.

440 a 26. ἀκίνητον—when not set in motion. The surface colour sets in motion the medium and so affects the sense (cf. *De An.* II. ch. 7, 418 a 31 : πᾶν δὲ χρῶμα κινητικόν ἐστι τοῦ κατ᾽ ἐνέργειαν διαφανοῦς). But Aristotle thinks that the action of the surface colour would be different if it itself were acted on by an underlying tint.

E M Y read κινητὸν, which would imply that the surface colour was independently itself in motion ; but this is not an Aristotelian doctrine.

440 a 30–31. The common reading is καὶ αὕτη τις ἂν εἴη χρωμάτων μίξις. Alexander interprets this to mean that Aristotle admits that the superposition theory is one which accounts for one way of mingling colours. But it is strange that, after rejecting the juxtaposition theory of mixture, Aristotle should say καὶ αὕτη—'this *too* is a theory which accounts for the mixture of colours.' Simon, thinking that the difficulty about μεγέθη ἀόρατα still applies to the superposition theory, suggests the punctuation and accentuation I have adopted and contends that here Aristotle is calling in question this second theory as well. If this is not so, he says, Aristotle must be convicted of carelessness, for he nowhere else points out the defect in the theory.

Without accepting his argument (which seems to be unfounded) I think we can still accept his interpretation of the intention of the clause. Aristotle calls the ἐπιπόλασις theory in question because it really is not an account of the μίξις of the colours. The two colours are simply juxtaposed, in this case one on the top of the other instead of in minute parts side by side. This is merely a case of the σύνθεσις of the colours, not of their true mixture. We may anticipate the doctrine which Aristotle refers to further down and which is expounded in *De Gen. et Corr.* I. ch. 10, 327 b 32 sqq.

There are two spurious kinds of mixture, μίξις merely πρὸς αἴσθησιν, *i.e.* the substances appear to sense to be mixed but are really not so. (1) First there is the juxtaposition of things that can be resolved into ultimate individual parts, *e.g.* grains of corn, men, etc. (εἰς τὰ ἐλάχιστα 440 b 5 sq. below); ὅταν...οὕτως εἰς μικρὰ διαιρεθῇ τὰ μιγνύμενα, καὶ τεθῇ παρ᾽ ἄλληλα τοῦτον τὸν τρόπον ὥστε μὴ δῆλον ἕκαστον εἶναι τῇ αἰσθήσει. This is the kind of μίξις referred to in 440 b 4 below, which explains the χρόαν κοινὴν (440 a 32) of distant objects, which vanishes when we approach them. This is a case in which σύνθεσις and μίξις are identical in the sense that σύνθεσις is the only μίξις of which the objects are capable. (2) Secondly, when there is no limit to the minuteness of the parts (*e.g.* in liquids), the mere juxtaposition of minute parts is merely apparent mixture (πρὸς αἴσθησιν). To more accurate vision the appearance of mixture ceases to exist. In true mixture (which seems to be analogous to what we should call chemical combination; cf. Mr Joachim in *Journal of Philol.* XXIX.) every part of the compound produced by the union of two substances must be homogeneous with the whole: cf. 328 a 10: τὸ μιχθὲν ὁμοιομερὲς εἶναι and below 440 b 3: πάντη πάντως. Each part of the one must completely interpenetrate the other, or rather, in union the two substances must completely change their nature so as to be incapable of being found in actuality in any part however minute. (This implies a still closer union than that of chemical combination, according to which the atoms are juxtaposed in the molecule, which is not homogeneous in every part.)

Now superposition of colours one over the other does not imply their mixture in the true sense.

440 a 31. κἀκείνως must mean 'on the former,' *i.e.* the juxtaposition theory, not 'in this way' (referring to the ἐπιπόλασις account) as Hammond has it.

The argument is, that the one colour shines through the other and that at close quarters the duality of the tint can possibly be detected, though at a distance the two produce a certain 'common' (κοινὴν) tint. But, says Aristotle, this general indeterminate tint can equally well be produced by the juxtaposition of parts of different colour provided they are minute enough or we are far enough away. But it is not this neutral tint, which varies with the accuracy of the vision, that has to be accounted for. Composite colours are on a different footing, and neither of the two theories has succeeded in accounting for them, cf. 440 b 16–19 beneath.

440 a 33. There is no need for substituting δ' for γὰρ with Susemihl (*Philol.* 1885).

The fact that no magnitude is invisible is the reason why we can account for the juxtaposition of minute parts differently coloured producing a common tint. If the parts were really invisible they would not produce any colour sensation either alone or together.

Compare chapter 6 below and notes.

The theory of juxtaposition is then rejected in so far as it implies the existence of invisible magnitudes, and retained to explain the production of neutral tints relative to the keenness of our vision, in so far as it is conceded that the parts do produce an effect upon our sight. The parts, as we shall see, are perceived ἐνεργείᾳ only in the whole (ἐν τῷ ὅλῳ); individually taken they are only δυνάμει perceptible.

440 a 34. From εἰ δ' 440 a 34 to b 14 is one long protasis.

440 b 2. τῶν ἐλαχίστων. Cf. *De Gen. et Corr.*, *loc. cit.* and note to 440 a 30–31. τὰ ἐλάχιστα are not infinitely minute parts, but the smallest parts that can be treated as individuals. Many things on division do not present such parts, *e.g.* water and other continuous substances are specially εὐδιαίρετα and prone to mix. Cf. beneath ll. 10 sqq., *De Gen. et Corr.* 328 b 3: τὰ ὑγρὰ μικτὰ μάλιστα τῶν σωμάτων· εὐόριστον γὰρ μάλιστα τὸ ὑγρὸν τῶν διαιρετῶν, since μικρὰ... μικροῖς παρατιθέμενα μίγνυται μᾶλλον, 328 a 33.

440 b 3. πάντῃ πάντως. Cf. *De Gen. et Corr.* 328 a 11.

ἐν τοῖς περὶ μίξεως. Probably only the passages referred to above.

440 b 10. ὅσα δὲ μὴ κ.τ.λ. *e.g.* water. Cf. above.

The modern atomic theory holds that there is a limit to the process of resolution and that that is found when the atom is reached. But there is a difficulty here, for the atom, if anything occupying space, must be divisible into smaller components.

440 b 16. κυρίαν. This is the reason of the real constant colour of objects.

440 b 22–23. τὸν αὐτὸν τρόπον κ.τ.λ. *i.e.* the mathematical development of all three is alike.

440 b 25. ὡρισμένα. How Aristotle reconciles this with the undoubted continuous graduation between colour and colour will be discussed when we come to chapter 6.

440 b 26. ὕστερον. Chapter 6.

CHAPTER IV.

440 b 28. This is the only place where Aristotle mentions the omissions in the *De Sensu*. Hence Biehl conjectures ἀφῆς instead of φωνῆς (as otherwise the absence of any other treatment of touch will be unnoticed). φωνή is defined in *De An*. II. ch. 8, 420 b 32 as σημαντικός τις ψόφος and again in 420 b 5 as ψόφος τις ἐμψύχου. It is significant sound uttered by a living creature (cf. above chapter 1, 437 a 11 and note).

ψόφος, of which φωνή is thus a species, is defined in *De An*. 420 b 11 as ἀέρος κίνησίς τις: cf. below ch. 6, 446 b 34: δοκεῖ δ' ὁ ψόφος εἶναι φερομένου τινὸς κίνησις. This movement of the air is of the nature of a rebound. The air rebounds when struck in the same way as smooth bodies rebound from a smooth surface (cf. *De An*. 420 a 21 sqq.).

440 b 29. ἐν τοῖς περὶ ψυχῆς. *De An*. II. ch. 8.

440 b 30. πάθος (cf. note to chapter 1, 436 b 5 above) may mean phenomenon or affection generally, though it is not phenomenon in the widest sense in which that term is employed by modern thought, viz. as including concrete substances. πάθος is phenomenon in the sense in which that means an affection, event or attribute ascribed to any concrete subject. Now πάθος is often used for a peculiarly psychical affection and so perhaps the subject to which, as πάθη, smell and taste are relative, is the perceiving soul. Hence it will be as subjective phenomena that they are almost identical. This seems to be borne out by a passage in the *De An*. II. ch. 9, 421 a 31 sqq.: διὰ τὸ μὴ σφόδρα διαδήλους εἶναι τὰς ὀσμὰς ὥσπερ τοὺς χυμούς, ἀπὸ τούτων εἴληφε τὰ ὀνόματα καθ' ὁμοιότητα τῶν πραγμάτων: odours not being distinctly presented like flavours have borrowed their names from the latter owing to the resemblance of the actual experience in the two cases. This is to follow Alexander and render τῶν πραγμάτων by 'the sensation.' Cf. Rodier, *Traité de l'Âme*, Vol. II. pp. 309–311.

For the connection between taste and smell cf. also *De An.* II.
ch. 9, 421 a 16: ἔοικε μὲν γὰρ ἀνάλογον ἔχειν πρὸς τὴν γεῦσιν καὶ
ὁμοίως τὰ εἴδη τῶν χυμῶν τοῖς τῆς ὀσμῆς and 421 a 26 ὥσπερ χυμὸς
ὁ μὲν γλυκὺς ὁ δὲ πικρός, οὕτω καὶ ὀσμαί.

Alexander, Thomas and Simon, however, seem to interpret
πάθος here not as subjective affection but as objective quality. It
is true that this subjective similarity rests upon an objective
foundation. Alexander explains the identity by means of the
passage in ch. 5 beneath, 442 b 29 sqq. Odour is produced by the
further modification of a substance in which flavour has been
already developed; τὸ ξηρόν is needed as a basis for both and the
effect produced in the first case by τὸ ξηρόν is obtained by disso-
lution (ἐναποπλύνειν), the same process as that by which τὸ ἔγχυμον
ὑγρόν produces odour both in air and water: cf. Rodier, *op. cit.*
Vol. II. pp. 309–316, Alex. *De Sens.* pp. 66, 67, 88–91 (W.).
But though the similarity has an objective foundation it does not
cease to be a subjective phenomenon, and it is as such that we
should infer τὸ αὐτὸ πάθος to be understood in antithesis to οὐκ ἐν
τοῖς αὐτοῖς, which must be interpreted as 'non in eisdem subjectis,' as
Simon renders it, following Thomas and Alexander. The vehicle of
taste is water, that of smell is air and water alike, or rather that
common nature which both have, named by Theophrastus τὸ δίοσμον (cf. chapter 5 beneath). St Hilaire and Hammond think that
οὐκ ἐν τοῖς αὐτοῖς refers to the diversity of the organs of the two
senses. But χυμός and ὀσμή could hardly be said to exist ἐν τοῖς
αἰσθητηρίοις, and if Aristotle meant here to refer to the organs his
statement is singularly obscure.

441 a 1. αἴτιον κ.τ.λ. This is the explanation of a difference
in function by a difference in faculty, a method much derided in
modern psychology. But when one remembers that the 'faculty'
is a determinate structure or disposition of the sense organ, and was
so to Aristotle, the explanation, though not a genetic one, is seen to
be adequate to the purpose in hand.

441 a 3. ἀκριβεστάτην. ἀκρίβεια contains at once the notions of
complexity and delicacy, or precision. The emphasis is probably on
the former in the famous passage in *De An.* I. ch. 1, 402 a 2, where
Psychology is said to rank among the first of the sciences in point
of ἀκρίβεια. For the want of definiteness in our sense of smell
cf. *De An.* II. ch. 9, 421 a 9 sqq.: τὴν αἴσθησιν ταύτην οὐκ ἔχομεν
ἀκριβῆ, ἀλλὰ χείρω πολλῶν ζῴων. The reason is—φαύλως ἄνθρωπος

ὀσμᾶται, καὶ οὐθενὸς ὀσφραίνεται τῶν ὀσφραντῶν ἄνευ τοῦ λυπηροῦ ἢ τοῦ ἡδέος. That is to say, where feeling-tone enters largely into the sensation there can be no exactitude in our perception, as modern Psychology teaches is in most cases true   But the final reason for both phenomena is the indefiniteness of the structure of the sense organ (ὡς οὐκ ὄντος ἀκριβοῦς τοῦ αἰσθητηρίου). Compare *De An.* II. ch. 9, 421 a 21 : κατὰ δὲ τὴν ἀφὴν πολλῷ τῶν ἄλλων διαφερόντως ἀκριβοῖ.

The reason for the superiority of touch in man is the greater softness of his flesh. Softness of flesh is an index not only of tactual discriminativeness but of intellectual endowment. Cf. *De An., loc. cit.* 421 a 26 and *De Part. An.* II. ch. 16, 660 a 11 : μαλακω-τάτη δ᾽ ἡ σὰρξ ἡ τῶν ἀνθρώπων ὑπῆρχεν. τοῦτο δὲ διὰ τὸ αἰσθητικώ-τατον εἶναι τῶν ζῴων τὴν διὰ τῆς ἀφῆς αἴσθησιν.

Aristotle's ideal of a εὐφυής would, on this showing, be the skilful surgeon or mechanician.   But we must remember that τὸ θερμὸν καὶ τὸ ψυχρόν were among τὰ ἁπτά, and probably by softness of flesh he means sensitiveness to these influences as much as anything else and hence merely delicacy of constitution in general.   At least so Alex-ander understands him.   Would this be an argument for the mental superiority of the female sex ?   If so, Aristotle is forgetting himself.

441 a 3–4. ἡ δὲ γεῦσις ἁφή τις ἐστίν, and hence is more ἀκριβής than smell.   Cf. *De An.* II. ch. 9, 421 a 18–20, also ch. 10, 422 a 8 : τὸ δὲ γευστόν ἐστιν ἁπτόν τι and *De Sens.* ch. 2, 439 a 1 : τὸ δὲ γευστικὸν εἶδός τι ἀφῆς ἐστίν.   Compare also *De An.* II. ch. 3, 414 b 11 and III. ch. 12, 434 b 18, likewise *De Part. An.* II. ch. 10, 656 b 37 and ch. 17, 660 a 21.

The chief arguments to prove the identity of taste and touch are (1) that by taste we are sensible of the presence of food which is an object of tactual sensation (414 b 7 sqq., 434 b 18–19), (2) that τὸ ὑγρόν is the ὕλη, the vehicle of taste, and it is ἁπτόν τι (422 a 11). But (3) Aristotle finds strong confirmation for his theory in the fact that neither requires an external medium for its operation as the others do (422 a 8 sqq.).   The flavoured substance impinges directly upon the sense organ—the tongue.   Again (4) the division into right and left parts, which is not to be detected in the case of the organ of touch, is almost unnoticeable in the tongue (656 b 33 sqq.) and (5) the softness of the human tongue causes its greater sensi-tiveness, just as softness of the flesh generally causes delicacy of touch (660 a, 17–21, cf. *De An.* II. ch. 9, 421 a 20 sqq. and last note). For this doctrine compare also the passage beneath, 441 b 26 sqq.

441 a 6–7. Cf. Zeller, *Presocratic Phil.* (Eng. Trans.), II. p. 166, Burnet, *Early Greek Phil.* p. 231, Empedocles v. 312 (Stein). But cf. Theophrastus *De Sens.* 7 (*Dox.* 500, *R.P.* 177 b), who says that Empedocles did not push his investigation of taste or touch further than to say that in them too sensation was caused by particles fitting into the pores of the sense organ.

441 a 7–8. The meaning of πανσπερμία is best illustrated by a passage in the *De Gen. Animal.* IV. ch. 3, 769 a 26 sqq., where he explains a theory that the various qualities of animals all lie commingled in the semen which forms as it were a πανσπερμία of all characteristics, by comparing the γονή to a liquid in which many different flavours are dissolved. πανσπερμία then evidently means a substance in which the germs of all things lie.

Trendelenburg (*De An.* p. 214) thinks that the word is a Democritean term. It certainly is employed by Aristotle three times (*Physics*, III. ch. 4, 203 a 21, *De Coelo*, III. ch. 4, 303 a 16 and *De An.* I. ch. 2, 404 a 4) to describe the mixture of atoms out of which, Democritus asserted, the world was fashioned. It is however once employed with reference to the theory of Anaxagoras (cf. *De Gen. et Corr.* I. ch. 1, 314 a 18 sqq.), according to which bone and flesh were the simple elements out of which air, fire, earth and water were constructed: οἱ δὲ (sc. οἱ περὶ Ἀναξαγόραν) ταῦτα μὲν ἁπλᾶ καὶ στοιχεῖα (λέγουσι), γῆν δὲ καὶ πῦρ καὶ ὕδωρ καὶ ἀέρα σύνθετα· πανσπερμίαν γὰρ εἶναι τούτων: *i.e.* 'for they—flesh and bone—constitute that in which the latter all lie in germ.' Cf. Zeller, *Presocratic Phil.* II. p. 332, Burnet, *Early Greek Phil.* p. 290 and note. It is quite likely that the term originated with Anaxagoras, whose interests lay more in biological phenomena than those of his predecessors, but there seems to be no doubt that Democritus, however inconsistent it may have been with the general drift of his mechanical philosophy, also employed it.

This special theory—that water is οἷον πανσπερμία χυμῶν—must be assigned to Democritus, at least in the first form in which it is stated (see next note). As Alexander (p. 68) points out, we must assume a spatial difference to be responsible for the difference of flavour in different parts, and this, says Alexander, stamps the theory as Democritean.

The first theory differs from the second in that it supposes that

11—2

flavours exist in water ἐνεργείᾳ—in actual fact though imperceptible to sense, while the second gives them only potential existence; according to it they exist in water only in germ. This second theory is then contrasted with a third, according to which water is qualitatively identical in every part, and any flavour can be derived from any portion of it, the differences which we actually find being caused τῷ μᾶλλον ἢ ἧττον θερμαίνειν—by the different amounts of heat to which different portions of water are exposed. Simon acutely conjectures that this third theory must be assigned to Anaxagoras owing to its compliance with his doctrine of πάντα ἐν πᾶσιν. It still comprises the doctrine that water is οἷον πανσπερμία in which tastes lie in germ, but assigns their actual differentiation out to an active external cause. (Note that Aristotle says τὸ ποιοῦν not ποιοῦν τι. All theories may have recognised the agency of heat in producing taste but not in producing differences in flavour.)

441 a 14. This passage causes difficulty, for at first sight it seems strange that, if Aristotle meant that the fruits were plucked, he should not have said καρπῶν instead of περικαρπίων. Hence Thurot and Susemihl (*Philol.* 1885) propose to read καρπῶν. But though the word properly means σκέπασμα καρποῦ, yet there are passages in which it can only mean the fruit as a whole, *e.g. Meteor.* IV. ch. 3, 380 a 11 and *Problems*, 25, 925 b 30, and cf. below 441 b 1. Alexander suggests that it is possible to use περικάρπιον in its literal sense and, in that case, the point will be that fruits change in taste independently of the removal or permanence of the husk or peel.

But this is hardly the meaning required. The other interpretation is possible, and the point is that, as the connection with the root has been severed, the water drawn up by the plant through its roots (τὸ ἐκτὸς ὕδωρ) does not give the change in taste.

πυρουμένων is the MS. reading, but it should mean, on the whole, 'ignited': cf. *De Part. Animal.* II. ch. 2, 649 b 5, where πυροῦν is distinguished from θερμαίνειν and identified with φλόγα ποιεῖν. Where it does not mean actually to ignite, it at least denotes such intense heating as occurs in roasting or baking (cf. *De Gen. Animal.* III. ch. 2, 753 b 4, and *Problems*, 927 b 39 sqq.). Now, here, in the case of the sun's action, no such intense degree of heating is involved. Hence I propose to read πυρρουμένων which means 'reddened,' and suggest that Aristotle is thinking of the reddening effect the sun produces on many fruits as it ripens them. He is here then referring to the ripening effect of the sun which actually makes fruits become sweet. (Mere cooking without adding a sweetening ingredient does not.) In the next clause he contrasts it with the effect produced by drying and withering which makes them bitter (cf. *Problems* 925 b 36: ἐλαῖαι καὶ βάλανοι παλαιούμεναι πικραὶ γίνονται). It is in the final clause—l. 18, καὶ ἑψομένους κ.τ.λ.—that he talks of the effect of cooking.

441 a 20. The sense is the same whether we read πανσπερμίας (which is grammatically preferable) or πανσπερμίαν. The water is a material in which the germs of the flavours lie commingled.

441 a 21-22. ὡς τροφῆς. Alexander, who reads ὡς ἐκ τῆς αὐτῆς τροφῆς, explains that many tastes arise out of the same water, as many different parts of the body —bones, flesh etc., are formed out of the same nourishment, and again different trees are nourished by the same water; and thus similarly each part of the same tree, root, bark and fruit, has a characteristic flavour though feeding on the same moisture. He is followed by Thomas who nevertheless used the early Latin translation which gives the equivalent of our reading. Both readings no doubt render such an interpretation possible, but ours rather suggests the translation I have given. In that case the sense is simpler. There is no parallel between water and food in general. Aristotle simply says that different tastes are developed by plants that live upon the same water; he may mean either the different tastes found in bark and fruit or the different flavours of different fruits. The latter is more probable since he has just been talking of fruits. He means that the same water can be supplied to different trees, yet you get different flavours, which ought not to be the case if one definite flavour resides in one definite portion of water as the second—the Democritean—theory would make out. The πανσπερμία theory in its first form is thus refuted and Aristotle passes on to the opinion of Anaxagoras.

441 a 24. δύναμις, in this line and again in the next, is practically equivalent to φύσις; cf. above ch. 3, 439 a 25: κοινὴ φύσις καὶ δύναμις. Cf. also *De Mem.* ch. 2, 452 a 31 and note.

441 a 25. λεπτότατον. The argument is directed merely against the proposition that water acted on by heat, without any other determinant, will develop flavour. Water alone when heated does not thicken, but all flavours reside in substances that show traces of thickening to a greater or less degree. Hence water plus heat is not alone the cause of flavours. That which causes the thickening in fluids must be the cause. This is earth (γῆ) or rather one of the qualities of γῆ—τὸ ξηρόν. Cf. *De Gen. et Corr.* II. ch. 2, 330 a 4: τὸ δὲ παχὺ τοῦ ξηροῦ.

The whole of the above discussion is a good example of the 'dialectical' development of an Aristotelian argument. Previous theories are dealt with in an order relative to the amount they contribute to the final solution of the problem. Though each is in turn set aside, some part of it remains unabrogated in the next, and the last to be discussed is that which approaches most nearly to the true account of the matter.

441 a 32. πάχος ἔχουσι. It is not sufficient for the argument to say that flavours thicken when heated, but that at all times they show traces of density.

441 a 33. συναίτιον. Cf. *De An.* II. ch. 4, 416 a 14 where πῦρ is likewise said to be the συναίτιον of the growth of bodies. *The* αἴτιον is ψυχή. (συναίτιον μέν πώς ἐστιν, οὐ μὴν ἁπλῶς γε αἴτιον.)

Some translators render φαίνονται 'apparently,' but with the participle it should mean 'evidently.' The sense also requires it, for this to Aristotle's mind is not merely an apparent fact, but a real fact which furnishes the proof positive that χυμός is dependent on τὸ ξηρόν. The previous proofs have been merely negative and directed against the claims of other circumstances to fill the position of cause.

This reasoning will support the reading διὸ εὐλόγως in 441 b 8 below.

441 b 5. γῆς τι εἶδος. Cf. *Meteor.* IV. ch. 7, 383 b 20 sqq. The πολλοί in 441 b 2 above are Metrodorus and Anaxagoras, according to Alexander.

441 b 8. διὸ εὐλόγως is the reading of MSS. L S U and evidently of the ancient Latin translation. Alexander also interprets as though this were the reading : διὰ τοῦτο οὖν φησὶν εὐλόγως καὶ τοὺς χυμοὺς ἐν τοῖς ἐκ τῆς γῆς φυομένοις, τουτέστιν ἐν τοῖς φυτοῖς, καὶ ταύτῃ τρεφομένοις μετὰ ὑγρότητος ἐγγίνεσθαι μάλιστα : the vet. tr. renders 'terra nascentibus' as though it actually read ἐκ τῆς γῆς. Whatever the reading, Alexander's must be the correct interpretation (cf. note to 441 a 33). It is on account of the savours being primarily in earth that they can enter into plants. Aristotle does not say εὐλόγως without being able to produce reasons.

441 b 10. ὥσπερ καὶ τἆλλα. Aristotle is no doubt thinking in particular of the other elementary qualities—τὸ ξηρόν etc., but this statement is with him a universal principle.

441 b 14. ἐν τοῖς περὶ στοιχείων. Cf. *De Gen. et Corr.* II. ch. 1 sqq. The fuller discussion (ἐν ἑτέροις ἀκριβέστερον, 329 a 27) referred to there seems to be lost, as all other references to the subject are more brief.

Up to this point the argument is clear. Aristotle is explaining what he has already proved as a fact. Earth in possessing the quality of dryness can act on τὸ ὑγρόν, since opposites modify each other. It is a case of explaining the qualities presented to the other senses by the interaction of the tactual properties of things. Cf. *De An.* II. ch. 5, 417 a 6, where he talks of the other αἰσθητά as the συμβεβηκότα of fire, earth, air and water. (Though he insists that in one way the former are prior to the latter, cf. *De Gen. et Corr.* II. ch. 2, 329 b 14: καίτοι πρότερον ὄψις ἁφῆς.)

The difficulty which now ensues is in connection with the function of τὸ θερμόν in helping to produce flavour.

441 b 15. οὐδὲν πέφυκε κ.τ.λ. This statement seems to conflict with that in *De Gen. et Corr.* II. ch. 2, 329 b 22: δεῖ δὲ ποιητικὰ ἀλλήλων καὶ παθητικὰ τὰ στοιχεῖα, μίγνυται γὰρ καὶ μεταβάλλει εἰς ἄλληλα. But probably there Aristotle is simply stating his doctrine in a rough provisional way. Really as σώματα and hence οὐσίαι the elements cannot be opposed to each other and act on each other. (So Alexander explains.) Cf. *Categ.* 3 b 24: ὑπάρχει δὲ ταῖς οὐσίαις καὶ τὸ μηδὲν αὐταῖς ἐναντίον εἶναι, and it is ἐναντία that act on each other; οὐσία is merely δεκτικὴ τῶν ἐναντίων. The upshot of the matter is, that it is not as substances, but as possessed of opposite qualities, that the elements act on each other. This sentence is then inserted as a caution, but how it furthers the main argument here is not apparent, unless indeed we connect it with that preceding clause in which we find it stated that heat is the peculiar property of fire, dryness of earth. Liquidity (τὸ ὑγρόν) will thus be the special characteristic of water, and the implication will be that the latter element will be acted on in a more pronounced way by earth, the element which has in an especial degree the attribute most opposed to its most characteristic quality. Fire possessing τὸ ξηρόν in a less marked degree will act upon it also, but not in the pre-eminent way in which γῆ does.

When Aristotle says that τὸ θερμόν is the ἴδιον of πῦρ, this cannot be in the full sense of ἴδιον consistent with the rest of his doctrine, for τὸ θερμόν is also shared by ἀήρ and, as we have seen, πῦρ is also ξηρόν. He must mean, as Alexander explains in conformity with *De Gen. et Corr.* IV. ch. 4, 382 a 3: τῶν στοιχείων ἰδιαίτατα ξηροῦ μὲν γῆ, ὑγροῦ δὲ ὕδωρ, that earth is the principal illustration of dryness or possesses dryness in a special degree, as fire does heat, and so on. Cf. Alex. *De Sens.* pp. 72–73 (W.).   Cf. also *De Gen. et Corr.* IV. ch. 5, 382 b 3: ὑγροῦ σῶμα ὕδωρ.

441 b 17–18. ἐναποπλύνοντες. A cognate word πλύσις is used in 445 a 16 for the corresponding process which produces odour.

Susemihl (*Philol.* 1885 and *Burs. Jahresb.* 17) wishes to delete τοὺς χυμούς, but in mentioning flavours here Aristotle is not illustrating a thing by itself.   He compares the solution of the primitive ξηρόν which produces flavours to the solution of flavours actually produced.

441 b 19. ἡ φύσις. No personification of Nature is implied here. Aristotle merely means that this is a natural process.   The function of πῦρ in the process is obscure.   Alexander makes it the cause of the percolation as well as of the κίνησις which renders τὸ ὑγρόν determinate in quality; κινοῦσα he renders by ἀλλοιοῦσα, *i.e.* changing qualitatively.   But it is possible to understand it literally— of the motion involved in the percolation.   Some, *e.g.* Hammond and St Hilaire, translating κινοῦσα in different ways, will have it to be concerned only with the former process.   But, unless we adopt the conjecture that the function of τὸ θερμόν is to act on τὸ γεῶδες, we may as well understand it to bring about local motion in this case as beneath in 442 a 6, where it is said to cause the light particles in food to rise upwards.

441 b 23. Here πάθος is used in a wide sense, but still with the signification of being the attribute of a subject that is passively affected when it (the attribute) comes into being.

441 b 24. ἀλλοιωτικόν. Cf. *De An.* II. ch. 5, 416 b 34: δοκεῖ γὰρ (ἡ αἴσθησις) ἀλλοίωσίς τις εἶναι· ἀλλοίωσις is that kind of κίνησις denoting qualitative change.   ἀλλοιοῦσθαι is practically identical with πάσχειν (cf. *Phys.* VII. ch. 3, 245 b 13: τὸ πεπονθὸς καὶ ἠλλοιωμένον προσαγορεύομεν: cf. Alex. *De An.* 84, 12), and both words are employed indifferently in the *De Anima* for psychical modifications (cf. II. ch. 5, 418 a 2 and 417 b 14).   But Aristotle points out that, though they both are used as though they were the proper terms (ὡς κυρίοις) for all psychical changes, there are some operations to which they are really not applicable.

1.   In the first place, the transition from the state in which man possesses knowledge to the exercise of that knowledge is hardly a case of πάσχειν or ἀλλοίωσις in the usual sense.   The change is not

produced by anything external. To exercise his intelligence is in a man's own power—ἐπ' αὐτῷ—for the universals which are the objects of knowledge are in a way in the soul. Again it is a case not of φθορὰ ὑπὸ τοῦ ἐναντίου but of σωτηρία, i.e. the realisation of a predetermined end.

2. Secondly, change such even as that from a state of ignorance to a state of knowledge, where the alteration is in a definite direction and towards the establishment of a definite higher development, towards the realisation of the potentialities of the individual in question (ἐπὶ τὰς ἕξεις καὶ τὴν φύσιν 417 b 16), is hardly ἀλλοίωσις proper, even though in the acquisition of knowledge one requires an external agent—the teacher.

With these reservations Aristotle proposes still to use the terms ἀλλοίωσις and πάσχειν. They are no doubt, in one way, specially applicable to sensuous processes, because there must be an external agent—the individual object (cf. 417 b 25: ἀναγκαῖον γὰρ ὑπάρχειν τὸ αἰσθητόν, and cf. 417 a 6 sqq.). But Simon points out that even sense perception cannot be properly a case of πάσχειν, for agent and patient must be in the same genus (*De Gen. et Corr.* I. ch. 7, 323 b 32 sqq.), which the sense faculty and its object are not. Cf. Introduction, sec. IV.

441 b 25. It would be possible to make προϋπάρχον agree with the subject of ἄγει, namely τὸ...πάθος, and this interpretation would give a meaning consistent with Aristotle's general doctrine, for previous to the act of perception the object is only δυνάμει αἰσθητόν. The next clause, however, requires us to construe it with τὸ αἰσθητικόν (as Hammond, Bender, St Hilaire do), or still better with τοῦτο (Simon), for it is not the sense *faculty* which existed δυνάμει before the act of sensation, but its operation. The δύναμις, the faculty, *actually* exists before the sensational experience.

For the doctrine of this passage see *De An.* II. ch. 5, 417 b 19: καὶ τὸ κατ' ἐνέργειαν (αἰσθάνεσθαι) δὲ ὁμοίως λέγεται τῷ θεωρεῖν. In knowledge (cf. last note) there is a two-fold transition, (1) from a state of ignorance to the acquisition of a definite body of knowledge, i.e. from mere indeterminate δύναμις to a determinate one or ἕξις; (2) there is also the change from the possession to the exercise of this ἕξις (εἰς ἐντελέχειαν, b 7). There is a corresponding double transition in sensuous process. The first is effected by the parent (ὑπὸ τοῦ γεννῶντος, b 17) of the sensitive individual and is the creation of a being with fully developed sense faculties. The second, corresponding to the exercise of knowledge, is the actual exercise of the sense faculty and is produced by the object of sense. In sense, then, the formation of a permanent psychical disposition is due to natural agency, in knowledge to instruction ; actual exercise of a faculty is in both a higher process, originated in the first case externally, in the second internally.

441 b 26–27. οὐ παντὸς ξηροῦ. Alexander thinks that this statement is made in order to rule out odour, which also owes its existence to τὸ ξηρόν. But, as ὀσμή is produced by τὸ ἔγχυμον ξηρόν, it is clear that those words are not used for the purpose of excluding it. By τὸ ξηρόν Aristotle surely means dry substance, and it is the same substance as has flavour that is odorous. The intention is obviously to rule out all ξηρόν that is not μεμιγμένον, *i.e.* does not enter into a compound.

441 b 27–28. ἢ πάθος...ἢ στέρησις. The positive modification is τὸ γλυκύ, the negative τὸ πικρόν : cf. 442 a 7 sqq.

441 b 30. I read οὐχ ἓν μόνον instead of οὐδὲν αὐτῶν with Bekker and Biehl. Wendland restores οὐχ ἓν μόνον to the text of Alexander, p. 77, and the vet. tr. renders 'non est unum solum,' which, in spite of what Biehl says, can be a translation only of οὐχ ἓν μόνον. This version apparently read also οὐδὲ αὐτοῖς τοῖς φυτοῖς after ζῴοις for it inserts 'neque ipsis plantis.' οὐχ ἓν μόνον gives the best sense, but μόνον might be dispensed with.

441 b 31. τὰ μὲν ἁπτὰ κ.τ.λ. Alexander points out that αὐξάνειν and τρέφειν are not identical. Things so far as quantitative cause increase ; only in so far as potentially capable of forming the substance of the body which they nourish are they said to be nutritive. Cf. *De Gen. et Corr.* I. ch. 5, 322 a 20 sqq. and also *De An.* II. ch. 4, 416 b 12 sqq.: ἔστι δ' ἕτερον τροφῇ καὶ αὐξητικῷ εἶναι· ᾗ μὲν γὰρ ποσόν τι τὸ ἔμψυχον αὐξητικόν (sc. τὸ προσιὸν or τὸ προσφερόμενον : cf. Rodier, *op. cit.* II. p. 242), ᾗ δὲ τόδε τι καὶ οὐσία τροφή. That is to say, τροφή (the abstract term) or τρέφειν is the continuous renewal of the individual which preserves its identity as an individual of definite type, *i.e.* as an οὐσία ; αὔξησις is that renewal in its quantitative aspect.

The point here, however, seems to be not to hold αὔξησις and τροφή apart, but to show that that which has the function of causing growth must also have the properties of nutritive food, and reciprocally τὸ τρόφιμον is known to sense as τὸ γευστόν (442 a 2) and the fundamental positive characteristic of things that have flavour is sweetness.

But food, as that which causes growth, is that which can rise up (owing to the agency of heat—for fire is the lightest element) and so become incorporated in the body. Hence it is both warm and light (each of which is a tactual quality); but that which is light is sweet, and hence that which causes growth is just that which has the gustatory quality of nutriment.

The whole argument rests upon the identification of τὸ κοῦφον (one of the ἁπτά) and τὸ γλυκύ, the basal quality of τὸ γευστόν, and hence of τὸ τρόφιμον.

442 a 1. τρέφει κ.τ.λ. This is treated simply as a statement to be verified by observation. It is not a proposition established by any special proof elsewhere. It gives the first obvious definition of τὸ τρόφιμον.

For the facts cf. *Problems*, 930 a 34 and *Meteor.* II. ch. 2, 355 b 7, also cf. note to l. 5 below.

442 a 3. ἢ ἁπλῶς κ.τ.λ. We must not translate '*whether* pure or mixed,' as thus we should assume that it was indifferent whether the sweetness was pure or mixed. As a matter of fact Aristotle, below in l. 12, says that pure sweetness makes the food indigestible.

442 a 4. ἐν τοῖς περὶ γενέσεως. *De Gen. et Corr.* I. ch. 5, pp. 350–352. Alexander also refers to the *De Gen. Animal.*, but it is difficult to find any strictly relevant passage there.

442 a 5. αὐξάνει must be used absolutely, much as it looks as though it should govern τροφήν along with δημιουργεῖ. Aristotle is discussing not the production of food but the growth of the body owing to feeding. For the process cf. *De Part. Animal.* II. ch. 3, 650 a 2 sqq.: ἐπεὶ δ' ἀνάγκη πᾶν τὸ αὐξανόμενον λαμβάνειν τροφήν, ἡ δὲ τροφὴ πᾶσιν ἐξ ὑγροῦ καὶ ξηροῦ, καὶ τούτων ἡ πέψις γίνεται καὶ ἡ μεταβολὴ διὰ τῆς τοῦ θερμοῦ δυνάμεως…διὰ ταύτην (τὴν αἰτίαν) ἀναγκαῖον ἔχειν ἀρχὴν θερμοῦ φυσικήν.

The ultimate ἀρχή of heat in the body of sanguineous animals is seated in the heart. Cf. *De Juvent.* ch. 4, 469 b 9: ἀναγκαῖον δὴ ταύτης τὴν ἀρχὴν τῆς θερμότητος ἐν τῇ καρδίᾳ τοῖς ἐναίμοις εἶναι.

For Neuhäuser's theory, that this σύμφυτον θερμόν, which seems to be the ultimate substratum both of the sensitive and nutritive soul, is also to be identified as the central organ of sensation, cf. Introduction, sec. VI.

For the connection of lightness and sweetness, bitterness and weight, cf. *Meteor.* II. ch. 2, 355 b 4 sqq.: τὸ μὲν ἁλμυρὸν ὑπομένει διὰ

τὸ βάρος, τὸ δὲ γλυκὺ καὶ πότιμον ἀνάγεται διὰ τὴν κουφότητα, καθάπερ
ἐν τοῖς ζῴων σώμασιν...τὸ γὰρ γλυκὺ καὶ πότιμον ὑπὸ τῆς ἐμφύτου
θερμότητος ἑλκυσθὲν εἰς τὰς σάρκας καὶ τὴν ἄλλην σύνταξιν ἦλθε τῶν
μερῶν κ.τ.λ.

The bodily heat is, however, only the συναίτιον in the production
of τὸ αὐξάνεσθαι καὶ τρέφεσθαι. The natural process due to heat is
indefinite and has no direction. Fire burns on until its material is
exhausted. But in living organisms there is a πέρας καὶ λόγος μεγέθους τε καὶ αὐξήσεως, *i.e.* there is a definite scheme and restriction in
the development and this is due to ψυχή which is the real αἴτιον.
Cf. *De An.* II. ch. 4, 416 a 8–18.

In *De Resp.* ch. 20, 480 a 8 we hear that the blood ἐν τῇ καρδίᾳ
δημιουργεῖται. Aristotle probably there refers to the very same
process. We read in *De Part. Animal.* II. ch. 4, 651 a 14 : τὸ
δ' αἷμα ἡ ἐσχάτη τροφή.

442 a 8. τὸ ἐν τῇ φύσει. Cf. *De Juvent.* ch. 4, 469 b 6 sqq. : πάντα
δὲ τὰ μόρια καὶ πᾶν τὸ σῶμα ἔχει τινὰ σύμφυτον θερμότητα φυσικήν :
cf. also above and the passage there quoted from *Meteor.* II.
Aristotle is there talking to begin with of the evaporation from
the sea, one of τὰ ἔξω σώματα. He expressly compares evaporation
by the sun to the process of animal nutrition. The sea remains salt
though the moisture which is evaporated from it and descends again
in rain is not salt.

442 a 9. Cf. quotation in note to 442 a 5 above. He has now
explained what was previously proved as a fact—that χυμὸς τοῦ τροφίμου ἐστίν, and he has done so by identifying flavour *par excellence*
with sweetness. Positive flavour is sweetness, just as positive
colour is white. Their opposites are στερήσεις--defects of being.

442 a 11. ταῦτα must refer to the latter—τὸ ἁλμυρὸν καὶ ὀξύ,
or else it means simply 'this fact.'

442 a 13. There is no one English word which will translate ἐπιπολαστικόν. It is almost the technical expression for ' indigestible,'
but it implied a theory of indigestibility—that the food tended to
rise too much. Cf. one of Aristotle's illustrations of final causality.
The final cause of taking a walk after eating is τὸ μὴ ἐπιπολάζειν τὰ
σιτία—*An. Post.* II. ch. 11, 94 b 11 sqq.

Biehl's reading ἀντὶ πάντων in l. 12 instead of ἀντισπᾶν τῷ
is doubtless correct. It does not, however, alter the general
meaning.

442 a 17. κινήσεως. It is not clear what exactly κίνησις refers to—the sense stimulus *caused by* χυμός or the κίνησις which *produces* χυμός.

442 a 18. L S U and all editions prior to Biehl's have οὗτοι ἐν ἀριθμοῖς μόνον· ὁ μὲν οὖν λιπαρὸς τοῦ γλυκέος κ.τ.λ. But there is no reason for making Aristotle say that the pleasant flavours alone were due to proportionate combination. On the analogy of the corresponding theory about colours they would rather be the class where the ratio of the ingredients was a simple one. Cf. ch. 3, 439 b 33 sqq. above.

442 a 22. All MSS. give ἑπτά but Susemihl (*Philol.* 1885) argues that it is quite impossible to reconcile this with the rest of the passage. Yellow is assigned to white, as oily is to sweet; hence, if the two lists are to square, the number must be either six or eight, as Alexander too maintains. (It is by distinguishing φαιόν from μέλαν and ἁλμυρόν from πικρόν that eight members are distinguished.) Hence, followed by Biehl, he boldly substitutes ἕξ for ἑπτά. The difficulty, however, disappears, when we recognise that τὸ ξανθὸν is included in the list, though, as an afterthought, assigned to white.

In other passages the different position of grey from that of the true chromatic tones is not noticed. They are both said to be ἀνὰ μέσον τοῦ λευκοῦ καὶ μέλανος : cf. *Categ.* ch. 10, 12 a 18, *Top.* I. ch. 15, 106 b 5, *Metaph.* x. ch. 5, 1056 a 27 sqq. The reason doubtless for ascribing grey to black rather than white when it is relative to both (cf. *Physics*, v. ch. 1, 224 b 31 sqq., and ch. 5, 229 b 17 sqq.) is that it is less positive than white, in a way a στέρησις of white, as black also is.

442 a 24. λείπεται κ.τ.λ. The ascription of yellow to white seems to be a recognition of its higher luminosity than that of the other colours. Cf. Plato, *Timaeus* 68 B, who brings in τὸ λαμπρόν into its composition. For the correspondence of the tastes and the colours generally and the ascription to sweet and bitter of τὸ λιπαρόν and τὸ ἁλμυρόν respectively, cf. *De An.* II. ch. 10, 422 b 10 sqq. The ground for the identification of τὸ λιπαρόν and τὸ γλυκύ seems to be the lightness of both. Cf. *De Part. Animal.* III. ch. 9, 672 a 8 sqq. τὸ λιπαρὸν κοῦφόν ἐστι καὶ ἐπιπολάζει ἐν τοῖς ὑγροῖς. τὸ λιπαρόν is light because it is warm. Cf. also *De Gen. Animal.* II. ch. 2, 735 b 25. Similarly τὸ ἁλμυρόν and τὸ πικρόν are both heavy.

442 a 25. φοινικοῦν κ.τ.λ. Three of these are the colours of the rainbow (with ξανθόν intermediate between φοινικοῦν and πράσινον : cf. *Meteor.* III. ch. 2, 372 a 8 sqq.). They alone are said not to be obtained by mixing (other chromatic tones presumably); κυανοῦν is less frequently mentioned.

442 a 27. τούτων should naturally refer to τοῦ λευκοῦ καὶ μέλανος, but it is generally held to signify the other colours. Both statements would be in conformity with Aristotle's teaching.

442 a 31. τὸ πότιμον. Cf. *De An.* II. ch. 10, 422 a 31 : τὸ ποτὸν καὶ ἄποτον are equivalents for γλυκύ and πικρόν. For the doctrine cf. Theophrastus, *De Causis Plantarum*, VI. 1, 2.

442 b 1. ἁπτά. Cf. Theophrastus, *De Sensu*, 60–82, R.P. 199. Zeller, *Presocratic Phil.* II. pp. 265–270. This is part of the doctrine of ἀπόρροιαι; the atoms which emanate from bodies actually impinge upon our sense organs and so cause sensation by contact. It is against this that Aristotle wishes to argue in the first place.

The transition to this discussion is not mediated by the distinction between αὐξάνειν and τρέφειν as Alexander thinks, but by the connection between taste and touch which suggests the Democritean theory that all sensation is effected by contact.

442 b 4. ἀδύνατον. Alexander (p. 83 [W.]) gives four separate reasons which might be employed. But the most important consideration is the fact that the other senses require an external medium. It is the absence of this that makes taste a kind of touch. The other senses do not act by contact (cf. *De An.* II. ch. 7, 419 a 26 : οὐθὲν γὰρ αὐτῶν (sc. ψόφον, ὀσμῆς κ.τ.λ.) ἁπτόμενον τοῦ αἰσθητηρίου ποιεῖ τὴν αἴσθησιν).

τοῖς κοινοῖς. For the distinction between the κοινά and the ἴδια αἰσθητά cf. *De An.* II. ch. 6, 418 a 17, III. ch. 1, 425 a 14, III. ch. 3, 428 b 22 and above 437 a 8, etc. The former comprise motion and rest, figure, magnitude, number and unity. The latter are the qualities, *e.g.* colour etc., reported by the special sense organs. The κοινὰ αἰσθητά are known however in modern philosophy as the primary qualities of bodies (cf. Hamilton's *Reid*, note D). They must be distinguished from what the commentators call the 'primae qualitates' in the Aristotelian scheme viz. θερμόν, ψυχρόν, ξηρόν, ὑγρόν. It has been pointed out (*e.g.* by Hamilton, p. 829) that these κοινά are hardly sense qualities at all and confirmation for this contention is drawn from Aristotle himself (cf. *De An.* II. ch. 6, 418 a 24 : τὰ ἴδια κυρίως ἐστὶν αἰσθητά; and below b 14–15 : ἢ οὐδεμίας...τὰ κοινὰ γνωρίζειν). They may be all described as the mathematical and dynamical qualities of body and, according to the Atomistic philosophers, these were the only objective attributes of things, all the rest being merely changes in our sensibility. (Cf. Theophrastus, *De Sens.* 63: τῶν δ' ἄλλων αἰσθητῶν οὐδενὸς εἶναι φύσιν, ἀλλὰ πάντα πάθη τῆς αἰσθήσεως ἀλλοιουμένης.)

This holds good without qualification of four of the senses, but to some tactual qualifications they did assign objective existence, *e.g.* τὸ μαλακόν, τὸ σκληρόν, τὸ βαρύ and τὸ κοῦφον, deriving these however ultimately from μέγεθος and σχῆμα; things that are light have more of void space in them than others. τὸ τραχύ and τὸ λεῖον with τὸ ὀξύ and τὸ ἀμβλύ seem to have been modifications of σχῆμα. Here Aristotle also treats the latter four attributes as belonging to the category of τὰ κοινά. He takes care to define τὸ ὀξύ and τὸ ἀμβλύ as τὸ ἐν τοῖς ὄγκοις (the word commonly employed also for the atoms themselves as well as for mass in general) as these are also the names for determinations of such ἴδια as ψοφός and χυμός. He commonly puts τραχύτης and λειότης along with other σωματικαὶ διαφοραί or σωματικὰ πάθη as μαλακόν and σκληρόν which are *consequent* upon the primary determinations— θερμόν, ψυχρόν etc. Cf. *De Part. Animal.* II. ch. 1, 646 a 17 sqq.: αἱ δ' ἄλλαι διαφοραὶ ταύταις ἀκολουθοῦσιν, οἷον βάρος...καὶ λειότης κ.τ.λ.

Among such, even μέγεθος is included in 644 b 14; but this is simply one of his rough general classifications. Aristotle did not, of course, mean to imply that σχῆμα and μέγεθος are in themselves tactual differentiae of the same nature as hard and soft, but it was his view that you do not have the concept of body without some characteristically tactual datum. It is impossible to construct bodies out of merely mathematical determinations, a point which modern Atomists do not sufficiently consider. You cannot analyse body into something that has no sensuous qualities, not even tactual ones.

If μέγεθος and σχῆμα are to be regarded as the ultimate characteristics of bodies, they must be treated as though they already possessed a tactual content, as though they were merely tactual differentiae, and this is exactly Aristotle's point here. The Atomists treat determinations of figure as though they in themselves contained a reference to tactual experience—as though they were given by one special sense, that of touch, whereas as a fact they, though given in connection with tactual experience, are not simply to be identified with it, and in fact can be discerned by means of other senses, notably that of sight.

In the *De Anima*, III. ch. 1, 425 b 4 sqq., Aristotle points out that it is owing to the fact that these mathematical and dynamical qualities of objects are given by more than one sense that they can be readily discriminated. Otherwise they would be confused with the special data of the single sense to which they were attached, just as he contends that, if the whole surface of the body gave the same sensations as the tongue (which discriminates both flavour and tactual properties) taste and touch would seem to be the same sense. For a discussion of ἀφή cf. *De An.* II. ch. 11. Aristotle does not there fully debate the question of the plurality of the ἐναντιώσεις, *e.g.* θερμόν and ψυχρόν, ξηρόν and ὑγρόν, μαλακόν and σκληρόν, which touch presents to us, nor does he consider to what extent determinations like ὀξύ and βαρύ, τραχύ and λεῖον, which appear in φωνή apparently as ἴδια, must be treated as κοινά in the case of touch. His definition of τραχύ and λεῖον in *Categ.* 8, 10 a 22 sqq. confirms his inclusion of them here in the list of the κοινά—λεῖον μὲν τῷ ἐπ᾽ εὐθείας πως τὰ μόρια κεῖσθαι· τραχὺ δὲ τῷ τὸ μὲν ὑπερέχειν τὸ δὲ ἐλλείπειν; *i.e.* these qualities are due to variations in figure.

442 b 8. εἰ δὲ μὴ πασῶν. Cf. *De An.* II. ch. 6, 418 a 10 κοινὸν πασῶν, where however he illustrates only in the case of ἀφή and ὄψις. Number and unity seem to be given by the exercise of any sense (cf. 425 a 20 : ἑκάστη γὰρ ἓν αἰσθάνεται αἴσθησις). On the other hand all are said to be perceived by means of κίνησις (425 a 17) and, in the case of the mathematical qualities such as are mentioned here, the κίνησις which discriminates them can be nothing else than the motion of the only two sense organs which have a surface continuously graded in sensitiveness, the eye and the surfaces of the bodily members. Aristotle does not work this out, but hence, probably, the reason why the discrimination of size and figure is limited to sight and touch.

442 b 9. Cf. *De An.* II. ch. 6, 418 a 15 ; III. ch. 3, 428 b 18, 25, where he qualifies the statement that ἰδία αἴσθησις is true, by the expression ἢ ὅτι ὀλίγιστον ἔχουσα τὸ ψεῦδος. Apparently he did not know of colour blindness.

442 b 11. οἱ δὲ cannot mean another set of people as Simon and St Hilaire think. It is part of the *same* doctrine as the preceding one to reduce the ἴδια to the κοινά. The error is (1) to assume that all sensation takes place by means of contact; (2) not to discriminate universal qualities of objects from the purely tactual, *i.e.* to treat them all as the data of a single sense ; (3) to reduce all the sense qualities to these quasi-tactual determinations.

442 b 13. σχήματα. Cf. Theophrastus, *de Sensu*, 65: τὸν μὲν ὀξὺν εἶναι τῷ σχήματι γωνιοειδῆ τε καὶ πολυκαμπῆ καὶ μικρὸν καὶ λεπτόν,...τραχὺν δ᾽ ὄντα καὶ γωνιοειδῆ...τὸν δὲ γλυκὺν ἐκ περιφερῶν συγκεῖσθαι σχημάτων, οὐκ ἄγαν μικρῶν κ.τ.λ.

Angularity was a characteristic of the atoms which caused acid and harsh tastes, roundness of those that caused the sensation of sweetness; but their size and their difference of impact on the body together with the heat supposed to be thus caused (*vid. loc. cit.*) played a part also.

For the Democritean theory of colour cf. Theophrastus, 73 and 80. The behaviour of the atoms relative to the πόροι (cf. above on Empedocles, ch. 2, 437 b 12) also was a determinant, as well as the density of the atmosphere, according to Democritus.

442 b 14. Alexander says that the preference is given to sight rather than touch because the latter does not perceive διάστημα (distance outward) and πλῆθος (a multitude of units). But surely the clause τὰ γοῦν κ.τ.λ. contains the reason. The illative force of γοῦν is continually backwards. The clause τὰ γοῦν κ.τ.λ. cannot, of course, be a consequence of εἰ δ᾽ ἄρα...τῆς γεύσεως μᾶλλον. It must be the ground for it. Hence the construction is loose; after μᾶλλον should follow ἐχρῆν without ὥστε and the τὰ γοῦν κ.τ.λ. clause should succeed. But that would make the argument too long and lumbering. Hence the τὰ γοῦν clause is brought up and has the additional function of confirming the καίτοι ἢ οὐδεμιᾶς κ.τ.λ. clause. It is clear that if it confirm the εἰ δ᾽ ἄρα clause, it will, whether intended or not, support the previous one. Aristotle argues 'if it is the function of taste to discriminate the κοινά,' and this we should infer from the atomist theory that taste discriminates the most minute spatial difference—τὸ τραχύ and τὸ λεῖον in particles imperceptible to the other senses, then it must in addition to perceiving the other κοινά be the best judge of figure.

But if the claim of taste to perceive best the κοινά rest on the fineness of its discrimination (falsely asserted), surely the real delicacy of the sense of sight is the cause of its justifiable claim.

The superiority of the sense of sight is as a rule assigned to its intellectual character: cf. ch. 1, 437 a, *Metaph.* i. ch. 1, 980 a 25, *De An.* iii. ch. 3, 429 a 3, ch. 13, 435 b 21. In the *Problems*, 886 b 35, we read that sight is ἐναργεστέρα than hearing, which comes to much the same thing as ἀκριβεστέρα in the sense of distinct. It is not said that touch generally is the most delicate of the senses; it is only contended that relatively to the senses of the other animals it is most delicate in man (441 a 2–3).

It looks, of course, strange to assign the discernment of the common sensibles to one sense when they are said to be common. Aristotle no doubt means their *accurate* discrimination. Simple experience would show that this is best obtained by sight.

442 b 20. ἐναντίωσιν. Cf. *De An.* II. ch. 11 and below ch. 6, 445 b 26 sqq.

442 b 22–26. Surely an account of proportionate elements in figure could be given analogous to the theory of proportionate numbers which he accepts.

442 b 28. Aristotle's treatise on plants is not extant. Two by Theophrastus survive, *De Causis Plantarum* and *Historia Plantarum*.

CHAPTER V.

442 b 29. Τὸν αὐτὸν κ.τ.λ. Alexander maintains that this refers to ch. 4, 440 b 30, where smell and taste are said to be σχεδὸν τὸ αὐτὸ πάθος. He is now to explain the analogy between the two. Its objective basis is the fact that the process involved in the genesis of each is the same; it is οἷον βαφή τις καὶ πλύσις (445 a 15); it is a process of infusion or solution. Add to this the fact that in both cases τὸ ξηρόν is the agent, with the sole difference that in taste it is not already modified, but in producing odour it must have been previously mingled with liquid. Further, as the vehicle of taste is τὸ ὑγρόν, so that of odour is ὑγρόν, for, as pointed out in 443 b 6, air as well as water is ὑγρός. Heat also seems to be operative or rather co-operative in the production of both (cf. 443 b 17 and note).

Here Aristotle calls the agent operative in the production of odour τὸ ἔγχυμον ὑγρόν. Elsewhere he names it τὸ ἔγχυμον ξηρόν, and cf. *De An.* II. ch. 9, 422 a 6: ἔστι δ᾽ ἡ ὀσμὴ τοῦ ξηροῦ. Hence Thurot, Torstrik, *De An.* p. 158, and Neuhäuser (*Aristoteles' Lehre von dem sinnlichen Erkenntnissvermögen und s. Organen,* p. 25) propose to read ξηρόν here instead of ὑγρόν, and Susemihl (*Burs. Jahresb.* XVII. p. 266) has lent his support to this conjecture. But, as Alexander points out, it makes no difference whether we call the agent here ξηρόν or ὑγρόν. We can call it either dry substance mixed with liquid or liquid mixed with dry. The main point is, that it must be μεμιγμένον τι *i.e.* τὸ ἤδη χυμὸν ἔχον.

442 b 30-31. ἐν ἄλλῳ γένει. The new γένος is the identical element in air and water of which it is the function to form a vehicle and medium for odour. Alexander (p. 89, l. 2 [W.]) has named this τὸ δίοσμον (following Theophrastus) on the analogy of the term τὸ διαφανές which is applied to the common constitution of air and water which enables them to form media for light. Cf. *De An.* II. ch. 7, 419 a 22 sqq., where however he says (l. 32) that the medium of smell has no special name.

The expression ἐν ἄλλῳ γένει is, however, quite vague and may mean merely ἐν τῷ ὀσφραντῷ—'in the domain of odorous quality.' τὸ ὀσφραντόν is the object of smell as τὸ ἀκουστόν is the object of hearing.

443 a 1–2. ᾗ πλυντικὸν ἢ ῥυπτικόν. Cf. ch. 4 ἐναποπλύνοντες 441 b 17, and beneath 443 b 8 ἀποπλύνομεν and 445 a 16 πλύσις. πλύνω is to wash; ῥύπτειν seems to contain more definitely the idea of scouring; the Latin rendering for it is *abstergere*. In the examples of its use in Aristotle (*e.g. Problems*, 935 b 35) it takes the accusative of the thing cleansed. Hence evidently ῥυπτικὸν ξηρότητος means 'able to cleanse, by scouring off and absorbing the surface of dry substance.' St Hilaire translates ᾗ πλυντικὸν ἢ ῥυπτικόν 'en tant qu'il peut transmettre et retenir,' Hammond, 'by virtue of its capacity to exude and throw off (dry savour).' But these renderings are impossible.

443 a 3. καὶ ἐν ὕδατι. Cf. *De An.* II. ch. 9, 421 b 10: καὶ γὰρ τὰ ἔνυδρα δοκοῦσιν ὀσμῆς αἰσθάνεσθαι, and beneath *passim*.

443 a 4. ὀστρακοδέρμων. Testacea must not be taken as a modern zoological designation. Any animal with a shell from the turtle to the sea-urchin is ranked under the ὀστρακόδερμα: cf. *Hist. Animal.* VIII. ch. 2, 590 a 19 sqq. Aristotle is, no doubt, thinking here of shell-fish. An example is afterwards given in 444 b 13— (αἱ πορφύραι) the purple-murex which, he asserts in *Hist. Animal.* VIII. ch. 2, 590 b, goes in pursuit of its prey and feeds on minute fishes.

443 a 5. ἐπιπολάζει. Air rises upwards by a 'natural' motion. Cf. *Meteor.* IV. ch. 7, 383 b 26: καὶ γὰρ ὁ ἀὴρ φέρεται ἄνω.

443 a 6. οὔτ' αὐτὰ κ.τ.λ. Aristotle thought the motion fishes make with their gills was not breathing. It is the expulsion of the water, which is taken in with their food, and which performs the 'cooling' function effected in respiring animals by the air. Cf. Zeller, *Aristotle*, II. pp. 43, 44, and Aristotle, *De Resp.* 476 a 1 sqq. especially 10: τὰ δὲ βράγχια πρὸς τὴν ἀπὸ τοῦ ὕδατος κατάψυξιν.

443 a 7. ὑγρά. Cf. *De Gen. et Corr.* II. ch. 3, 330 b 4, 331 a 5, etc.

443 a 8. φύσις. Cf. note to 442 b 30–31. Mr Cook Wilson (*Journal of Philol.* XI. p. 119) conjectures πλύσις instead of φύσις. This is possible but not necessary. τὸ ὀσφραντόν is indifferently the πάθος of the thing that smells and the odorous thing itself.

443 a 11. ἄοσμα. Cf. 437 a 22, 441 b 14 and notes. For the sources of the whole discussion cf. *Meteor.* IV.

443 a 12. For the doctrine contained in this statement cf. *De Gen. et Corr.* II. ch. 2, 329 b 11; the elements differ only κατὰ ἁπτὴν ἐναντίωσιν.

443 a 14. χυμὸν καὶ ξηρότητα. Cf. *De Gen. Animal.* 761 b 9: ἡ θάλαττα ὑγρά τε καὶ σωματώδης. The dry element is of course the salt contained in it; cf. 441 b 4: οἱ γὰρ ἅλες γῆς τι εἶδός εἰσιν. The reference for λίθος below is *Meteor.* IV. ch. 7, 383 b 20: (λίθος) γῆς μᾶλλον, for ξύλα also ch. 7 and for χρυσός etc. chs. 8, 9, 10.

443 a 15. ἔλαιον. Either the oil said to be extracted from salt has more smell than that which comes from natron and so the previous statement is directly verified, or there is a greater quantity of this product derived from salt and thus the strong smell of salt is explained by the fact that it contains more ὑγρόν than the other substance.

What the process referred to is, one can hardly tell. Aristotle in *Prob.* 935 a 8, talks of τὸ ἐν τοῖς ἅλασιν ὑφιστάμενον ἔλαιον, and this should mean a deposit or sediment. ἐξικμάζον should point to some process in which heat was employed. νίτρον was compounded with oil to form soap. Perhaps something similar was done with salt. Impure salt and oil may have been boiled together, and the product which distilled over collected. This would rather confirm the suggestion that Aristotle is referring to the stronger smell of the one compound than of the other.

νίτρον is any salt of sodium or potassium that has a strong alkaline reaction. It is not potassium nitrate—our salt-petre.

443 a 20. τὸ ὑγρόν. For ἄργυρος, καττίτερος cf. *Meteor.* IV. ch. 10, 389 a 8. Anything that melted with heat was held to be aqueous. We must remember however that the concepts of τὸ ὑγρόν and ὕδωρ are wider than what we understand by moisture and water. They correspond more nearly to the modern concept of the fluid *state* of matter. Hence Aristotle could talk of τὸ ὑγρόν in metals without meaning exactly that water, the actual particular substance known as such, was found in them. He was under the necessity of using popular terms with a more or less restricted denotation and a particular intension, for wide and far reaching scientific generalisations. To our mind this inevitably suggests both a fancifulness in the generalisation and a vagueness in the concept of the particular substance which permitted the name for it to be so widely applied. Both those characteristics are true of all primitive theories for, as Aristotle himself remarks (*Phys.* I. ch. 1, 184 a 21): ἔστι δ᾽ ἡμῖν πρῶτον δῆλα καὶ σαφῆ τὰ συγκεχυμένα μᾶλλον. τὸ ὑγρόν is fluidity or the fluid element generally, of which ὕδωρ is the typical example. The concept corresponds, as modern science shows, to an important objective distinction in the *condition* of matter. The peculiarity of the Aristotelian theory lies in regarding τὸ ὑγρόν not as a state into which matter may pass but as a quality which certain species of matter (ἀήρ and ὕδωρ) always possess.

443 a 23. Cf. above ch. 2, 438 b 26 sqq. and notes. ἀναθυμίασις (cognate of Latin *fumus*) is used in two senses: (1) in its generic meaning it corresponds more exactly to our word reek; it is any vapour which rises up and is wafted upwards from a substance. As such it has two species (cf. especially *Meteor.* ii. ch. 4, 359 b 27 sqq.) which are distinguished as being respectively moist and dry or at least as containing a greater proportion of ὑγρόν or ξηρόν respectively. The former is steam or moist vapour, the latter is more accurately described as smoke. Aristotle expressly proposes to use the general term to represent the latter variety (as he does in i. ch. 3, 340 b 27 sqq.) and this (2) is its second and more restricted meaning. Both species of ἀναθυμίασις are hot by nature. The dryness of the smoky kind comes from the earth which enters into its composition (340 b 26).

443 a 24–25. καὶ πάντες...ὀσμῆς. This seems to be a case of dittographia of the passage beneath l. 27. In consequence of the scribe's mistake l. 27 was mutilated and hence we must restore to it, with Christ, the ἐπὶ τοῦτο which appears here.

443 a 25. Heraclitus, fragment 37 in Bywater's edition: cf. Burnet, *Early Greek Phil.* p. 136. Hence Heraclitus must have held that odour was smoke.

443 a 28. ἀτμίδα. Cf. *Meteor.* i. ch. 9, 346 b 32 : ἔστι δ' ἡ μὲν ἐξ ὕδατος ἀναθυμίασις ἄτμις. Cf. also note to 443 a 23.

443 a 34. ὀσμᾶται κ.τ.λ. Cf. *De An.* ii. ch. 9, 421 b 10 sqq.

443 b 2. ἀπορροίαις. If the sense of smell were stimulated by effluxes it would be really a sense of touch, cf. 440 a 21 and note. Another reason against the efflux theory (noticed by Alexander) is given in *Problems*, 907 a 33. If that theory were true, odorous objects would evaporate away in time. Aristotle does not deny that smoke and vapour are odorous (cf. above ch. 2, 438 b 26 and *Prob.* 906 a 21 sqq. where he talks of the odorous qualities of θυμιάματα); he only means that exhalations are not the mechanism for transmitting odour. The sensation of smell is not caused by the evaporated substance impinging on the sense organs (cf. *De An.* 421 b 16). The μεταξύ in respiring animals is the air, and when that enters the nostrils it can be described as an ἀναθυμίασις indeed, but it is πνευματώδης (cf. below 445 a 29)—a waft of air.

Aristotle has, however, great difficulty in not regarding odour as a gas or the analogous diffusion of a solid in a liquid. Cf. 438 b 26 and below ἀτμίδος 444 b 33, *De An.* 421 b 24, and below 444 a 24 sqq.

443 b 4. πνεῦμα—air or wind—is more especially the air we breathe.

443 b 7. ὁμοίως. Between what is the similarity? Aristotle is explaining the correspondence between tastes and odours; he has already pointed out one identity—the ὑγρότης of the vehicle of both. Now he asserts that the process which generates the two is identical—ἀπόπλυσις. The argument is 'If in this case—the production of odour—the action of dry substance on moist is the same as in the production of taste—ἀπόπλυσις, then we can explain the analogy of the two.' He is not comparing the effect of τὸ ξηρόν on air with its effects on the fluids proper, otherwise he would have said ἐν τοῖς ἄλλοις ὑγροῖς after just pointing out that ἀὴρ ὑγρὸν τὴν φύσιν ἐστίν. He means τοῖς ὑγροῖς to include air and then gives air as the example of τὰ ὑγρά which is most important for present purposes. It is a very common function of καί in Aristotle to coordinate the generic and the specific, the latter coming second and illustrating the former or defining it more exactly (cf. Bonitz, *Ind.* p. 357). Cf. in this treatise 439 a 18 sq.: τὴν αἴσθησιν καὶ τὴν ἐνέργειαν, 441 a 10 sq.: τὸ θερμὸν καὶ τὸν ἥλιον, 441 b 19 sq.: τὸ ξηρὸν καὶ τὸ γεῶδες, etc.

The above is Alexander's interpretation, but he suggests that the argument may be intended to compare the action of τὸ ἔγχυμον ξηρόν in producing odour in air and in the fluids proper. If it is the same, then, assuming already that odour is produced by flavoured substance, we could explain why the odours we are cognisant of (which are propagated in air) correspond *singillatim* to flavours (which exist in liquid), Alex. 94, l. 20 (W.): κατὰ γὰρ τὰς τῶν χυμῶν διαφορὰς ἔσονται καὶ ὀσμῶν διαφοραί, εἴ γε ὑπὸ τούτων ἐκεῖναι γίνονται, ὡς ἕπεσθαι ἐκείνῳ ὃ φίλον ἐκείνῳ, εἰ οὕτως ἔχοι.

One thing seems certain, that Aristotle is *not* comparing the action of τὸ ξηρόν in producing tastes in water, with its action in diffusing odours in air, for in that case all mention of the propagation of odour in water would be omitted, and it would be natural to infer that it did not exist in water: but this is the reverse of the theory for which he contends.

443 b 8. ἀνάλογον κ.τ.λ. Cf. *De An.* ii. ch. 9, 421 a 16–18: ἔοικε μὲν γὰρ ἀνάλογον ἔχειν πρὸς τὴν γεῦσιν καὶ ὁμοίως τὰ εἴδη τῶν χυμῶν τοῖς τῆς ὀσμῆς. But further on (*loc. cit.*), in 26 sqq. he points out that though smells are distinguished as γλυκύ, πικρόν, δριμύ etc., the epithets applied to taste, yet not all objects have the taste and smell designated by the same name—τὴν ἀνάλογον ὀσμὴν καὶ χυμόν. Some are sweet, both to taste and smell, others not.

443 b 15–16. Cf. *Meteor.* iv. ch. 3, 380 b 2, where unripe flavours are said to be ψυχροί. Cold generally is the principle which counteracts heat (ἀντίστροφον τῇ θερμότητι *De Gen. Animal.* ii. ch. 6, 743 b 28), which is the great principle of life or activity according to the Aristotelian philosophy.

443 b 17. κινοῦν καὶ δημιουργοῦν. Cf. the similar *rôle* played by heat in the development of taste and nutrition (chapter 4 especially 442 a 5). Its function in producing odour is not brought into such prominence; but cf. 444 a 26: ἡ γὰρ τῆς ὀσμῆς δύναμις θερμὴ τὴν φύσιν ἐστίν and 438 b 27 and also *Problems*, 906 b 37 : ἡ ὀσμὴ θερμότης τίς ἐστι, and elsewhere for the influence of heat in producing smell.

443 b 19. εἴδη...δύο. It is unlikely that Aristotle here refers to τὸ ἡδὺ καὶ τὸ λυπηρόν as Hammond (p. 173) thinks. If that were so it would mean that odour *per se* was exhaustively divided into two species, the pleasant and the unpleasant, but nothing is said to confirm this. Aristotle certainly implies that all odours are either pleasant or unpleasant, but he does not elevate those epithets into specific differences. Alexander (*De Sens.* p. 97, l. 23 sqq. [W.]) conjectures that perhaps τὸ ἡδύ and τὸ λυπηρόν are the primary species of that kind of odour which is independent of taste, and that the others are subsequent to them and, possessing no names of their own, correspond to the particular flavours and perfumes from which they originate.

This would make the classification of odours *per se* pleasant and the reverse correspond on the whole to the classification of the species of the other sense qualities. But it is hardly possible that τὸ ἡδύ and τὸ λυπηρόν can be regarded as objective determinations like γλυκύ and πικρόν. Besides, it is clear from *De An.* ii. ch. 9, 421 b 1 sqq. that the same epithets mark the species of odour *per se* pleasant as those which distinguish the varieties dependent on taste. Among odours *per se* pleasant are included the scents of flowers

(l. 30 below) and to these in the *De Anima* are applied the terms γλυκύ, δριμύ etc.—ἡ μὲν γὰρ γλυκεῖα [ἀπὸ τοῦ] κρόκου καὶ μέλιτος, ἡ δὲ δριμεῖα θύμου καὶ τῶν τοιούτων.

The smell of honey is, no doubt, one of the class of odours which follow the taste. That of crocus or saffron is a scent *per se* pleasant, for the taste of the substance is not sweet. Probably Aristotle would have explained the phenomenon that many things did not have the corresponding odour and flavour by this distinction between the two different orders of smell. The problem is, however, not worked out.

Alexander, though lending some colour to the suggestion that τὸ ἡδὺ καὶ τὸ λυπηρόν are the species of odour *per se* pleasant and the reverse, yet does not hold that εἴδη...δύο here refers to them. Aristotle is referring to the two great divisions of odour—ὀσμὴ καθ' αὑτὴν ἡδεῖα, and that which is only κατὰ συμβεβηκὸς ἡδεῖα. The latter is called τὸ θρεπτικὸν εἶδος in 444 b 10. It is true it should rather be a γένος and that term is employed in 444 a 32 and b 4, but Aristotle frequently uses γένος and εἶδος indifferently to designate a class.

Here it certainly looks strange that Aristotle after using εἶδος to denote a wide group should in the next line employ it to refer to *infimae* species, but this is characteristic of the carelessness of his style. He says 'There are two species of odour' meaning by that two divisions, and then the word 'species' suggests to him the fact that some people have denied the existence of any species at all in odour.

443 b 23. κατὰ συμβεβηκὸς, i.e. indirectly: cf. note on κατὰ συμβεβηκός chapter 1, 437 a 5, 11.

443 b 33. Εὐριπίδην. Euripides is criticised by the comic poet for sickening over-refinement of style. Cf. Meineke, *Frag. Com. Graec. Strattis*, p. 298.

Perhaps there may be a hit in comparing to φακῆ what would be left if the meretricious additions were removed. μύρον is a perfume, not a spice. Cf. Cic. *ad Att.* 1. 19, 2.

Perhaps the force of the taunt may be thus rendered: 'Don't put hair-oil in your soup!'

444 a 1. νῦν. Aristotle is not necessarily to be regarded as mourning the degeneracy of his own time. The νῦν need not have that signification.

444 a 2. βιάζονται. Anything contrary to nature (φύσις) is βίαιος: cf. the famous βίαιός τις or βίᾳ ὅστις in *Nic. Eth.* I. ch. 3, 1096 a 6.

The idea here seems to be that gourmands get a pleasure from odour which appears to arise from taste. It is in the exercise of the latter sense (along with that of touch) that men are intemperate. Cf. *Prob.* 949 b 6, etc. and Sir A. Grant, *Ethics of Aristotle*, II. p. 49.

444 a 4. ἴδιον here and in l. 9 below is interpreted as μάλιστα ἴδιον by Alexander who, influenced by 21–24 below (*q.v.*), thinks that other respiring animals also perceived, though in a less degree, this kind of odour. But in 21–24 Aristotle is talking merely of odour in general and explaining why it is perceived by means of inhaling the breath. It is because of its higher function in man that odour is drawn in with the breath, and the same mechanism is provided for animals (in which the higher functions are lacking) in order that Nature might not have to devise a new organ for them (444 b 5).

Independently, however, of the influence of ll. 21–24, there was some reason for Alexander interpreting ἴδιον as μάλιστα ἴδιον, for otherwise Aristotle appears to make an absolute qualitative distinction in sensation depend upon a mere quantitative difference— the greater size of the human brain as compared with that of other animals.

444 a 10–11. Cf. *De Gen. Animal.* II. ch. 6, 743 b 28 sqq.

444 a 13–15. This is obviously the same account of the origin of catarrh as is given in *De Somno*, ch. 3, 458 a 2. The ἀναθυμίασις is not an exhalation from food as it exists outside the body; it arises from the food that has been eaten. The process by which the nutritive element in food is diffused into the blood is called by Aristotle an ἀναθυμίασις—volatilisation—in 456 b 3. It is an excess of this exhalation which, when carried up to the brain, produces a flow of phlegm.

ὑγίεια is defined in *Phys.* VII. ch. 3, 246 b 5; *Prob.* 859 a 12, etc. as a συμμετρία—balanced proportion—of heat and cold (cf. beneath l. 36).

444 a 18 sqq. Cf. above ch. 4, 441 b 30. Food is always a mixture. Alexander explains that it is always the cold associated with the liquid element in food which is the cause of its unhealthiness. He, however, identifies the ἀναθυμίασις from food which causes catarrh with the odour which is connected with taste. There is, however, nothing in the text to justify this and Aristotle has just refused to identify odour with ἀναθυμίασις. Probably in order to get my translation οὖσα should be inserted after ὑγρά. This is ugly but possible. If we render 'whether dry or cold' there is no point and, indeed, there is disagreement with the doctrine that all food has both characteristics.

Aristotle is probably thinking of the supposed efficacy of some perfumes in expelling colds and warding off infectious diseases.

444 a 20. ἡδεῖα must be understood, if not read, after ἡ καθ' αὑτήν. It appears after εὐώδους in MSS. L S U. Alexander interprets ἡδεῖα ὀσμή and Aristotle does not elsewhere talk of ἡ καθ' αὑτὴν ὀσμή, but of ἡ καθ' αὑτὴν ἡδεῖα (ὀσμή): cf. 443 b 30. Bekker's text is ἡ δ' ἀπὸ τῆς ὀσμῆς τῆς καθ' αὑτὴν εὐώδους ὁπωσοῦν κ.τ.λ.

If we retain this reading the missing substantive after εὐώδους cannot be τροφή as Bonitz (*Ind.* p. 533 a 3) suggests. Aristotle is discussing not the food but the odour which is ὠφέλιμος. Hayduck (*Prog. Kön. Gym. zu Meldorf*, 1877) suggests ἡδονή after εὐώδους, as also does Mr Cook Wilson (*Journal of Philol.* XI. pp. 119–120); but it is doubtful whether ἡδονή could designate the objective quality of odour which is supposed to promote health. The latter also suggests ἡ δ' ἀπὸ τῆς ὀσμῆς τῆς καθ' αὑτὴν ἡδείας εὐωδία.

I suggest ἡ δ' ἀπὸ τῆς ὀσμῆς καθ' αὑτὴν εὐωδία. Cf. 445 a 1 : αὐτῆς δὲ καθ' αὑτὴν τῆς δυσωδίας οὐδὲν φροντίζουσιν.

Aristotle could quite well talk of εὐωδία καθ' αὑτήν and δυσωδία καθ' αὑτήν. ἡ καθ' αὑτὴν εὐωδία would mean odour essentially pleasant, whereas ἡ καθ' αὑτὴν ὀσμή would mean smell which is essentially smell. But Aristotle does not wish to show that the opposite kind of odour is not essentially odour, but that it is not essentially pleasant.

444 a 21. διὰ τοῦτο. Because of its function in maintaining health in man who is the final aim and end of all the endeavour of nature. Aristotle is talking of smell in general; he does not mean that its higher function is shared by any of the animals.

444 a 23. μετέχει κ.τ.λ. Aristotle seems to think of the air as entering into the constitution of the body. Certain organs *e.g.* that of hearing (cf. ch. 2, 438 b 21 and *De Gen. Animal.* v. ch. 2, 781 a 24 sqq.) seem to contain air. Animals that do not breathe have a σύμφυτον πνεῦμα which performs the same function as the breath. (Cf. *De Somno*, 2, 456 a 12.) The probably spurious writings περὶ πνεύματος and περὶ ζῴων κινήσεως also declare that there is a σύμφυτον πνεῦμα in the lungs of respiring animals and in the heart. This doctrine may be a legitimate deduction from such passages as the present. Cf. 481 a 1, 27, 482 a 34, 703 a 15 etc. Cf. Introduction, sec. VI. and the passage there quoted where the σύμφυτον θερμόν is also called πνεῦμα.

444 a 26–27. ἡ γὰρ τῆς ὀσμῆς κ.τ.λ. Cf. *Prob.* 907 b 9 : ὅλως ἡ ὀσμὴ διὰ θερμότητα γίνεται and cf. note to 443 b 17.

444 a 27–31. There is no reason for considering that κατακέχρηται...κίνησιν should be postponed till 444 b 7 as Susemihl (*Philol.* 1885) and Hammond think, or for deleting it as Hayduck (*op. cit.*) wishes. It is certainly better to postpone it than to delete it and it comes in quite well at b 7, but it may stand here quite well as a note to amplify what has been already said. It points out the double function of ἀναπνοή, the operation which has just been under discussion.

ὡς παρέργῳ. Cf. *De Resp.* 473 a 24. The windpipe is the essential organ for conveying the breath. When it is closed death ensues. Not so in the other case.

444 a 34. κατὰ μέγεθος. Cf. *De Part. Animal.* II. ch. 14, 658 b 8.

444 a 35. χαίρει. St Hilaire (p. 61) has a marvellous notion that Aristotle in distinguishing the higher kind of odour is erecting a personal liking into a theory. But for evidence that the distinction was widely recognised cf. *Eth. Eud.* III. ch. 2, 1231 a 11 : διὸ ἐμμελῶς ἔφη Στρατόνικος τὰς μὲν καλὸν ὄζειν, τὰς δὲ ἡδύ.

444 b 3. Biehl and Bekker read διὰ τὸ ἀναπνεῖν which, of course, must be taken along with ὅσα πλεύμονα ἔχει. In that case we must understand διὰ τὸ ἀναπνεῖν to be equivalent to ἀναπνοῆς ἕνεκεν because we learn from *De Resp.* 476 a 7 that breathing is the *final* cause of the existence of the lung (ὁ μὲν πλεύμων τῆς ὑπὸ τοῦ πνεύματος καταψύξεως ἕνεκέν ἐστιν); the determining cause in the ordinary sense both of the existence of the lung and of ἀναπνοή alike is rather the greater vital heat of respiring animals (cf. 477 a 14).

But if we take this reading, the sense becomes very difficult. The sentence τοῖς δ᾽ ἄλλοις...δύο ποιῇ ll. 2–5 will mean that Nature gave the rest of the respiring animals the kind of smell not necessarily connected (for health reasons) with the head, in order not to make two organs and one of them have no functions. The thought will be that the animals, having nostrils, may as well smell by them. This is to make ὅπως μὴ αἰσθητήρια δύο ποιῇ equivalent to the well known Aristotelian doctrine that Nature does nothing in vain. But this doctrine may be variously interpreted ; here it would mean that, having once made a thing, Nature must assign it a use. But such a maxim is hardly to be identified with the principle of parcimony —'entia non sunt multiplicanda praeter necessitatem'—which is surely the true import of the Aristotelian doctrine. If Nature really does nothing in vain and does not wish to make a superfluity of organs, it would surely be better not to give the lower animals nostrils at all if the species of smell connected with food has no necessary connection with the upper part of the head. A still greater objection to the above interpretation is, that αἰσθητήρια has to be taken as referring (1) to the organ of smell and (2) to the organ of breathing—the windpipe which is not an αἰσθητήριον at all (Alexander notices this).

It is as above that St Hilaire, following most commentators, takes this passage, but Simon proposes to detach διὰ τὸ ἀναπνεῖν from what precedes and connect it with what follows translating as I have done. The reading must thus, of course, be διὰ τοῦ ἀναπνεῖν which is the version found in MSS. P U pr. S. This is also supported by Mr Cook Wilson (*Journal of Philol.* XI. p. 120). Cf. *De Resp.* 475 b 19: (τὴν κατάψυξιν ποιεῖται) διὰ τοῦ ἀναπνεῖν καὶ ἐκπνεῖν. The argument then is, that Nature made respiration the means of perceiving odour in the case of the other respiring animals in order to avoid making a separate sense organ for them. The αἰσθητήρια δύο are the nostrils in man and the problematical new organ of sensation in the other animals. Nature, in making the lower respiring animals perceive odour by means of the nostrils, avoided making a second sense organ of a new type—a type not found in man, her chief creation. But in the case of the non-respiring animals, as he goes on to say, probably some other contrivance has to be resorted to. It is thus that Alexander interprets from ἀπόχρη onwards; hence it is strange he does not notice the ineptitude of the reading διὰ τὸ ἀναπνεῖν.

444 b 5. ἀπόχρη κ.τ.λ. Biehl, following E M Y, strikes out ἐπείπερ before and ὡς after the καὶ which precedes ἀναπνέουσιν. These stand in Bekker's text, which if retained will hardly give the sense required. St Hilaire renders—'et il leur suffit, quoiqu'ils respirent les deux espèces d'odeurs comme les hommes, d'avoir uniquement la perception de l'une des deux,'—a mistranslation.

Hammond—'It is enough for these respiring animals that they have the sensation of only one class of smells' etc. But this is merely an obvious and insipid deduction from what has been said about the greater size of the human brain, and besides it throws no light, as it should, on the previous clause.

444 b 8. Cf. *De An.* II. ch. 9, 421 b 26.

444 b 9. ἐντόμων. Though insects live in air they do not respire, thinks Aristotle. He had not the means at our disposal for observation, which show that the opposite is the case; cf. Packard, *The Study of Insects*, p. 40; Owen, *Compar. Anatom. and Physiol. of the Invertebrate Animals*, p. 368. Cf. οὐκ ἀναπνεῖ τὰ ἔντομα, *De Resp.* 475 a 29. But they employ τὸ σύμφυτον πνεῦμα in a way analogous to respiration: cf. *De Somno*, ch. 2, 456 a 11 sqq. Cf. Hammond, p. 305.

444 b 13. κνῖπας. Not the species known by the name *knipes* in modern Zoology, which is a 'beetle allied to the Cryptarcha.' Cf. Hammond, p. 176.

444 b 13–14. αἱ πορφύραι. Not 'purple sea-fish' nor 'les rougets de mer.' Aristotle asserts in *Hist. Animal.* VIII. ch. 2, 590 b 2 sqq., that ἡ πορφύρα is among the class of shell-fish that move and that it is caught by a bait, as it feeds on small fishes.

444 b 21. ἑτέρα. Cf. *De An.*, *loc. cit.* 421 b 20.

τοῦ γὰρ κ.τ.λ. Cf. *De An.*, *loc. cit.* 21–23. It is strange that Wallace (*Aristotle's Psychology*, p. 246) should think that Aristotle did not really mean that the *manner* of perceiving smells was different in respiring and non-respiring animals when he quotes (§ 7) the passage from the *De Sensu* here beginning οὐ τὸν αὐτὸν τρόπον.

By a difference in 'manner' Wallace must mean a difference in the quality of the sensation. He blames Aristotle for being 'misled by language' in assuming that odorous quality should be perceived by the sense of odour.

But Aristotle throughout proceeds on the principle that the only way for establishing the identity of sensations is the identity of their objective ground. It is really impossible to tell whether the qualitative character of the mere subjective affection is identical in any two people or any two species. We have to assume that, where the objective content is the same, the quality of the sensation is the same. Thus I believe that my sensation when I enjoy the perfume of a rose is the same as my neighbour's. We apprehend something that is chemically identical.

Now, though Aristotle knew nothing of chemical qualities in our sense, he tries to prove the objective identity of that which is perceived both by respiring and non-respiring animals. He points out in *De An.*, *loc. cit.* 23, that it has the same physiological effect. Strong odours—and he meant by odours practically chemicals diffused either in air or water (cf. note to 443 b 2 and Introduction, sec. VII.) have a destructive action upon both classes alike and hence are the same. This inference was all the more easily made because he conceived their effect to be exercised upon the organ of smell or, at least the head, the region in which it is situated and out of the material of which it is formed (cf. beneath l. 34 καρηβαροῦσι).

That there should be chemical qualities apart from taste or smell, and qualities of any kind which are not perceived by some of the senses, would have appeared strange to Aristotle and the normal Greek mind, for which had not been shattered the harmony between Nature and man, in whom evolution has developed senses to give warning of most of the ordinary collocations of qualities which affect his well-being. But, if Aristotle had discovered that any quality, not distinguishable directly by man, still had an effect upon the sentience of some other form of life (*e.g.* the ultra-violet rays on ants), he would have been bound by his own principles to assume the existence of a new sense in these creatures, if the quality which affected them had a sufficient amount of objective difference from the qualities which stimulate human sensibility.

444 b 24–25. ἀφαιρεῖ κ.τ.λ. Cf. *De An.* 421 b 26–422 a 6, for a closely parallel account. 422 a 1 : τοῖς δὲ τὸν ἀέρα δεχομένοις ἔχειν ἐπικάλυμμα, ὃ ἀναπνεόντων ἀποκαλύπτεσθαι.

μὴ ἀναπνέοντα Cf. *De An.* 421 b 14 : μὴ ἀναπνέων δὲ ἀλλ' ἐκπνέων ἢ κατέχων τὸ πνεῦμα οὐκ ὀσμᾶται.

444 b 26. Cf. *De An.* 421 b 28 : τὰ μὲν γὰρ ἔχει φράγμα καὶ ὥσπερ ἔλυτρον τὰ βλέφαρα, ἃ μὴ κινήσας μηδ' ἀνασπάσας οὐχ ὁρᾷ.

444 b 28–29. Cf. *De An.*, *loc. cit.* (continuing): τὰ δὲ σκληρόφθαλμα οὐδὲν ἔχει τοιοῦτον ἀλλ' εὐθέως ὁρᾷ τὰ γινόμενα ἐν τῷ διαφανεῖ.

Alexander and all other editors read ἐκ τοῦ δυνατοῦ ὁρᾶν αὐτῷ εὐθύς. In that case the meaning would be 'from the possession of the faculty' or 'from the time when the faculty (of seeing) exists.' The ancient Latin translation has 'a facultate existente.'

444 b 31. δυσχεραίνει. In *Hist. Animal.* IX. ch. 40, 626 a 26 he points out that bees dislike unpleasant smells. He probably is thinking of this here and below in l. 35—θείου.

But in the *De An.* III. ch. 13, we hear that excessively strong odours, colours, sounds do not destroy life except κατὰ συμβεβηκός, 435 b 10.

444 b 35. θείου. Cf. *De An.* 421 b 25.

445 a 8. δι' ἄλλου. Cf. above ch. 1, 436 b 20: αἱ δὲ διὰ τῶν ἔξωθεν αἰσθήσεις.

The flesh (cf. *De An.* II. ch. 11, especially 423 b 26) really forms a medium for touch. But the difference between this and an external medium forms an important basis for classifying the senses. Cf. *De An.* III. ch. 12, 434 b 15, and ch. 13, 435 a 16 sqq.

445 a 11. καὶ ἐν ἀέρι κ.τ.λ. Because the objects of sight and hearing exist in air and water. Alexander says that so far as the γένεσις of ὀσμή is due to ξηρότης it is related to taste and touch, so far as ἐν ὑγροῖς γίνεται it is related to the externally mediated senses.

Note below τῷ διαφανεῖ = τῷ ὁρατῷ: cf. chapter 3.

445 a 15. οἷον βαφή τις. Note that Aristotle does not say that this is anything more than an analogue to the process which produces odour.

445 a 18-19. Cf. *De An.* III. ch. 12, 434 b 20: ψόφος δὲ καὶ χρῶμα καὶ ὀσμὴ οὐ τρέφει. The Pythagoreans may have observed the stimulating effect of some odours. Cf. Alex. *De Sens.* p. 108 (W).

445 a 21. Alexander thinks that Aristotle means that, because περιττώματα (περίττωμα = excrement) are both dry and liquid, they show that the food from which they are secreted is composite, *i.e.* consisting of both γῆ and ὕδωρ. (This must be so indeed according to the doctrine of the Περὶ μακροβιότητος, ch. 3, 465 b 18-19, where περίττωμα is said to be ὑπόλειμμα τοῦ προτέρου, *i.e.* the food.)

But probably the argument does not run quite in this way. Aristotle says that food must be composite. But probably he means a little more than merely μεμιγμένον as in chapter 4, 441 b 30 sqq. σύνθετος when applied to the objects of sense tends to mean more than merely composite, but refers continually to things that have density: cf. *Meteor.* IV. ch. 5, 382 a 26 sqq.: ἅπαντα ἂν εἴη τὰ σώματα τὰ σύνθετα καὶ ὡρισμένα οὐκ ἄνευ πήξεως. τὸ σύνθετον = τὸ συνεστηκός. Cf. συστησόμενον below. σῶμα once more tends to have the same application: cf. beneath l. 25: ἔτι πολὺ ἧττον εὔλογον τὸν ἀέρα σωματοῦσθαι, and σωματῶδες above. Though all the four elements, fire and air included, are σώματα, yet we hear in *Prob.* 932 b 2: πυκνότερον ἡ θάλαττα καὶ μᾶλλον σῶμα. σωματώδης and γεώδης are constantly conjoined: cf. Bonitz, *Ind.* p. 745 b 21 sqq.

Now ὀσμή is nothing crassly material in this sense; cf. *Prob.*

865 a 21 : ἡ ὀσμὴ οὐ σωματώδης. Hence he must prove that γῆ, the most bodily of the elements, is an essential constituent of τροφή. Hence he is probably thinking of περίττωμα as something solid (it is the heavy element in food (cf. 442 a 7), and hence is to be identified with γῆ, the heaviest element; cf. *De An.* III. ch. 13), and more or less γεῶδες, and γῆ is ξηρά. The argument is—the excrement proves that in the compound of which food consists there must be solid matter. But it might be objected that the water in it (and water is one of the media of odour) is the really nutritive element. No, says Aristotle, water alone does not nourish; some of the more solid elements must be mingled with it and, if that is so, still less likely is it that air, which cannot be solidified, should support life. The reasoning is very much condensed. Water, ἄμικτον ὄν, cannot nourish a solid body. But cannot it be solidified? Not unless something γεῶδες is mixed with it. This would be true (cf. 441 a 30: θερμαινόμενον οὐδὲν φαίνεται παχυνόμενον τὸ ὕδωρ) except in the case of freezing, which would certainly not produce a nutritive solid! Still less likely is it that air could be solidified. On this interpretation there is no need to insert εἰ after ἔτι δ᾽, l. 22, as Hayduck, *op. cit.*, suggests.

The waste residue in plants is, Alexander explains, such substance as gum, the bark and in a way the leaves, etc.

445 a 26. τόπος δεκτικὸς, *i.e.* ἡ κοιλία : cf. *De Somno,* 3, 456 b 2, 3 : τῆς μὲν οὖν θύραθεν τροφῆς εἰσιούσης εἰς τοὺς δεκτικοὺς τόπους.

445 a 29. ἀναθυμιάσεως. Cf. note to 443 a 23 and cf. 444 a 24. Aristotle allows the ἀναθυμίασις theory in this modified form. The medium may be described as an ἀναθυμίασις. Just as in the previous chapters, here also he adopts something from previous theories. The medium is a gas, in the case of breathing animals at least, but not an exhalation from the odorous substance. But he can only explain odour as a quasi-diffusion of substance in this gas. With Aristotle, however, it is difficult to distinguish medium and object (cf. above 445 a 14 where he identifies τὸ ὁρατόν and τὸ διαφανές), and so we should be bound to say odour *was* an ἀναθυμίασις of some sort; cf. Introduction, sec. VII. That is however not quite accurate, as it is some nature common to both gases and liquids that is τὸ δίοσμον or the κοινὴ φύσις of the two to Aristotle.

He seems here to have in a way anticipated the discovery of the truth that the diffusion of a substance in a liquid is analogous to its behaviour as a gas. Once more he differs from modern theory in regarding τὸ δίοσμον as a κοινὴ φύσις which had a permanent existence of its own instead of as a mere state, or disposition to act, of matter which may cease to be so characterized.

445 a 32. αἰσθήσεως. This perhaps points to some subjective experience of his own.

445 b 1. As Biehl suggests, περὶ τῶν αἰσθητῶν must have fallen out or must at least be presupposed before καθ᾽ ἕκαστον αἰσθητήριον. Aristotle has not discussed the αἰσθητήρια since chap. 2, except incidentally in chap. 5, and at the beginning of chap. 3 (439 a 7) he proposes to give an objective account περὶ τῶν αἰσθητῶν τῶν καθ᾽ ἕκαστον αἰσθητήριον.

CHAPTER VI.

445 b 3. εἰ πᾶν σῶμα κ.τ.λ. This is a principle with Aristotle. Cf. *De Coelo*, I. ch. I *ad init.* σῶμα is μέγεθος ἐπὶ τρία—a tridimensional magnitude. More strictly μέγεθος is the quantitative determination that all bodies possess. μέγεθος is that which is divisible into continuous parts (cf. *Metaph.* v. ch. 13, 1020 a 11: μέγεθος δὲ τὸ εἰς συνεχῆ (διαιρετόν)). The continuous (τὸ συνεχές) is that which is infinitely divisible. Compare *De Coelo*, 268 a 6: συνεχὲς μέν ἐστι τὸ διαιρετὸν εἰς ἀεὶ διαιρετά, σῶμα δὲ τὸ πάντῃ διαιρετόν. Cf. also *Phys.* III. chs. 6, 7. There Aristotle tells us that μεγέθη are infinitely *divisible* only; *i.e.* though the process of division can be carried *ad infinitum* there are no actually existing infinitely small parts. Compare μέγεθος l. 10 below, συνεχές l. 29, etc.

445 b 4. παθήματα, a variant for πάθη: cf. Bonitz, *Ind.* p. 554. In *De Coelo*, I. ch. I Aristotle tells us that the objects of physical science are μεγέθη καὶ σώματα with their πάθη and κινήσεις, and the ἀρχαί, *i.e.* the elements.

445 b 7. ποιητικόν. Cf. ch. 3, 439 a 18: ποιήσει τὴν αἴσθησιν etc. This is not intended as an argument for the alternative ἀδύνατον, but is rather a development of the positive thesis that infinite divisibility of the σῶμα entails infinite divisibility of the πάθος.

445 b 9. τήν τε αἴσθησιν. Infinite divisibility of the παθήματα αἰσθητά means infinite divisibility of the αἴσθησις. Hence all bodies, however minute, will cause sensation and be perceptible.

445 b 10. ἀδύνατον κ.τ.λ. This looks as if it established not the proposition to be proved but its converse. But the reasoning no doubt is—'could we not have αἴσθησις, extremely minute, which is not the perception of a body?' 'No,' says Aristotle, 'we cannot have any perception, take colour for example, in which the content is not a quantum and hence a determination of σῶμα.'

Cf. below ch. 7, 449 a 22 : τὸ αἰσθητὸν πᾶν ἐστι μέγεθος κ.τ.λ.

445 b 16. τῶν μαθηματικῶν, *e.g.* lines, points, planes etc. It had been part of the Pythagorean doctrine to give these substantial existence and to make everything consist of them. (Cf. *Metaph.* I. ch. 8,

989 b 29 sqq., and also *Metaph.* XIII. ch. 1.) Aristotle distinguishes the objects of mathematics from those of physics in *Phys.* II. ch. 2, and elsewhere. They are determinations of number and magnitude taken in abstraction from the concrete—τὰ ἐξ ἀφαιρέσεως (cf. *De An.* I. ch. 1, 403 b 15) and more particularly considered apart from the motion or change of the objects to which they belong. Compare also *Metaph.* VI. ch. 1, 1026 a 7 sqq. They are not really separable from the things of sense like the object of metaphysics but are considered as such. Cf. *De An.* III. ch. 7, 431 b 15: τὰ μαθηματικὰ οὐ κεχωρισμένα ὡς κεχωρισμένα νοεῖ (ὁ μαθηματικός). The argument is that if the constituents of sensible objects are not themselves sensible, the only alternative left is that they are mathematical entities.

ἔτι κ.τ.λ. We must take this as a further argument *against* the existence of imperceptible bodies.

It has been conceded that if sensation is not divisible *ad infinitum* the ultimate constituents of bodies are not objects of sense, and further they cannot be objects of consciousness at all, as they cannot be merely mental entities—νοητά. We know objects either by αἴσθησις or by νοῦς or, as in the case of mathematical entities (already ruled out of court), by a union of the two.

445 b 17. νοῦς is that faculty of the soul which is peculiar to man among mortal creatures and which receives the εἴδη—forms or intelligible character—of things without their matter (ὕλη). Cf. *De An.* III. chs. 4–8. The objects of νοῦς are νοητά and these evidently are simply conceptual contents, as they are said to have their concrete existence in the sensible forms of things. Cf. *De An.* III. ch. 8, 432 a 2 sqq. νοῦς in operation (ἐι ἐργείᾳ) is identical with its objects (431 b 17, *Metaph.* XII. ch. 7, 1072 b 21).

οὐδὲ νοεῖ κ.τ.λ. These insensible objects are the constituents of external bodies and hence must be external. They must be σώματα and contain ὕλη, and αἴσθησις is indispensable for the apprehension of such objects. Cf. *Metaph.* VIII. ch. 1, 1042 a 25: αἱ δ᾽ αἰσθηταὶ οὐσίαι πᾶσαι ὕλην ἔχουσιν. They must be καθ᾽ ἕκαστα, and these are the objects of αἴσθησις: cf. *De An.* II. ch. 5, 417 b 22, etc.

Though Aristotle does not employ this argument here against the existence of imperceptible magnitudes, it raises a difficulty which besets all modern theories of atoms, ether etc. Physical scientists of a certain school continually talk of the atom as a mere concept. They do not explain how it is possible for solid bodies to be composed of concepts. Cf. Karl Pearson, *Grammar of Science*, ch. VII. *passim*.

445 b 19. The theory of atoms lies at the basis of the doctrine of ἀπόρροιαι previously discussed, chapter 4 *ad fin.* It consists in finding the reality of physical bodies not in their sensuous characteristics, but in some quantitative determination of their minute parts. But Aristotle refuses to entertain the theory that there are bodies with no sensible and only mathematical qualities, and in particular that they are atoms in the strict sense of bodies perfectly indivisible.

445 b 21. τοῖς περὶ κινήσεως. The reference is to the *Physics*— frequently styled τὰ περὶ κινήσεως, and in particular, as Alexander says, to the last books. Thomas is still more explicit and says the sixth, where indeed the chief discussion of the doctrine of indivisible magnitudes is to be found. The theory that magnitude is infinitely divisible will be found in the third book, chs. 6 and 7 (cf. note to 445 b 3) and the definition of continuity which, being the characteristic of all magnitude, entails its infinite divisibility, is to be found in Book v. ch. 3. Things that are continuous have a common boundary—ὅταν ταὐτὸ γένηται καὶ ἓν τὸ ἑκατέρου πέρας οἷς ἅπτονται (227 a 11). This is practically repeated in vi. ch. 1: συνεχῆ μὲν ὧν τὰ ἔσχατα ἕν (231 a 22), where he goes on to show that nothing continuous can be made up of indivisible parts. Indivisible parts must be either entirely discrete or entirely coincident, and so cannot compose the continuous.

Hence Aristotle arrives at another definition of the continuous. It is that which is divisible into parts themselves infinitely divisible— λέγω δὲ τὸ συνεχὲς τὸ διαιρετὸν εἰς ἀεὶ διαιρετά (232 b 24). Since continuity is the universal characteristic of magnitude, this yields us the further proposition that magnitude is that which is divisible into magnitudes—πᾶν μέγεθος εἰς μεγέθη διαιρετόν (232 a 23). Aristotle shows in addition that, if magnitudes were composed of indivisible parts, motions would be impossible; every distance would be traversed as soon as entered upon if motion, like magnitude, were made up of indivisible parts. Motion is continuous and likewise time.

Those proofs, it is obvious, affect only atoms that are held to be spatially indivisible. To the modern theory which recognises that the atom must have a definite bulk and even a composite structure Aristotle's refutation does not apply. The atoms are only physically not spatially discontinuous, and there is no more difficulty in imagining minute discrete bodies than in the perception of discrete masses appreciable to sight. Aristotle's other objections to an atomic theory are to be found mostly in the *De Coelo* and the *De Generatione et Corruptione* (cf. Zeller, *Aristotle and the Earlier Peripatetics*, Vol. I. pp. 430 sqq., pp. 445 sqq.). As Zeller says, without the modern theories of chemical, molecular and gravitational attraction, it was difficult to see how discrete atoms could cohere in a solid body, and hence Aristotle's criticism of the ancient atomists was justified. At the same time also, the arguments in the *Physics* form a valuable corrective to such modern thought as regards all the individual things of sense as *really* discrete in structure and only *apparently* continuous. They are only discrete from one point of view; relatively to the molecule or the atom they are discrete, but relatively to other composite structures water and iron are continuous. To be continuous is to be thought of merely as a magnitude so far as internal structure is concerned. So elastic balls may have many properties and many forms of action on each other and on other things; but these are relations to external things that affect them as a whole; when regarded in this way they are considered as being internally merely magnitudes, *i.e.* as continuous. The atom itself relatively to which they are discrete must itself relatively to them be regarded as merely a magnitude, *i.e.* as continuous. One does not inquire what makes the parts of the atom cohere together and, if one did, one would have to think of the atom as being composed of smaller atoms which again must be continuous. But there comes a point where this continual division and subdivision of matter ceases to have interest. Hence we cannot look to the discreteness of matter for its reality. The reality of objects must lie, as Aristotle said, in the 'form' or, as modern theory would put it, in the law of the combination of their elements and the qualitative difference to which that gives rise.

445 b 24. ὧν μὲν γὰρ κ.τ.λ. The passage where we find the doctrine expounded is in the *Posterior Analytics* I. ch. 20, 82 a 21 sqq. (Cf. also ch. 22, 84 a 29.) There, however, it is set forth in another connection. Aristotle shows that the number of terms to be interposed between the subject and predicate of any proposition which we desire to demonstrate, is not infinite. If it were, the proposition could never be proved, as it is impossible to traverse the infinite. All the terms in the series must be *contiguous*, with nothing intervening between them...ἐχόμενα ἀλλήλων ὥστε μὴ εἶναι μεταξύ (82 a 31). If there were an infinity of terms to be inserted at any point in the series, it would constitute a break and the terms would not be contiguous. (For the definition of ἐχόμενον cf. *Phys.* v. ch. 3, 227 a 6—ἐχόμενον δὲ ὃ ἂν ἐφεξῆς ὂν ἅπτηται, and 226 b 23—ἅπτεσθαι δὲ ὧν τὰ ἄκρα ἅμα.)

There is some difference, however, between a series of terms bound together by the identity of the subject of which they are predicated and a number of specifically diverse but generically identical qualities. According to Aristotle, in both cases they are to be considered as a series arranged between two extremes. In the case of qualities these extremes are the members of the series with least specific resemblance and, if one takes seriously the spatial designation (τὰ ἐντός or τὰ ἀνὰ μέσον) applied to them, the intermediate members of the group must be thought of as being arranged in accordance with the amount of the resemblance they each possess to the extremes. We have seen, however, (chapters 3 and 4) that Aristotle does not prefer to think of them as forming a continuum like a line, but as being formed by different proportions in the admixture of the two fundamental extreme qualities, *e.g.* black and white, sweet and bitter. Though forming a linear series, they do not constitute a uniformly continuous line. Thus though he may, as here, talk of opposites (ἐναντία) in terms of spatial relation and call them ἔσχατα (cf. *Categ.* ch. 6, 6 a 17: τὰ πλεῖστον ἀλλήλων διεστηκότα τῶν ἐν τῷ αὐτῷ γένει ἐναντία ὁρίζονται) qualitative difference is really other than spatial diversity. It is this that causes the number of species in a genus to be limited in number. If a genus were really a spatial whole, its parts, the species, would need not merely to be ἐχόμενα— contiguous, but συνεχῆ—continuous, and hence capable of resolution into an infinite number of subdivisions (cf. note to 445 b 21). If the members of the series were not merely contiguous but had a common boundary, as things continuous have, it would mean that there was no reason for drawing the boundary between any two at one point rather than another. The only common boundaries are spatial existences—point, line and surface, and these can be drawn anywhere. It is magnitude that is *per se* continuous, but in so far as genera are not magnitudes they are not *per se* continuous (καθ' αὑτὸ συνεχὲς, l. 30) and besides do not present this aspect of infinite divisibility.

445 b 25. ἔσχατα. Cf. notes to ll. 21 and 24 above.

πᾶν δὲ κ.τ.λ. Cf. 442 b 20.

445 b 28–30. Division into unequal parts is, Alexander tells us, progressive division of the parts which the first division yields into the same fraction as that which they are of the whole, *e.g.* the division

of a line into two and again of the half into two and so on. This is the special example of 'unequal division' which Aristotle, in *Phys.* VIII. ch. 8, 263 a 3 sqq. in reply to Zeno, shows to be infinite—ἐν δὲ τῷ συνεχεῖ ἔνεστι μὲν ἄπειρα ἡμίση, ἀλλ᾽ οὐκ ἐντελεχείᾳ ἀλλὰ δυνάμει (263 b 28). Any actual division of a continuum into distinct parts is finite. In order for the parts to be distinct the termini of adjacent parts must be, at least, reckoned as distinct. Hence the whole, which was continuous, by the division ceases to be so and *ipso facto* loses that capacity for infinite division which, as continuous, it possessed.

True the parts again can be divided, but any division of them into distinct elements which can actually be realised is once more finite.

All this seems to point to the conclusion that the very spatial determinant by which we are able to construct a continuum, *e.g.* a line, and to consider it as resoluble into distinct parts, is itself a qualitative distinction (*e.g.* direction right or left) which exists over and above the characteristic of magnitude, which is the universal attribute of spatial quantity. Aristotle goes so far as to say (263 b 7) συμβέβηκε γὰρ τῇ γραμμῇ ἄπειρα ἡμίσεα εἶναι, ἡ δ᾽ οὐσία ἐστὶν ἑτέρα καὶ τὸ εἶναι. Thus, not only has a line (with all other figures) a non-quantitative aspect, but the possibility of determining it as a quantity depends upon this qualitative character. (Cf. also for the general doctrine III. ch. 7, 207 b 10: ἄπειροι γὰρ αἱ διχοτομίαι τοῦ μεγέθους.) The result, however, of this is that anything considered as a continuum divides into a limited number of units (ἴσα can mean little else than units; all things considered as units are held to be equal) but an infinite number of diminishing fractions. Units are the constituents of a continuum, species of a genus.

445 b 30. τὸ δὲ μὴ κ.τ.λ. Cf. note to l. 24 above.

445 b 31. ὑπάρχει δὲ κ.τ.λ. Cf. above 445 b 10 sq.: ἀδύνατον λευκὸν μὲν ὁρᾶν, μὴ ποσὸν δέ. Spatial quantity or μέγεθος = τὸ συνεχές. Cf. also *De An.* III. ch. 3, 428 b 24: κίνησις καὶ μέγεθος ἃ συμβέβηκε τοῖς αἰσθητοῖς.

445 b 32 sqq. There is a somewhat similar passage in *Phys.* VII. ch. 5, 250 a 20 sqq. The sound which one single grain of millet makes in falling exists as a separate sound (καθ᾽ αὑτό) only potentially in the whole, *i.e.* it is not actually a separate sound—οὐδὲ γὰρ οὐδέν ἐστιν ἀλλ᾽ ἢ δυνάμει ἐν τῷ ὅλῳ (250 a 24). For the general question as to how far Aristotle by his distinction between potential and actual settles the difficulty about *petites perceptions* and sub-consciousness generally, cf. Introduction, sec. VIII.

446 a 2. διέσει. A quarter of a tone was the least interval taken notice of in Greek music. Hence, I fancy, ὁ ἐν τῇ διέσει φθόγγος must be a sound with difference in pitch from that of the one before it within, *i.e.* less than, a quarter-tone. Aristotle means that the interval of a quarter of a tone is not thought of as resoluble into parts, as larger intervals are. The parts of an interval are not however sensations. Hence this phenomenon is hardly parallel to that in the illustration from sight or that quoted in note to 445 b 32 above from the *Physics*. In those instances we have sensations which *per se* are not actually appreciable when existing concomitantly, being merged in the whole of which they are elements.

For δίεσις cf. *Anal. Post.* I. ch. 23, 84 b 38: ἡ ἀρχή (*i.e.* ultimate simple (ἁπλοῦν) constituent) ἐν μέλει δίεσις. In *Metaph.* XIV. ch. 1, 1087 b 35 it is called ὑποκείμενον ἐν ἁρμονίᾳ.

446 a 3. συνεχοῦς ὄντος. The notes are still continuous in time.

446 a 4. λανθάνει. Hence there seems to be no μεταξύ; the notes seem to be ἐχόμενα ἀλλήλων, *i.e.* contiguous but separate, and hence the continuity of the scale is broken up.

446 a 6. δυνάμει κ.τ.λ. The difficulty in this obscure passage is increased by the discrepancy between the MSS. E M Y read ὅταν μὴ χωρὶς ᾖ; ὅταν χωρισθῇ is the reading given by most others and by Alexander. I have followed that of E M Y, which is supported by the ancient Latin translation, because of the difficulty of giving any sensible interpretation to the following sentence, καὶ γάρ...διαιρεθεῖσα, if we read χωρισθῇ; the sense it gives does not really conflict with what is said later on.

Aristotle says that the very minute parts of the objects of sense, if not separated, are perceived only potentially and not actually. But this does not commit him to the statement that, if severed from the whole, they are actually perceptible. This is no doubt the general rule; an object like a one-foot measure which has only potential existence in a larger whole is made actual by being marked off. It then becomes an explicit object of consciousness, not merely a potential one. But, he goes on to say, very minute fractions cannot exist in isolation from the whole, as the larger parts of a whole can when broken off. They lose their identity (cf. note to 446 a 9 below, *De Gen. et Corr.* I. ch. 10, 328 a 24 sqq.) and become parts of the new substance into which they are absorbed, and increase its bulk.

As such they cannot be even merely potentially perceptible as parts of the substance to which they belonged originally. They are, no doubt, potentially perceptible parts of the new substance but, if they have lost their εἶδος, as Aristotle says in *De Gen. et Corr., loc. cit.*, they cannot be on the same footing as elements which have entered into a true mixture and which, on resolution of the mixture, become actually what they were before.

These considerations make it clear that, when in l. 11 ἡ τῆς αἰσθήσεως ὑπεροχή is mentioned, Aristotle means the minute sensation which can be even potentially *per se* perceptible only when coming from a part of the object which is *not* separated from the whole. He argues—the minute αἴσθησις which has only existence in a more distinct sensation (ἐν τῇ ἀκριβεστέρᾳ) and, as such, is only potentially in its individuality a sensation, is not *per se* actually perceptible and hence capable of isolation ; hence the similarly minute object of sense (τὸ τηλικοῦτον αἰσθητόν), which causes it, must be in the same case. It is not *per se* actually perceptible, but added to and taken along with the other parts of the whole it is actually perceptible and, since that is so, it, even in its individuality, must be thought of as being only potentially an object of sense.

It is, I suppose, προσγενόμενον (l. 16) which has prompted some interpreters to think that Aristotle is considering the fortunes of the minute part of the grain of millet in actual isolation. But, if it were *per se* potentially perceptible when in actual isolation from the whole to which it belongs, one would expect that the change caused by addition to the whole would be to raise it, as such, to actual perceptibility; but this Aristotle will not allow. προσγενόμενον, as we see from l. 20 below and *Phys.* 250 a 24, just means ἐν τῷ ὅλῳ. There is no reason why it should not be used of intellectual as well as of actual addition.

τὸ αἰσθητὸν χωριστὸν αἰσθάνεσθαι (l. 14) does not imply that the αἰσθητόν exists χωρίς; it means, practically, to perceive it καθ᾽ αὑτό. Similarly things that exist χωρίς—χωριστά—are identified with οὐσίαι, the independent existences which are the subjects of predication, and which Aristotle in *Anal. Post.* I. ch. 4, 73 b 9 calls καθ᾽ αὑτά. Cf. *Metaph.* VII. ch. 3, 1029 a 28: τὸ χωριστὸν καὶ τὸ τόδε τι ὑπάρχειν δοκεῖ μάλιστα τῇ οὐσίᾳ.

We can easily explain the substitution of χωρισθῇ for μὴ χωρὶς ᾖ by an editor who read on and found that χωρίς the minute parts of objects were not actually perceptible, and indeed could not exist and retain their previous character, if his logic led him to believe that 'if not separate then not actually perceptible' contradicted the statement 'if separate not perceived' (χωριζόμεναι κ.τ.λ.). Such statements are only apparently in opposition. If we retain χωρισθῇ, we shall have to translate 'they are potentially perceptible but not, when in isolation, actually so. [This is different from the case of] the one-foot measure which exists potentially in the two-foot rule and actually when bisection is made.' But the ellipse to be supplied is so extraordinary that one might justly, with Biehl, suspect the authenticity of the whole clause if χωρισθῇ is to be read. Its genuineness, if we adopt the better attested reading, is confirmed by the force of καὶ γὰρ. Aristotle is pointing out that even in the case of large objects like the one-foot rule the same thing holds good as of τὰ μικρὰ πάμπαν.

446 a 8. διαιρεθεῖσα is here equivalent to ἀφαιρεθεῖσα if it is to make any sense. It is not the one-foot rule which is bisected but the two-foot measure. Hence one would expect διαιρεθείσῃ (Bywater, *J. of P.* XVIII. p. 243) or διαιρεθείσης ταύτης. But perhaps this sense of διαιρεῖν is idiomatic. Cf. note to ch. 3, 439 b 20 διελομένους.

446 a 9. καὶ διαλύοιντο. *In addition* to being so very minute as to surpass (ὑπερέχειν) the discrimination of the sense, these minute particles lose their self-identity on being isolated.

ὑπεροχή is, as the commentators notice, employed in rather a different sense from the usual. It naturally means excess in greatness: cf. chapter 3, 439 b 31.

For the doctrine cf. *De Gen. et Corr.* I. ch. 10, 328 a 24 sqq.: ὅσα εὐδιαίρετα, πολλὰ μὲν ὀλίγοις καὶ μεγάλα μικροῖς συντιθέμενα οὐ ποιεῖ μίξιν, ἀλλ' αὔξησιν τοῦ κρατοῦντος· μεταβάλλει γὰρ θάτερον εἰς τὸ κρατοῦν, οἷον σταλαγμὸς οἴνου μυρίοις χοεῦσιν ὕδατος οὐ μίγνυται· λύεται γὰρ τὸ εἶδος καὶ μεταβάλλει εἰς τὸ πᾶν ὕδωρ.

446 a 11. The minute fraction of substance in isolation from the rest is not perceptible at all. Aristotle goes on to discuss what happens when we do perceive it in some way—when ἐπελήλυθεν ἡ ὄψις.

446 a 12. δυνάμει γάρ. We are not now discussing the separate existence, but the separate perceptibility of the object—τὸ αἰσθητόν, but in the sensation (αἴσθησις) to exist and to be perceptible is the same; hence it is indifferent which of the two we assert to be potential.

446 a 18. ἐνυπάρχειν means practically to form a constituent; cf. *Metaph.* V. ch. 13, 1020 a 7: ποσὸν λέγεται τὸ διαιρετὸν εἰς ἐνυπάρχοντα and *Anal. Post.* I. ch. 22, 84 a 14 sqq.; 'odd' ἐνυπάρχει in the definition of number, while number ὑπάρχει—belongs to, or is a predicate of, odd. Cf. also the definition of ὕλη—ἐξ οὗ γίνεταί τι ἐνυπάρχοντος, etc., cf. Bonitz, *Ind.* p. 257. Hence it is probable that Aristotle is thinking of the μεγέθη which compose finite bodies as the subject here, as ἐνυπάρχειν is generally used of that which stands to anything in the relation of ὕλη.

Perhaps, however, he is thinking of χρώματα etc. as the subject. In that case the translation will run—'But when determinations of colour, taste or sound, existing in the concrete are so related to each other as to be also actually perceptible and perceptible, not merely in the whole but individually, they must be limited in number.'

This would mean that he is talking once more of the πεπερασμένα εἴδη of sense qualities. But they have already been accounted for, and this seems to touch on the only case left undescribed—the distinguishable parts of a continuum, which are ἐνεργείᾳ perceptible not merely in combination but in isolation. If this be the interpretation, the argument is that, in the case when the constituents of the objects perceived are distinct and individually perceptible and hence limited in number, the qualities presented by them must have the same limitation. χρώματα etc. are but items of sensuous determination, though, no doubt, Aristotle is thinking of the different colours and sounds etc., as presented in the form of segments in a continuum.

446 a 19 πρὸς αὐτά. Alexander reads τοσαῦτα which perhaps, if understood as meaning 'of sufficient size or intensity,' *i.e.* τοσαῦτα τὸ μέγεθος, improves the sense. We must not understand 'sufficiently numerous,' *i.e.* τοσαῦτα τὸ πλῆθος, as no multiplication of the numbers of the insensible parts of objects makes *the parts* any the more perceptible *per se.* πρὸς αὐτά can, however, quite well mean 'in relation to each other.' Cf. ἑαυταῖς below ch. 7, 447 b 32.

446 a 24. ὅταν ἐνεργῶσιν may be taken either with the clause before or with ἀφικνοῦνται.

τὸ μέσον = τὸ μεταξύ, which is defined in terms of this phenomenon in local movement in *Phys.* v. ch. 3, 226 b 23: μεταξὺ δὲ εἰς ὃ πέφυκε πρῶτον ἀφικνεῖσθαι τὸ μεταβάλλον, ἢ εἰς ὃ ἔσχατον μεταβάλλει κατὰ φύσιν συνεχῶς μεταβάλλον.

446 a 28. Ἐμπεδοκλῆς. Cf. *De An.* II. ch. 7, 418 b 20: καὶ οὐκ ὀρθῶς Ἐμπεδοκλῆς...ὡς φερομένου τοῦ φωτὸς καὶ τεινομένου ποτὲ μεταξὺ τῆς γῆς καὶ τοῦ περιέχοντος, ἡμᾶς δὲ λανθάνοντος.

Aristotle goes on to say that it is asking too much to wish us to believe that light passes from east to west across the whole sky without the movement being detected. It was, of course, impossible without modern scientific instruments and methods to discover the movement of light. For the Empedoclean theory cf. chapter 3. Cf. also *R. P.* § 177, Zeller's *Presocratic Phil.* (Eng. Trans.), II. p. 158. According to Philoponus, on this theory light was a σῶμα issuing from the illuminating body, *vide* below 446 b 30.

446 a 32. ποθέν ποι. Cf. *Metaph.* XII. ch. 2, 1069 b 26 and *Nic. Ethics*, X. ch. 3, 1174 a 30, and *Phys.* VII. ch. 1, 242 a 31 : τὸ κινούμενον πᾶν ἔκ τινος εἰς τι κινεῖται.

446 b 1. Time is infinitely divisible like motion and magnitude; cf. *Phys.* IV. chs. 11, 12 ; VI. 1, 2, 3 etc. ; VIII. ch. 8, 263 b 27 : οὐχ οἷόν τε εἰς ἀτόμους χρόνους διαιρεῖσθαι τὸν χρόνον.

446 b 3. ἅμα κ.τ.λ. This is equivalent to saying it is instantaneous. An act of perception is in this characteristic distinct from local movement, which cannot be instantaneous : cf. *Phys.* VI. ch. 1, 231 b 30: εἰ Θήβαζέ τις βαδίζει, ἀδύνατον ἅμα βαδίζειν Θήβαζε καὶ βεβαδικέναι Θήβαζε. Perception is an ἐνέργεια, which as such has no γένεσις : cf. Alex. *De Sens.* p. 126 (W.) and above, Introduction, sec. IV.

446 b 5. The construction here seems to be defective. As I have translated, instead of οὐδὲν ἧττον, οὐδὲν μᾶλλον should have been written ; but it was natural to say ἧττον when denying that they *possessed* the aspect of process any the less on account of the instantaneousness of the act of perception considered as a psychical event. Perhaps, indeed, Aristotle wrote μᾶλλον, for which by a blunder ἧττον was substituted ; or he may have written ἀλλ' οὐκ εἰσιν.

Thomas and Simon, however, punctuate after γίγνεσθαι, making the apodosis begin at ὅμως. In this case we must regard δηλοῖ... ἀέρα, ll. 7–10, as a parenthesis and translate from l. 4 καὶ μή κ.τ.λ.—'and if sensations have no genesis, but exist without coming to be, yet, as sound, etc...., is not the same true of colour and light?' Cf. *Phys.* VIII. ch. 6, 258 b 17, *De Coelo*, I. ch. 11, 280 b 27.

Aristotle means that the instantaneousness of the psychic act does not detract from the lapse of time in the physical process. Though there is no γένεσις in the former, there is in the latter. Hammond conjectures ὁμοίως for ὅμως and translates, 'Also if everything at the same moment hears and has heard, and in a word perceives and has perceived, and there is no time process in sensations, nevertheless they lack this process in the same way in which sound, after the blow has been struck, has not yet reached the ear.' But I fail to see how a sound which is on its passage to the ear can be said to 'lack process' and how, if this were so, it would help Aristotle's argument. Moreover Aristotle does not say that we are unaware of the lapse of time which takes place while a sound is being transmitted. He implies the opposite. He only says that in the psychical act there is no process.

446 b 8. μετασχημάτισις is a change of shape: cf. *De Coelo*, II. ch. 7, 305 b 29 (γίγνεσθαι) τῇ μετασχηματίσει, καθάπερ ἐκ τοῦ αὐτοῦ κηροῦ γίγνοιτ' ἂν σφαῖρα καὶ κύβος. μετασχηματίζεσθαι is also conjoined with (though differentiated from) ἀλλοιοῦσθαι. It consists in the rearrangement of elements which retain the same nature, while ἀλλοιοῦσθαι indicates qualitative change.

μετασχηματίζεσθαι is that form of γένεσις that would specially suit an atomic theory and hence Aristotle applies it to the propagation of sound, which he conceives of in quite a mechanical way. He evidently thinks of the air taking on a different σχῆμα for every different articulate sound. These are subject to alteration in proportion to the distance we are from the person with whom we are talking. He is evidently thinking mainly of mistakes in following some one's words, not merely of inability to hear at all. That would rather be accounted for by the absence of definite σχῆμα than by change of σχῆμα in the air which communicates the motion or in the motion transmitted.

446 b 11. τῷ πως ἔχειν. Alexander interprets—τῷ κατὰ σχέσιν εἶναι. He distinguishes three classes of relata:

(1) Those which are κατὰ σχέσιν, *e.g.* ἴσα, ὅμοια etc., in which the mode of their relation (the σχέσις) does not depend upon their relative position in space.

(2) Those which are κατὰ σχέσιν, but where the σχέσις consists in spatial relation (ἐν ποιᾷ θέσει), *e.g.* δεξιόν.

(3) Those, *e.g.* αἴσθησις and αἰσθητόν, which, though requiring some σχέσις which consists in spatial relation (οὐχ...ᾧ μηδὲν αὐτῇ (sc. τῇ ὄψει) διαφέρειν τὴν θέσιν τῶν ὁρωμένων καὶ τὸ διάστημα πρὸς τὸ ὁρᾶν) are not strictly ἐν σχέσει, like τὸ δεξιόν, but require a δύναμις ἀντιληπτική on the part of the αἴσθησις. Light might travel from object to eye on account of the spatial relation of the two, but vision would not result unless the eye were endowed with a certain faculty. This, in the minds of certain other commentators, *e.g.* Simon and

Thomas, seems to connect with the distinction drawn between certain classes of relata in *Metaph.* v. ch. 15, 1020 b 26 sqq.

In this chapter there are likewise three main divisions of relata:

(1) τὰ κατ᾽ ἀριθμὸν λεγόμεια, e.g. τὰ ἴσα. Things are equal of which the quantity is *one* (ἴσα δὲ ὧν τὸ ποσὸν ἕν, 1021 a 12).

(2) τὰ κατὰ δύναμιν λεγόμενα, e.g. τὸ θερμαῖνον πρὸς τὸ θερμαινόμενον.

(3) Such as τὸ ἐπιστητόν and ἐπιστήμη, αἰσθητόν and αἴσθησις.

In the first two classes (cf. Bonitz, *Metaph.* p. 261) the whole notion of the relata can be discovered in the relation. *A* is understood by being referred to *B*, and *B* by being referred to *A*. In the third class, however, the relation is not mutual; one of the terms requires independent explanation; τὸ αἰσθητόν can be ·explained by referring αἴσθησις to it, but αἴσθησις requires other definition than reference to τὸ αἰσθητόν. We advance no further by saying that vision is relative to those things of which there is vision, δὶς γὰρ ταὐτὸν εἰρημένον ἂν εἴη (1021 a 32).

Aristotle's meaning, however, is no more than this, that ὄψις is not explained by being regarded as relative to τὸ ὁρώμενον, but if we refer it to χρῶμα it can very well be defined and we obviate any useless repetition. Hence the distinction does not affect the real relation of the object of vision (χρῶμα) to vision (ὄψις), but only the mental way of relating them when the former is styled not χρῶμα but the object of vision—τὸ ὁρώμενον.

Thus there is no justification for Simon's attempt to connect this distinction with that here. He says, the 'ratio' in a relation of this kind *pendet ab alio*, and hence there must be activity on the part of τὸ αἰσθητόν which, hence, must be at a distance.

Nor is there necessarily a reference to the δύναμις ἀντιληπτική of sense, as Alexander conjectures.

Aristotle simply states that seer and thing seen must occupy definite positions; their relation must depend to some extent at least upon their relative θέσις. They are not like things of which the relation is purely non-spatial like equals. It is not the *manner* and *mode* of their being which relates them, as in the case of equal quantities, but something else which entails a definite spatial position.

We cannot translate πως purely indefinitely as 'anyhow.' Things that are equal do not exist 'anyhow' but 'somehow.'

The result of the argument is to establish the necessity of determinate spatial position for seer and thing seen and hence it advances a plea in favour of the transmission of light in the same way as sound is carried to the ear. The last argument had shown that the object which sounds and the hearer must be in determinate spatial positions.

446 b 12. If we do not read ἄν before ἔδει the clause will refer to ἴσα not to τὸ ὁρῶν καὶ τὸ ὁρώμενον, and becomes identical in meaning with the following one and πως above will have to be translated as 'utcunque.' 'It is not by being *anywhere* etc.' But this is not possible.

446 b 16. The air which is ψαθυρός (as water also is: cf. above ch. 4, 441 a 28) is *made* continuous by being struck by an object that is smooth of surface and so continuous; it is thus that sound is transmitted : cf. *De An.* II. ch. 8 *passim.* Sound is caused by a movement (a blow, which involves φορά or spatial movement, occasions it, cf. 419 b 10–13) which is quick enough to strike the air and make it continuous. If the movement is too slow the air disperses (419 b 20 sqq.). It is hard and smooth bodies which, when struck, have this effect upon the air, though apparently the air itself when imprisoned in any closed or partially closed space can function in the same way—as in the case of the echo (419 b 25 sqq.).

Sound is this movement (ἔστι γὰρ ὁ ψόφος κίνησις τοῦ δυναμένου κινεῖσθαι τὸν τρόπον τοῦτον ὄνπερ τὰ ἀφαλλόμενα ἀπὸ τῶν λείων, ὅταν τις κρούσῃ, 420 a 21), or rather this movement is sound, for Aristotle does not, like the modern physicists, think of sound as being merely a movement when outside the ear; its peculiar quality seems to exist objectively though entirely relative to the act of hearing (cf. Introduction, sec. IV. and *De An.* III. ch. 2, 425 b 26 sqq.).

At the same time it will not do to go so far as Rodier (*Traité de l'Âme*, Vol. II. p. 286) and say that sound is not to be identified with the motion that causes it but is an objective quality in the same way as, according to Aristotle, colour is to be regarded, and that its transmission to the ear is not a movement any more than the transmission of light is.

(Rodier appears to me to misunderstand μετασχημάτισις; it (cf. note to 446 b 8) is not qualitative change and, even if it were, his argument would not be advanced any the further. Aristotle distinctly says above (l. 10) that, in the transmission of sound, the air experiences φορά, and if in 7–10 Aristotle were describing the increase in faintness in sound (which he is not) it would be only caused by a transition of the air from a state of motion to some other condition.)

At the same time there is a difficulty here. In the *De Anima* Aristotle describes the φορά, the movement which causes us to hear, as a rebound and quivering of the air all in one mass—ὥστε τὸν ἀέρα ἀθροῦν ἀφάλλεσθαι καὶ σείεσθαι (420 a 25) and again in 420 a 1 he says τότε δὲ (when struck) εἰς γίνεται ἅμα. That would make this φορά have the same characteristics as that species of ἀλλοίωσις which, below, in 446 b 32 sqq., he wishes to distinguish from φοραί (and among them the φορά which constitutes sound) as being instantaneous — ἐνδέχεται γὰρ ἀθρόον ἀλλοιοῦσθαι, καὶ μὴ τὸ ἥμισυ πρότερον, οἷον τὸ ὕδωρ ἅμα πᾶν πήγνυσθαι (447 a 2 sqq.). It seems then that in the *De An.* Aristotle is simply emphasising the assertion that the air is rendered one and continuous throughout the whole extent of the space between the sonorous object and the ear—ἑνὸς ἀέρος συνεχείᾳ μέχρις ἀκοῆς. ἀθροῦν need mean no more than this; but ἅμα, if by ἅμα is meant 'at the same moment' (*vide* Rodier, *ad loc. cit.*), is putting the point too strongly. Here he plainly affirms that though the medium is continuous, the movement (in which it becomes continuous) falls into successive parts, just as qualitative change may also betray succession, as appears from the passage below and *Phys.* VII. chs. 4 and 5 esp. 250 a 31 sqq.: καὶ τὸ ἀλλοιοῦν καὶ τὸ ἀλλοιούμενον ὡσαύτως τὶ καὶ ποσὸν κατὰ τὸ μᾶλλον καὶ ἧττον ἠλλοίωται, καὶ ἐν ποσῷ χρόνῳ, ἐν διπλασίῳ διπλάσιον κ.τ.λ.

It is indeed necessary to grant this, as ὀσμή is an ἀλλοίωσις and occupies successive times in propagation.

446 b 17–18. τὸ αὐτὸ κ.τ.λ. On a theory which reduced all the senses to ἀφή this could not be so; each person would perceive only the tangible things that impinged upon his own sense organs.

ἔστι μὲν ὡς...ἔστι δ' ὡς. This continually means 'in one sense...and another' not 'at one time and at another' as Bender and Hammond take it. Cf. *Meteor.* III. ch. 6, 378 a 32 and cf. πῶς μὲν ... πῶς δὲ, *Phys.* III. ch. 6, 206 a 13, πῶς...πῶς above 446 a 17–18; cf. also *Phys.* VIII. ch. 8, 263 b 5, etc.

If the κίνησις has μέρη, then the πρῶτος is in contact with one μέρος, ὁ ὕστερος with another. Hence in one sense it is not τὸ αὐτό which they perceive.

446 b 19. ἀπορία. Hammond seems to regard this as a new problem. But τούτων naturally refers to what has just been said.

R. 14

446 b 20. There is no need for adding 'in the same way' as Hammond does; ἄλλῳ cannot bear such a meaning. The doctrine controverted is the unqualified assertion that the same thing can be perceived by only one person. It seems to be an echo of nominalism. It was left to Aristotle to resolve the difficulty by pointing out that there are different ways of perceiving the same thing.

446 b 25–26. τοῦ δὲ δὴ ἰδίου. Alexander explains this as τὸ προσεχὲς καὶ ἴδιον μέρος τοῦ ἀέρος ἢ τοῦ ὕδατος, and so Simon also. It is the part of the medium in contact with the sense organ—what he might have called τὸ ἔσχατον κινούμενον (cf. *De An.* III. ch. 12, 434 b 33) as opposed to the sense object which is τὸ πρῶτον κινοῦν (ἔσχατον can, however, be used in both senses, that of nearest and of farthest; cf. *Phys.* VII. ch. 2, 244 b 1 sqq. and *De Gen. et Corr.* I. ch. 7, 324 a 26 sqq.). The meaning is, that this nearest part of the medium is numerically different in each case, though it is qualitatively identical in all; the qualitative change or motion produced in the medium by propagation outward from the sense object must be numerically a different πάθος or a different μέρος of the κίνησις when issuing to the right and to the left and when near and far, but it is of the same kind. Aristotle, it must be remembered, thinks of the sense quality, and that is to him an αἰσθητόν, as existing objectively in the medium. The word to be supplied after ἰδίου is no doubt αἰσθητοῦ and, as a sense quality is an αἰσθητόν to him, perhaps he is thinking of τοῦ ἰδίου more as quality—the quality relative to the special sense, than as the portion of the medium which is nearest. We might paraphrase his meaning thus—'The qualitative affection of sense proper (ἰδία αἴσθησις) is numerically different for each person though specifically, *i.e. quâ* quality, identical, while an object numerically one and identical is perceived by all.' ἀριθμός and ἕν are among the contributions of κοινὴ αἴσθησις. Hence perhaps Aristotle is obscurely hinting that, as ἰδία αἴσθησις gives an object numerically different in each individual, it is the function of κοινὴ αἴσθησις to introduce numerical identity and hence real objectivity into the perceptible world.

446 b 26–27. ἅμα πολλοί. This is an additional point; if perception is due to κίνησις of the medium, and numerical difference in the κίνησις directly affecting the sense does not necessitate difference of τὸ πρῶτον κινοῦν, perception of it—τὸ πρῶτον κινοῦν—may be simultaneous in different people.

446 b 28. If sound etc. were σώματα then, in perception, the object would really be 'divided from itself' as a body can only be in one place at the same time. According to the ἀπόρροιαι theory, the sound, scent and light *are* σώματα—material particles.

446 b 29. οὐδ' ἄνευ σώματος, *i.e.* the κίνησις or ἀλλοίωσις which is propagated in different parts must be the πάθος of a σῶμα (which has μόρια). The plurality of the sense experiences depends upon the medium having μόρια and hence being a σῶμα. Thus this sentence refers merely to what goes before. As we shall see it makes no sense if taken with what follows.

446 b 30. τῷ ἐνεῖναι γάρ τι φῶς ἐστίν. I have here followed Alexander and cod. P, as no other reading seems to give an adequate meaning. Alexander connects this with the doctrine in *De An.* II. ch. 7, 418 b 16 sqq. where light is defined as the παρουσία...πυρὸς ἢ τοιούτου τινός. Cf. also above ch. 3, 439a 21 sq.: ὅταν γὰρ ἐνῇ τι πυρῶδες ἐν διαφανεῖ, ἡ μὲν παρουσία φῶς. The argument, then, is, that though light is due to the presence of something, yet it is not, as one might expect, a movement set up by it. It is hence, if not a movement, an ἐνέργεια as said before (418 b 9). ἐνέργεια in the proper sense is not κίνησις (cf. *De An.* II. ch. 5, 417 a 16) nor even ἀλλοίωσις. Compare also *Phys.* VII. ch. 3, 246 a 10 where it is said that bodily and mental ἕξεις are not ἀλλοιώσεις. Light is described as a ἕξις in *De An.* II. ch. 7, 418 b 19 and III. ch. 5, 430 a 15. The change from δύναμις to ἐνέργεια in the proper sense is not mere alteration from one quality to its opposite, but is a movement ἐπὶ τὰς ἕξεις καὶ τὴν φύσιν. A positive ἕξις like virtue is a τελείωσις, or state which reveals the true nature of the thing which possesses it. It is Alexander's contention that light is something of this kind and is not to be described as an ἀλλοίωσις like odour. Hence it does not require time for its propagation. Cf. Introduction, sec. VII.

If we read τῷ εἶναι we shall have to render with the vet. tr.—'per esse enim aliquod lumen est' which Thomas expands into—'per unum aliquod esse, id est, per hoc quod totum medium sicut unum mobile, movetur uno motu a corpore illuminante.' Or else we must suppose that there is some contrast between being and motion. This, however, is not an Aristotelian doctrine, though there were other theories which identified motion with τὸ μὴ ὄν: cf. *Phys.* III. ch. 2, 201 b 20: ἔνιοι, ἑτερότητα καὶ ἀνισότητα καὶ τὸ μὴ ὂν φάσκοντες εἶναι τὴν κίνησιν.

Bender (p. 29) renders 'das Licht ist Licht durch ein gewisses Sein,' which seems to require some such explanation as the above.

St Hilaire (p. 81) gives rather a different interpretation. Light exists because it is 'un être particulier.' Hammond (p. 184) seems to follow him in rendering 'Light has a substantial nature.' εἶναί τι may mean to be an οὐσία—something χωριστόν. Cf. *Phys.* IV. ch. 6, 213 a 31—οὔκουν τοῦτο δεῖ δεικνύναι, ὅτι ἔστι τι ὁ ἀήρ. But, if it meant that here, it would imply that light was something concrete, a σῶμα, which it is not. To imagine, then, that Aristotle here declares that light is a σῶμα as opposed to sound and smell which he has just declared not to be σώματα, is quite unwarranted and besides it does not in the least help us to understand how the transmission of light is instantaneous.

Perhaps we might translate τῷ εἶναι (it should possibly be τὸ εἶναι) as frequently elsewhere (cf. 449 a 19) by 'in aspect' and render 'In aspect light is something real' *i.e.* 'light may be regarded as something real'; it is not concrete—οὐσία—in the ordinary sense, but οὐσία ὡς εἶδος (as the soul is said to be in *De An.* II. ch. 2, 414 a 13 sqq.). Light is an εἶδος or ἐνέργεια. If this be the interpretation and we adhere to the reading τῷ εἶναι it will give exactly the same meaning as Alexander requires, who gets it by other means.

The difficulty remaining, however, is how what is said in the first clause should lead one to expect that light is a movement. The presence of οὐ in the ἀλλά clause gives the Greek this sense. On Alexander's reading there is some ground for expecting light to be a κίνησις, which it is then denied to be; not so much according to my interpretation of the other reading.

I suggest τῷ κινεῖν γάρ τι φῶς ἐστίν τι, *i.e.* light shows its reality by stimulating something. Light κινεῖ—stimulates—something—τι—viz. the sense, but is not a movement itself.

446 b 31. ἀλλ' οὐ κίνησις. The question here is—What does Aristotle mean by κίνησις? Does he mean 'un simple mouvement' (St Hilaire) *i.e.* φορά, or motion generically, *i.e.* μεταβολή? It is quite impossible, from Aristotle's use of the term, to decide whether he employs it here in its specific or its generic signification. In the *Physics* κίνησις is continually used in the sense of φορά but, where he has occasion to distinguish the various kinds of change, he employs the specific terms if there is any likelihood of confusion arising. Cf.

Phys. III. ch. 1 for the distinction between the four kinds of change—γένεσις καὶ φθορά, ἀλλοίωσις, αὔξησις καὶ φθίσις, φορά. They are divided according to the categories respectively of οὐσία, ποιόν, ποσόν and ποῦ, which have nothing in common. Hence the diversity alluded to here—ὅλως κ.τ.λ. l. 31. If the light is to be identified as a kind of ἀλλοίωσις, as Thomas thinks, then this latter statement is brought forward in support of the former. The argument runs— light is an ἀλλοίωσις, which may be (cf. below 447 a 1–2) instantaneous, and hence not φορά and hence not κίνησις, for κίνησις *proper* is φορά. Cf. *Phys.* VIII. ch. 7, where it is contended that φορά is πρώτη τῶν κινήσεων.

On the other hand, as we have seen, if Aristotle is in earnest about light being an ἐνέργεια, it cannot be even ἀλλοίωσις. This is Alexander's contention and according to his interpretation, ὅλως... φορᾶς must come as a reply to a possible objection—'Is it not true that ἀλλοίωσις is different from φορά, *i.e.* κίνησις κατὰ τόπον, and that hence light may be an ἀλλοίωσις?' Aristotle replies 'It is true that they are distinct, for ἀλλοίωσις may take place in all parts at once ; however (οὐ μὴν ἀλλ᾽, 447 a 3 sq.), when the quantity is large (of substance to be changed) this is impossible. Hence light is not an ἀλλοίωσις and hence not a κίνησις at all.'

As against this theory and in support of the former view we have these statements in the *De Anima*, viz.—the medium κινεῖται by the object of vision and again itself κινεῖ the sense. There κίνησις is apparently used vaguely in its generic sense without distinction from ἀλλοίωσις, so that it seems necessary to hold that, if, in the stimulation of the sense by the object of vision, a κίνησις, in the strict sense of φορά, is not set up in the medium, at least ἀλλοίωσις is. Cf. *De An.* II. ch. 7, 419 a 13 sqq. : ἀλλὰ τὸ μὲν χρῶμα κινεῖ τὸ διαφανές, οἷον τὸν ἀέρα, ὑπὸ τούτου δὲ συνεχοῦς ὄντος κινεῖται τὸ αἰσθητήριον ; III. ch. 12, 434 b 30 sqq. : ὥσπερ γὰρ τὸ κινοῦν κατὰ τόπον...οὕτω καὶ ἐπ᾽ ἀλλοιώσεως and 435 a 4 : ὁ δ᾽ ἀὴρ ἐπὶ πλεῖστον κινεῖται καὶ ποιεῖ καὶ πάσχει...βέλτιον...τὸν ἀέρα πάσχειν ὑπὸ τοῦ σχήματος καὶ χρώματος...διὸ πάλιν οὗτος τὴν ὄψιν κινεῖ. Cf. also *Phys.* VII. ch. 2, 244 b 10 sqq. esp. 245 a 6.

The explanation of the difficulty seems to be that Aristotle regards light in two different ways which are not properly reconciled. (1)· According to his own peculiar conception it is the ἐνέργεια τοῦ διαφανοῦς caused by the presence of fire. This is the concept of the objective nature of light. It is a qualitative determination of certain objects and, considered as such, it has absolutely no connection with any such thing as motion or transmission. Light is the colour of the medium realised, its true activity, just as the soul is the true activity of the body. This is its teleological definition. But (2) Aristotle likewise inherited from previous philosophy and popular thought the theory that light was something passing between seen thing and seer or *vice versâ*. He allows that there must be some action whether mechanical or qualitative exerted by the object directly upon the medium and indirectly upon the sense.

According to the popular idea this exactly was light. So, when the question was raised—'does light take time to travel?,' Aristotle, if he had wished to identify light with the κίνησις or ἀλλοίωσις that stimulates sense, should have answered in the affirmative or admitted that it was at least possible. But, instead, he recoils upon the teleological definition of light to which the notion of movement is irrelevant. Hence his doctrine really is, not that it is an 'instantaneous movement' but rather (what that really is) no movement at all.

But, as his opponents mean by light a movement between the eye and the object, it appears as if, in denying that light is a movement, he were denying his own theory that an actual movement of some kind did take place between object and eye. Without doubt too there was a confusion in his own mind on the subject. His raising it in connection with sound and odour shows this. Naturally the fact that there is no noticeable interval between the production of any object and our seeing it led him practically to contradict his previous assertions.

447 a 2. ἀθρόον. Cf. *Phys.* I. ch. 3, 186 a 16 and VIII. ch. 3, 253 b 23 : οὐ γὰρ εἰ μεριστὸν εἰς ἄπειρον τὸ ἀλλοιούμενον, διὰ τοῦτο καὶ ἡ ἀλλοίωσις, ἀλλ᾽ ἀθρόα γίνεται πολλάκις, ὥσπερ ἡ πῆξις.

We cannot say that all qualitative change proceeds continuously (συνεχῶς) or is συνεχής in the full sense of the word which is explained in *Phys.* v. ch. 3, 226 b 27 sqq. It is not sufficient that the time should be continuous but that the action should be continuous also (μὴ τοῦ χρόνου (οὐδὲν γὰρ κωλύει διαλείποντα, καὶ εὐθὺς δὲ μετὰ τὴν ὑπάτην φθέγξασθαι τὴν νεάτην) ἀλλὰ τοῦ πράγματος, ἐν ᾧ κινεῖται). Themistius (Paraph. ad *Phys.*, *loc. cit.*) explains that movement such as the galloping of horses is not continuous, though the time in which the movement takes place is. Qualitative change seems to be more comparable to this and appears to take place by a series of successive bounds. There seem to be ultimate sections in the process which are instantaneous and not divisible into smaller sections each diverse in point of time.

So it is too with αὔξησις καὶ φθίσις. If a drop wears away so much of a stone in a given time, the half of it does not perform *so* much of the attrition in half the time. It does it in no time. What is washed away is divisible, but its parts were moved not separately but all together.

In *Phys.* vii. ch. 5, 250 a 28 sqq. it had been admitted (cf. above) that, in general, qualitative change falls into different time sections just like κίνησις proper, yet the half of the cause of change need not cause a change of half the extent. But this is true also of κίνησις proper. Though two men push a boat so far in a given time, one man need not be able to move it at all. The point here is different. It is, as said, that often change either in quality or bulk proceeds in sections.

447 a 3. πῆξις is congelation of any kind (cf. *Meteor.* iv. chs. 5–7) and is produced either by heating or cooling. θερμαίνεσθαι and ψύχεσθαι are examples of ἀλλοίωσις (cf. *Phys.* vii. ch. 3, 246 a 7 sqq.). Compare also *Phys.* 253 b 25 quoted above. By τὸ θερμαινόμενον καὶ πηγνύμενον (cf. note to 443 b 7 on the function of καὶ) no doubt the thickening of milk or some such substance by heat is indicated.

447 a 8. ὀσμή seems to be propagated by an ἀλλοίωσις and is admitted not to be instantaneous (l. 10 beneath). The instantaneousness of the sections of qualitative change does not make the ἀλλοίωσις as a whole instantaneous in this case. Obviously there is ' much ' to be changed. If light is conceived of as an ἀλλοίωσις, then the whole distance from object to eye must be thought of as being one section. How this can be reconciled with οὐ μὴν ἀλλ᾽ ἂν ᾖ πολὺ κ.τ.λ. it is difficult to see, for, if a considerable quantity of water cannot undergo qualitative alteration all in one moment, *a fortiori* the vast extent of medium intervening between eye and object should require a long time to transmit the light. If the words οὐ μὴν ἀλλ᾽ κ.τ.λ. only affect such qualitative changes as θέρμανσις, Aristotle should have pointed out in what respect those differ from the ἀλλοίωσις involved in light and should have ascribed the slowness of the change in these cases to those peculiarities. γεῦσις is brought in as a qualitative change too which would be perceived in the same way as odour if we were surrounded by water.

As we have seen, Aristotle does not distinguish between the diffusion of a quality in that which serves it as a vehicle and its transmission through a medium. The difference between the mediated sense qualities and the others is, that in the former their vehicle is a medium always in contact with the sense organs, while in the other cases it is not so. Special contact has to be effected between the body possessed of the quality and the sense. Hence one reason why the latter are both called tactual senses.

Aristotle's declaration here is interesting, because from it we may infer what we already know from ch. 4, 442 a 29 sqq., that he did not conceive even taste to be a diffusion of the actual particles of the flavoured substance, since he would not allow that to be the means of producing smell, and the only difference between taste and smell is due to the fact that we do not live in water.

Hence we must lay stress on the fact that diffusion is only a metaphorical term for the process by which odour and flavour alike are propagated; cf. 441 b 17 : ὥσπερ οὖν οἱ ἐναποπλύνοντες ; 443 b 7 sq. : οἷον ἀποπλυνόμενον ; 445 a 15 sq. : οἷον βαφή τις καὶ πλύσις.

447 a 9. μεταξύ. Cf. 445 a 8, 436 b 20, *De An.* III. ch. 12, 434 b 15 : αἱ γὰρ ἄλλαι αἰσθήσεις δι' ἑτέρων αἰσθάνονται, οἷον ὄσφρησις ὄψις ἀκοή, etc.

447 a 11–12. As we have seen, his customary way of stating the matter is, that χρῶμα causes sensation, while without φῶς, which is the ἐνέργεια of the medium, colour cannot stimulate the sense (*De An.* II. ch. 7 *passim*). That τὸ διαφανές should be illuminated is a precondition of the perception of colour. (Cf. Rodier, *op. cit.* Vol. II. p. 281.) In that sense it could be said ποιεῖν τὸ ὁρᾶν. From another point of view φῶς is the χρῶμα τοῦ διαφανοῦς and as such is the object of sense itself and ποιεῖ τὸ ὁρᾶν. Thus Aristotle might use this expression without thinking of light exactly as the κίνησις which produces sight (cf. above notes to 446 b 30 sqq.). τὸ αἰσθητόν means both the quality spread over the medium and τὸ πρῶτον κινοῦν itself. Cf. above note to 446 b 25 sq. But in so far as the sense object which causes sensation is a quality and hence an εἶδος and hence also an ἐνέργεια, process cannot be imputed to it. Though due to an ἀλλοίωσις it is not, itself, an ἀλλοίωσις ; it is an ἐνέργεια. But *all* sense qualities may be so regarded and hence there should be no grounds for supposing that in the case of one sense there was not to be found that process of transition by which the objective quality was realised in the particular consciousness in the case of the others.

CHAPTER VII.

447 a 15. ἀτόμῳ. Alexander explains that this is not an absolutely atomic time, for such according to Aristotle does not exist, but a time which, when divided, does not yield one part qualified by one sensation—another by another : cf. beneath 448 b 22.

447 a 16. ἐκκρούει. Cf. *De Gen. Animal.* v. ch. 1, 780 a 8, with reference to light stimuli, and for the general case *De Insom.* ch. 3, 460 b 32 sqq.

447 a 19. Cf. note to ch. 1, 436 a 5 for the interpretation of ὑποκείσθω.

μᾶλλον κ.τ.λ. This seems to be a self-evident principle with Aristotle, but perhaps it might be held to be in antagonism to such passages as *De An.* I. ch. 1, 402 b 21 sqq.: ἀλλὰ καὶ ἀνάπαλιν τὰ συμβεβηκότα συμβάλλεται μέγα μέρος πρὸς τὸ εἰδέναι τὸ τί ἐστιν. Aristotle would, however, distinguish between the two cases. The entering of one sensation into relation with another by means of combination alters the essential nature of the sensation. You no longer have the same sensation to investigate but a new one—a compound. Hence we may say that the original sensation may be more adequately perceived *per se* when in isolation than when in composition.

αἰσθάνεσθαι. αἴσθησις is a δύναμις κριτική (cf. *Anal. Post.* II. ch. 19, 99 b 35) and by it we recognise a thing as what it is. We must, as Alexander points out, remember that αἴσθησις has two aspects, one of πάθος the other of κρίσις. Its function as κρίσις is the function of mind in general and hence, as *e.g.* above in ch. 6, 445 b 16 sqq., we get the terms applicable to mind in general (κρινοῦμεν, γνωσόμεθα) applied in the special case of sense perception. Cf. also *De An.* III. ch. 9, 432 a 16 : τῷ τε κριτικῷ, ὃ διανοίας ἔργον ἐστὶ καὶ αἰσθήσεως.

447 a 23. τοῦτο, *i.e.* in the case of harmony when the two tones combine to form a third thing—a concord. Aristotle is arguing against the simultaneous perception of two things which remain diverse. His point is that, if they are to be perceptible at one and the same time, they must combine or, in some way, form a third thing. The combination is obvious in the case of harmonies.

εἰ δὴ κ.τ.λ. Aristotle goes on to argue that where the combination is not obvious, as it is in harmony, still the result of the simultaneous presentation of the two sensations must result in a modification of the stronger, if one is stronger than the other.

447 a 30. ὅπερ κ.τ.λ. Aristotle is arguing from the case of the objective mixture of things to the intermingling of subjective sensations. He may do this in virtue of his realism. To a modern sensationalist who holds that complex things are simply fused sensations this would not be possible; the argument would need to run the other way. For Aristotle's doctrine of μίξις cf. notes to ch. 3, 440 a 30 sqq.

447 a 31. ἐν ᾧ ἂν μιχθῶσιν. Alexander explains that he is excluding such cases as those mentioned in ch. 6, 446 a 8 sqq. where there is no proper mixture but an absorption of a minute volume of one thing into the substance of the other. ἐφ᾽ ᾧ would give the sense required more easily than ἐν ᾧ.

447 b 1. τοιαῦτα. Cf. below also in 449 a 6 sqq. esp. l. 9: οὐδὲν γὰρ ἐκ τούτων ἕν.

τούτων = objects of different senses. There is no qualitative union such as occurs in the combination of tones and, on his theory, of colours, tastes etc.; the union is κατὰ συμβεβηκός—co-existence in one thing (τὸ αὐτὸ καὶ ἐν ἀριθμῷ, l. 16). How the perception of such union is possible is discussed in that passage and in *De An.* III. ch. 2, 426 b 8—427 a 16.

μίγνυνται κ.τ.λ. Cf. *De Gen. et Corr.* I. ch. 10, esp. 328 a 32.

447 b 3. κατὰ συμβεβηκός. This is a case in which the perception of the object of one special sense may be effected indirectly, through the instrumentality of another. Cf. *De An.* III. ch. 1, 425 a 30 sqq.: τὰ δ᾽ ἀλλήλων ἴδια κατὰ συμβεβηκὸς αἰσθάνονται αἱ αἰσθήσεις,...οἷον χολὴ ὅτι πικρὰ καὶ ξανθή. The union is union in one thing, not a qualitative union of the sensations.

447 b 4. αἰσθάνεσθαι. He is arguing once more from the absence of objective unity to the absence of subjective unity.

447 b 7. Reading ἐπεί with Biehl we should have to regard this clause as an explanation of the reason why we can argue *a fortiori* from the case of objects falling under a single sense to the case of heterogeneous senses. It is not a confirmation merely of the previous clause.

If we read ἔτι with Alexander and L S U, the sequence of the argument is not so clear, but the possibility of connecting this with the previous clause too intimately is removed.

447 b 10. κίνησις. By the κίνησις is indifferently meant either the sense affection or the stimulus. We may therefore translate—'the stimuli are more closely located.' This clause forms a premiss on which the previous one rests. It, itself, seems to be an accepted topical maxim which connects the possibility of simultaneous functioning with the physical connectedness of the two elements; they are both κινήσεις in the same organ and hence ἅμα in space. Aristotle means more than that they are *similar*, as Alexander interprets.

447 b 12. ἂν μὴ μιχθῇ. This contention—that if not combined two things cannot be simultaneously perceived, *i.e.* if simultaneously perceived then combined—is not proved by the clauses which immediately follow but by the section from καὶ εἰ μία l. 16—αὐτά l. 18. Lines 12–16 rather prove the simple converse—that, if combined, sensations are perceived ἅμα.

The argument runs—A mixture is a unit. Perception of a unit is unitary and a unitary perception occurs in a unitary time, *i.e.* ἅμα. For support of the statement that perception of a unit is unitary (*i.e.* the last premiss) we get ὅτι μιᾷ...δύναμιν μία in lines 14–16. The perception of a unit with which we are concerned, the perception that occurs in unitary time, is explicit perception (ἐνεργείᾳ) and the explicit perception of a unit is numerically one, *i.e.* unitary; it is of a specific unity that the potential perception is single.

(This is the very idea of ἐνέργεια—to be complete in one and the same moment, not to be a κίνησις which varies from moment to moment. Cf. *De An.* II. ch. 5, 417 a 16–17 and Rodier, *ad loc. cit.*)

447 b 15. ἑνὸς κ.τ.λ. By saying that it is of the specifically single that the implicit perception is one, Aristotle means that the perception of various white objects is specifically identical. It is the same qualitative affection; but actual perception is the perception of this particular white object here and now; it is numerically different from the perception of any other white object. It is only as a faculty that the sense of white colour is a unity and its unity is the specific unity of the various sensations of white. Again, relatively to black and white taken as numerical units the sense of sight itself is a specific unity.

447 b 16. καὶ εἰ. Here the proof of the proposition first laid down begins. The sequence of the argument is best seen by beginning at the other end—l. 22, μία δὲ ἡ δύναμις. We are, by agreement, considering the case of a single faculty, *e.g.* sight. The act of vision must occur in a unitary time—l. 21 μιᾶς γὰρ εἰσάπαξ κ.τ.λ.; when the faculty is single and the time a unit, the act of sense or vision must be unitary—l. 19, ἀλλὰ κατὰ μίαν δύναμιν. Going back to l. 16, καὶ εἰ μία κ.τ.λ., we find it further stated that if the act is single the objects perceived by it must be single. We still lack the completing premiss that if two things are perceived as one they must be combined. This is not explicitly stated unless, instead of ἄρα before μὴ in l. 18, we read γὰρ. If we read γὰρ we make the train of reasoning complete and much improve what is at best a very ill-arranged argument.

447 b 24. ἀδύνατον. Cf. above l. 7 and beneath 449 a 4.

447 b 27. Consciousness is here an adequate interpretation of ψυχή, though the term ψυχή has generally a wider meaning.

This sentence—φαίνεται γὰρ κ.τ.λ.—seems merely to support the argument generally or rather one of the previous statements viz., that if you perceive simultaneously it is a unit which must be perceived.

447 b 28. εἶδει. Alexander will have it that here Aristotle includes generic identity. The different qualities falling under one sense are specifically distinct, merely generically identical (cf. l. 30), and according to Alexander it is these which have their relative identity recognised by the same sense, while it is a single sense functioning in a certain manner which recognises actual specific identity. This latter contention is correct, but Alexander can hardly be right in saying that here generic identity is included in specific. The train of thought is rather as follows—Specific identity is perceived by a single sense functioning in a certain manner (cf. *De An.* III. ch. 1, 425 a 20: ἑκάστη γὰρ ἓν αἰσθάνεται αἴσθησις). 'I add the latter qualification,' says Aristotle, 'because a single sense without specifying the manner of its functioning merely recognises generic identity (the identity *e.g.* of black and white) not specific; (the function of a single sense is to discriminate the specifically diverse. Cf. *De An.* III. ch. 2, 426 b 8 sqq. esp. 10: καὶ κρίνει τὰς τοῦ ὑποκειμένου αἰσθητοῦ διαφοράς); but, in recognising various white things as white, *i.e.* as possessing specific identity, it operates in a definite different mode, and one other than that by which it recognises the contrary quality black. There is a corresponding difference of mode in which each sense recognises the corresponding positive qualities *e.g.* white and sweet, and the corresponding negative qualities like black and bitter.'

Thus the conclusion is, that it is the same sense functioning in a definite manner which is different in the case of each of two contraries, though corresponding in the various senses according as the contraries are ἕξεις or στερήσεις. As Alexander points out, numerical difference of the sensations can be discerned only by temporal difference of the perception, specific difference by the difference of the manner, generic by the difference of the sense faculty.

447 b 32. σύστοιχα. Cf. beneath 448 a 17–18, cf. Bonitz, *Ind.* p. 736 b 61, σύστοιχα 'ea sunt, quae in eadem serie continentur.' The 'series' (συστοιχία) need not be a genus; generally it is not. Aristotle here ranks the opposed qualities of all the generically different senses under the two heads of ἕξις and στέρησις. It is these which form the titles of the two series. Cf. *Metaph.* IV. ch. 2, 1004 b 27 : τῶν ἐναντίων ἡ ἑτέρα συστοιχία στέρησις. Cf. also the Pythagorean distinction of two συστοιχίαι, the one headed by τὸ πέρας the other by τὸ ἄπειρον. *Metaph.* I. ch. 5, 986 a 23 sqq.

(The use of συστοιχία in *Metaph.* X. 1054 b 35 and 1058 a 13 seems to be somewhat different.)

For the use of ἑαυταῖς cf. above ch. 6, 446 a 19 : πρὸς αὐτά.

448 a 2. ἔτι. This section further shows that the opposition of the κινήσεις of the respective sense affections which are specifically distinct makes simultaneous perception of them impossible.

448 a 3. ἅμα κ.τ.λ. Cf. *De An.* III. ch. 2, 426 b 29 : ἀλλὰ μὴν ἀδύνατον ἅμα τὰς ἐναντίας κινήσεις κινεῖσθαι τὸ αὐτὸ ᾗ ἀδιαίρετον καὶ ἐν ἀδιαιρέτῳ χρόνῳ. εἰ γὰρ γλυκύ, ὡδὶ κινεῖ τὴν αἴσθησιν ἢ τὴν νόησιν, τὸ δὲ πικρὸν ἐναντίως. This comes in the *De Anima* in a different connection ; there he is proving that there must be something unitary which distinguishes the opposed sense modifications, something which is only in aspect divisible (cf. beneath at the end of the chapter). Cf. also *De Coelo*, II. ch. 13, 295 b 14 : ἅμα δ' ἀδύνατον εἰς τἀναντία ποιεῖσθαι τὴν κίνησιν.

Alexander understands χρόνῳ after αὐτῷ (l. 4). The whole discussion, he thinks, is one about time. We are not at present raising the question of the unity of what perceives as in the *De Anima*. But this restriction of τῷ αὐτῷ to time is impossible. It must be one thing that is diversely affected if there is to be any controversy as to the possibility of the two affections being simultaneous (ἅμα). Aristotle denies as a general principle that they can be so.

448 a 7. τὰ μὴ ἐναντία. These are evidently the intermediate qualities. It is not quite clear whether the theory about them here is quite the same as that presented in earlier chapters. There they are held to be mixtures of the two extreme qualities and, if by saying that some can be assigned to one extreme, others to the other, Aristotle simply means that there is a greater proportion of the one element in one case, of the opposite one in another, then the two theories can be reconciled. This is Alexander's explanation.

On the other hand τὰ μεμιγμένα seem to be introduced in l. 10 as a fresh class and are explicitly illustrated only by musical examples.

But probably there is no real discrepancy between this chapter and previous ones. By τὰ μὲν and τὰ δὲ in l. 7 he probably refers to τὸ ξανθόν and τὸ φαιόν which are assigned to white and black respectively, ἁλμυρόν and λιπαρόν which are claimed by πικρόν and γλυκύ (cf. ch. 4, 442 a 18 sqq.); and by τὰ μεμιγμένα to the other qualities.

448 a 9–10. Though τὰ μεμιγμένα are illustrated only by musical examples, Alexander thinks that the words in which he describes the ratio between the components of these compounds make it evident that he is thinking of colours and tastes as being composed by the intermixture of various *amounts* of two original components. Cf. l. 13: ὁ μὲν πολλοῦ πρὸς ὀλίγον...14: ὁ δ' ὀλίγου πρὸς πολύ. But this is to confuse the matter. When Aristotle says it is impossible to perceive τὰ μεμιγμένα ἅμα, unless as one, he does not mean to repeat that we cannot perceive *their components* simultaneously unless as one. He has already said that contraries cannot be perceived simultaneously unless perceived as one, *i.e.* unless they form an intermediate colour, taste, etc. Aristotle is here asserting that we cannot perceive two *intermediate* colours simultaneously unless they coalesce.

448 a 10–11. τὸ διὰ πασῶν κ.τ.λ. By this Aristotle surely means the harmony of the fifth with the tonic and of octave with tonic. It is difficult to see how the different notes of the scale could be regarded as mixtures.

This is, in fact, the case in connection with which a difficulty is raised beneath in 448 a 21 sqq.

The chords in question are, in modern terms, composed of two sets of vibrations, one of which is in the case of the octave concord, twice as rapid, in the case of the fifth, $1\frac{1}{2}$ times that of the other.

448 a 12. εἰς λόγος. Aristotle's point is that two blended sounds, *e.g.* the chord of the fifth or the octave, themselves depend upon a relation between tones of different pitch and hence cannot themselves be simultaneously perceived unless they form a new combination. If they do there is a single ratio formed once more, but if not we shall have the impossible task of presenting together two incompatible relations, that of the fifth—3 to 2—*i.e.* odd to even—and that of the octave—2 to 1 or even to odd, and this is impossible.

The only difficulty left is to explain why Aristotle seems to identify the former relation with that of much to little and the latter with that of little to much. But probably he does not mean to identify them. The explanation will be, as Alexander suggests, that by the mention of the ratio of much to little he is indicating the composition of some mixed colour, *e.g.* red, which contains a large proportion of one quality, *e.g.* white, and, by the relation of little to much, another colour, in which the proportion of white is small compared with the other component.

Alexander and most of the commentators seem to think that Aristotle is in this passage discussing, not the simultaneous perception of qualities themselves composite but of the components in composite qualities. This (cf. note to ll. 9-10 above) is erroneous and makes them distort the sense and take ἔσται γὰρ ἅμα κ.τ.λ., l. 13, as explaining the οὕτως...γίνεται, l. 12, not the ἄλλως δ' οὔ. They would translate 'Thus and not otherwise we get a ratio between the extremes, for there will be in the one case the simultaneous presentation of the relation of odd to even, etc., in the other case of even to odd, etc.' As Alexander explains, Aristotle is referring to the difference of the single ratio in each case. But the point is, that the simultaneous presentation of two such diverse ratios is impossible. Besides, the other interpretation requires us to take ἅμα as applying *separately* to both clauses ὁ μὲν κ.τ.λ. and ὁ δ' ὀλίγου. But there is no sense in saying that the relation of odd to even is simultaneous; the simultaneity must apply to the two ratios.

In my interpretation I am on the whole in agreement with Hammond.

448 a 16. γένει. It is wrong to confuse specific and generic difference as Hammond does. The point is that, if specific difference renders simultaneous perception impossible, *a fortiori* generic does.

448 a 19. πλείον κ.τ.λ. We now proceed to a still wider divergence. Sweet and white, though heterogeneous, are still in the same συστοιχία; sweet and black lack even that connection. Torstrik's conjecture of τοῦ λευκοῦ for τοῦ μέλανος and τὸ μέλαν for τοῦ λευκοῦ weakens the sense. It makes this clause merely a deduction from the principle quoted above and not an advance on it. Bekker's reading of τὸ λευκόν for τοῦ λευκοῦ brings a perfectly irrelevant premiss into the argument.

τῷ εἴδει, deleted by Torstrik, is unnecessary and, if allowed to stand, can only be translated vaguely in the manner given. Still it is quite in Aristotle's manner to change readily from the restricted to the wider use of a technical term, and we must bear in mind the essential identity of the notion of εἶδος as species, and εἶδος as form. We might render—'in ideal content.'

448 a 21 sqq. The case cited is apparently not the simultaneous perception of two different chords but of the two tones in one concord. The theory put forward is that really the perception is not simultaneous but only apparently so. With the first part of the conclusion Aristotle does not disagree, if it be meant that the two tones cannot be heard together as two separate units. But, on the other hand, when they form a συμφωνία they have coalesced and are heard simultaneously. Thus his argument becomes an attack on the doctrine that the coalescence is not real but apparent merely.

448 a 23. φαίνονται. The contention is, that the union of tones is merely apparent, just as it was contended in the juxtaposition theory of colour in ch. 4, 440 a 22 sqq. that the union of elementary tints which produced an intermediate one was of the same nature— that it was effected by a mixture πρὸς αἴσθησιν merely (cf. notes *ad loc. cit.*). The means by which such an apparent union can be obtained is in both cases the same; it is owing to the interval between the sensations being imperceptible that this happens. Without this being granted the theory will not hold, and, accordingly, Aristotle proceeds to argue against the existence of a χρόνος ἀναίσθητος.

448 a 25. If the theory, that imperceptible moments of time exist, is true, it will be as possible to have simultaneous sensations of sound and colour as of different tones. But this conclusion is repugnant to Aristotle. Sensations of different senses cannot combine—hence cannot be simultaneously presented.

This is the first ground on which he rejects the theory.

448 a 26–28. We must remember the principle laid down in *Physics* IV. ch. 14, 223 a 16 sqq., that apart from ψυχή time cannot exist. Hence a time in which we are not conscious is not time. A χρόνος ἀναίσθητος is strictly a time *in* which we are not conscious, for, as Alexander points out, time is not perceived καθ' αὐτό but by means of the events which happen in it. Aristotle expresses this frequently when he says, *e.g. De Gen. et Corr.* II. ch. 10, 337 a 23, that time does not exist apart from change.

The argument here is derived from the continuity of time (cf. *Physics* IV. ch. 11, 219 a 13, etc.), which itself depends upon the continuity of the change apart from which it cannot exist. If in a single continuous time there are sections in which no consciousness occurs, the continuity of the consciousness will be broken; but, when one is continuously conscious, one is not aware of breaks.

Alexander apparently reads εἰ ὁρᾷ καὶ οὐκ αἰσθάνεται (l. 32), the latter words merely repeating the sense of λανθάνοι ἂν (l. 32).

Simon follows the reading καὶ οὐκ αἰσθάνεται καὶ αἰσθάνεται, which simply states more explicitly the contradiction implied above.

448 b 1. The ancient Latin version does not translate καὶ εἰ αἰσθάνεται (l. 33), nor does Alexander read it. It is probably a gloss. In that case we should have to remove the comma after ἔτι, making the sentence start with that word.

If we retain the clause, the sense will be—" But if there are no breaks in our consciousness and we still perceive whatever object is before us during the whole of the time even though certain sections of it are imperceptible, then we shall have to say that perception throughout any whole time is really always effected by perception in some part of it only." Thus, as Alexander says, we do not perceive this time ἁπλῶς καὶ κυρίως, but only indirectly. We do not perceive a whole as a whole. The argument then goes on to show how by subtracting the χρόνοι ἀναίσθητοι from any whole and from the remainder successively *ad infinitum*, you could show that no time, however small, was, *per se*, an object of consciousness.

448 b 2. πρᾶγμα. Bound up with and illustrative of the proof we have just outlined (note to 448 a 26–28) of the non-existence of insensible moments of time, there runs a parallel proof of the non-existence of insensible material magnitudes. Alexander explains their conjunction by making out that it is the supposed σώματα ἀναίσθητα καὶ ἀμερῆ which have motions in imperceptible times. These have already been disposed of in chapter 6 and in the *Physics* etc. But it is obvious that this proof which shows that there are no χρόνοι ἀναίσθητοι, will equally well get rid of σώματα ἀναίσθητα, indeed of insensible magnitudes of all kinds, for the discussion is carried on wholly in terms of μέγεθος.

Here the two cases are argued out concurrently, and so closely interwoven that they seem to get confused.

448 b 5. τὴν ὅλην. It is absurd to make this refer to τὴν γῆν (l. 8) as Bender and Hammond do. How can CB be taken away from the whole earth? Alexander correctly explains that Aristotle is illustrating both magnitudes, the temporal and the spatial, by a line AB, and the feminine inflection here refers to the γραμμή.

The contention of the whole passage leads to the conclusion that here, as in many cases, our text consists of notes either written for or taken from a lecture in which there were many cursory explanations and asides, which have not come down to us. Probably by this stage in the proof Aristotle had already drawn the line on something analogous to our blackboard, and this explains the sudden appearance of the feminine inflection in the adjective without the previous introduction of any feminine substantive for it to agree with.

If we make the apodosis begin at καὶ we must say that Aristotle implicitly, if not explicitly, identifies perception of a whole time with perception during a continuous time, *i.e.* during the whole of it. That is in fact what he means by the latter, and what he frequently expresses, *e.g.* in 448 b 2 by αἰσθάνεσθαι ἐν: cf. also l. 9 ἐν τῷ ἐνιαυτῷ = during a whole year, and ἐν ᾗ οὐκ ᾐσθάνετο l. 7, 448 a 29 ἐν συνεχεῖ χρόνῳ.

For this way of translating τῶν νῦν τούτων, cf. *Phys.* VI. ch. 6, 237 a 16, IV. ch. 10, 218 a 15.

448 b 7. In order to carry on the parallel proof affecting an extended magnitude he should have added to ἐν ᾗ, ἢ ἧς. The reference to the extended magnitude appears once more, however, in the next clause—ἢ ταύτης τι.

448 b 8. ἐν ταύτης τινὶ ἢ ταύτης τι. We must remember that the same line is representing indifferently either a temporal or a spatial magnitude.

τὴν γῆν κ.τ.λ. Simon and St Hilaire rightly say that this is the *reductio ad absurdum* of the theory that, by perceiving a part, we can perceive the whole. On this interpretation we must render ἐν τῷ ἐνιαυτῷ—during the whole year, 'totum annum,' Simon, p. 257.

Alexander does not give quite the same interpretation. He thinks that ὥσπερ τὴν γῆν is an illustration of how we may have indirect (κατὰ μέρος) perception of a whole. We may, in an improper and unqualified way (ἁπλῶς), say that we perceive the whole earth by perceiving a part, or assign the Olympic contest to such and such a year because it occurs in a certain time falling within the year.

Whichever interpretation we follow, the result is the same. Such perception is only indirect perception of a whole, not of a whole *per se*, and, if there are imperceptible moments, it alone is possible, and we can never have perception of a whole as a whole.

448 b 10. οὐδὲν αἰσθάνεται. This is doubtless put in as a reply to an objection that the line AB by which he was illustrating was perceived as a whole

(A_____C |___B).

He reminds the objector that they have agreed that CB shall represent an imperceptible part.

448 b 14. ἅπαντα μὲν οὖν κ.τ.λ. We must understand that the conclusion reached in the previous clause is rejected. For the doctrine cf. chapter 6, 445 b 30 sqq. where he shows that the minute parts of objects, though not *per se* actually perceptible, are still perceptible ἐνεργείᾳ in the whole, *i.e.* when taken in conjunction with the other parts, and that even *per se* they are potentially perceptible (446 a 15 sq.: δυνάμει τε γάρ ἐστιν ἤδη, καὶ ἐνεργείᾳ ἔσται προσγενόμενον).

The doctrine involved in both passages is the same and the conclusion the same, viz. πᾶν μέγεθος αἰσθητόν.

448 b 16. ἀλλ' οὐ φαίνεται ὅσον—ἀλλ' ἐνίοτε ἀδιαίρετον, ὁρᾷ δ' οὐκ ἀδιαίρετον. This should probably be connected with what is said in *De An.* III. ch. 3, 428 b 29 sqq. about the falsity which may attach to φαντασία. φαντασία may be exercised along with sensation (παρούσης τῆς αἰσθήσεως). In the case of the perception of size (and the other κοινὰ αἰσθητά) which may itself be erroneous, the φαντασία which results from this perception may also be false, whether the perception is present or not, καὶ μάλιστα ὅταν πόρρω τὸ αἰσθητὸν ᾖ. If, with Freudenthal (*Ueber d. Beg. d. Wort.* φαντ. *b. Arist.*, p. 12), we take πόρρω as referring to spatial distance, as πόρρωθεν does here (but cf. Rodier, Vol. II. p. 433), then Aristotle is instancing the error which attaches to our idea of distant objects. Cf. also 428 b 3: οἷον φαίνεται μὲν ὁ ἥλιος ποδιαῖος and *De Insom.* ch. 1, 458 b 28, and ch. 2, 460 b 18. But though, in the above passages, the discrepancy between φαντασία and belief (πίστις) is discussed, we nowhere meet with an explanation of any conflict between imagination and perception of the common sensibles which goes so far as to assert that something which is imperceptible is yet imageable.

Hence we may conclude that, when Aristotle says that magnitudes sometimes appear to be indivisible, he would not probably refer the act of mind to φαντασία in the strict sense defined in *De An.* III. ch. 3 (κίνησις ὑπὸ τῆς αἰσθήσεως γιγνομένη 429 a 1) or as the faculty of images (cf. 428 a 1). It is rather to be classed as a mistaken opinion and to be ascribed to δόξα. In fact φαίνεται is here used vaguely, and κατὰ μεταφοράν (cf. 428 a 2), but in a sense which is very common (cf. above 448 a 23 and frequently elsewhere) as implying 'appearance' in the modern sense, as opposed to reality. (For a discussion of the *minimum visibile* cf. Introduction, sec. VIII.)

448 b 18. ἐν τοῖς ἔμπροσθεν. I hold (following Alexander's second alternative) that this refers to ch. 6, 445 b 11 : ἀδύνατον γὰρ λευκὸν μὲν ὁρᾶν, μὴ ποσὸν δέ, not to the subsequent discussion (cf. note to 448 b 14), for the principle involved is not πᾶν μέγεθος αἰσθητόν but πᾶν αἰσθητὸν μέγεθος, the simple converse, which is also discussed at the end of this chapter, 449 a 22 sqq.

448 b 19. This passage from 448 b 19 to 449 a 22 presents very serious difficulty. In the first part of it the text has been practically reconstructed by Biehl, who attaches great authority to MSS. E M Y. Consequently the interpretations of Alexander and most commentators who follow a very different version have to be in many places discarded. This in itself is small loss, as it can hardly be said that those interpretations were consistent either among themselves or with the previous part of the treatise. But the difficulty still remains of extracting the exact drift of the argument from the crabbed Greek of the reconstructed and, it is supposed, more ancient version. Down to 449 a 10 runs an argument to which we can find no strict parallel in the *De Anima*, and it is here that the textual reconstruction takes place. From this point onwards we can trace an identity between the reasonings here and those passages in *De An.* III. ch. 2, 426 b 8—427 a 16 and ch. 7, 431 a 19 sqq., which are themselves already so famous for their obscurity. Consequently the advantage resulting from a greater unanimity as to the text is annulled by a greater divergence of opinion as to the purport of the argument.

In order to arrive at a conclusion as to the general meaning of the passage we must, as it were, take our bearings and recapitulate the results attained in the previous part of the chapter together with the main conclusions arrived at in the *De Anima*.

The solution already given of τῆς πρότερον λεχθείσης ἀπορίας is, that consciousness of two sensations simultaneously is only possible when the two combine to form a unitary product (447 b 11 : τῇ μιᾷ δὲ [αἰσθήσει] ἅμα δυοῖν οὐκ ἔστιν αἰσθάνεσθαι ἂν μὴ μιχθῇ). Only sensations, however, belonging to the same sense can give a unitary product (447 a 32 sqq.), and, as an illustration of this unitary product, he gives the concord which two different tones compose and, though Aristotle does not explicitly mention them (cf. notes to 448 a 7 sqq.), everything points to his having in his mind the composite colours, odours and flavours which in previous chapters he asserted to be formed by the combination of the two qualities which in each sense are most opposed to each other (ἐκ μὲν ἐνίων γίνεταί τι...μίγνυνται γὰρ ὧν τὰ ἔσχατα ἐναντία). Qualities of diverse senses do not combine (ἐκ δ' ἐνίων οὐ γίνεται, τοιαῦτα δὲ τὰ ὑφ' ἑτέραν αἴσθησιν...οὐκ ἔστι δ' ἐκ λευκοῦ καὶ ὀξέος ἓν γενέσθαι ἀλλ' ἢ κατὰ συμβεβηκός). This statement is repeated again in the passage we are to discuss 449 a 9-10 : οὐδὲν γὰρ ἐκ τούτων [γλυκέος καὶ λευκοῦ] ἕν.

The conclusion then is, that sensations of different senses cannot be simultaneously present in consciousness, while those belonging to the same sense escape the same disability only by sacrificing their individuality and merging in a compound (μῖγμα) in which they are not ἐνεργείᾳ, actually, discernible.

Now, in view of the opposition between this conclusion and the passages in the *De Anima* as well as the solution finally come to at the end of this chapter (ὥστε καὶ αἰσθάνοιτ' ἂν ἅμα τῷ αὐτῷ καὶ ἑνί, 449 a 21), which is evidently Aristotle's final opinion, how are we to treat the arguments in the earlier part of the chapter? Are they merely dialectical? Or do they merely emphasise a point of view which, while so far legitimate, is modified and transcended by the final presentation of the subject? To us who have followed Aristotle's method of developing an argument in previous chapters, this seems the more likely answer, but whether he has made the relation between the two points of view quite plain, and whether indeed he was clear about it in his own mind, is another question.

In the passages in the *De Anima* there is no mention whatsoever of the sensations coalescing with each other. The question is raised how we distinguish the various sense qualities, and the word chiefly used for this action is κρίνειν, which is paraphrased once (426 b 14) by αἰσθάνεσθαι ὅτι διαφέρει [τὰ αἰσθητά]. The reply is, that they must be distinguished by something unitary and in a unitary moment of time (ἅμα). If the first condition were not fulfilled, consciousness would be divided into independent parts, separate like the minds of different individuals; if the moment of their distinction were not a unit, qualities could not be pronounced to be distinct at one and the same moment.

Obviously Aristotle is there not discussing qualities which have merged with each other and lie indistinguishably commingled in their product. It is noteworthy also that, apparently, he finds the greatest difficulty in explaining the simultaneous distinction of contrary qualities, not of those belonging to diverse senses. (Cf. Rodier, Vol. II. pp. 388 sqq. and pp. 501 sqq. On the whole I follow Rodier and Alexander.) (1) The first explanation proposed is, that what perceives is in aspect or mode of existence (τῷ εἶναι) diverse, though a numerical and spatial unit (τόπῳ δὲ καὶ ἀριθμῷ ἀδιαίρετον 427 a 5), just as things have various diverse qualities, but yet are numerically and spatially one (cf. beneath 449 a 16 : τὸ γὰρ αὐτὸ καὶ ἓν ἀριθμῷ λευκὸν καὶ γλυκύ ἐστι). (I agree with Rodier and Alexander in identifying the second solution in this chapter of the *De Sensu* with the former of the two explanations in the *De Anima* in III. ch. 2.)

But (2) it is only potentially that *contrary* qualities (as distinguished from those merely diverse) can form a unity. When actual they cannot be realised in the same subject. When forming a mixture they have potential existence and thus can be realised in the same subject. Hence we must think of the soul, not as being analogous in this case to a thing in which diverse qualities are combined, but rather to something incorporeal, *e.g.* a point, which is at one and the same time actually one or two, according to the way in which it is viewed. A point *per se* is a mere unit and indivisible, but, viewed as the end of one line and the starting point of another, it is two. In the line AB which is intersected at the point C

A   **|C**   **B**

C is employed in two ways at the same time, as the terminus of AC and the starting point of CB (δὶς γὰρ τῷ αὐτῷ χρῆται σημείῳ ἅμα 427 a 12).

This is, without doubt, the same solution as that mentioned briefly below in 449 a 12 sqq. 'In so far as that which perceives sweet and white is actually indivisible it is one, in so far as actually divisible it is diverse.'

Note that in the *De Sensu* Aristotle applies the explanation, which he had reserved in the *De Anima* for contraries, to mere differents like white and sweet, afterwards returning to the more general solution which he had given in the *De Anima* (ἢ ὥσπερ ἐπὶ τῶν πραγμάτων αὐτῶν ἐνδέχεται, οὕτως καὶ ἐπὶ τῆς ψυχῆς 449 a 14–15) and which seemed to be inadequate to account for the perception of *contraries*. This need not mean a recoil on Aristotle's part from the teaching in the *Psychology*. From the discussion there in III. ch. 7, it appears that he thought the cases of contraries and of differents not to be fundamentally diverse. (I follow here Rodier's text and interpretation.) *Vide* 431 a 21 : ἔστι γὰρ ἕν τι, οὕτω δὲ καὶ ὡς ὅρος. καὶ ταῦτα, ἐν τῷ ἀνάλογον καὶ τῷ ἀριθμῷ ὄν, ἔχει πρὸς ἑκάτερον, ὡς ἐκεῖνα πρὸς ἄλληλα· τί γὰρ διαφέρει τὸ ἀπορεῖν πῶς τὰ μὴ ὁμογενῆ κρίνει ἢ τὰ ἐναντία, οἷον λευκὸν καὶ μέλαν ; κ.τ.λ.

Here we find (1) that that which discerns the sensibles is ὡς ὅρος, as it were a limiting point (cf. πέρας in the previous passage) ; (2) that the sensations (ταῦτα) are, in virtue of this principle, related to each other as the qualities (ἐκεῖνα) are among themselves ; (3) that this numerically identical consciousness relates the various pairs of ἐναντία in an analogous fashion (as we can gather also from *De Sensu*, ch. 7, above 447 b 32 sqq.: ὡς δ' αὕτως ἑαυταῖς τὰ σύστοιχα κ.τ.λ.). Hence, if white bears to black the relation that sweet bears to bitter, the proportion will be transposable, as we may say that white is to sweet as black to bitter. Here now we are relating to each other τὰ μὴ ὁμογενῆ and hence it follows that the mode of distinguishing them is not essentially different from the way in which we discriminate contraries.

It follows, then, that Aristotle's final opinion contained both elements and that the two are really complementary to each other (cf. Rodier II. p. 501), viz., (1) that the relation of sensations in consciousness is the same as that of objective qualities in things, (2) that the only parallel we can find for the relating consciousness is the mathematical point with its double function of oneness and duality.

Notice that Aristotle is confident that this perception of two qualities *is* simultaneous, while it must be different from the only kind of simultaneous perception of qualities yet accounted for (up to 448 b 17) in the *De Sensu*. This was the perception of qualities in fusion ; that is the distinction (κρίσις) of the different sensations.

It is true that in *De Sensu*, ch. 7, 447 b 28 sqq. Aristotle says it is the function of a single sense to discriminate specifically different and opposite qualities like white and black. But there is no indication at that point that this discrimination must be instantaneous; the drift of the argument seems rather to be that what is perceived at a single instant must be a numerical unit. Alexander (*De Sensu*, p. 167, ll. 10 sqq. [W.], p. 352, ll. 10 sqq. [Thurot]) professes to find the account given of the perception of contraries here unsatisfactory. It is merely, he thinks, the same as that first hazarded in the *De Anima* and there set aside. The same thing cannot be both white and black, and hence, if the union of sensations in the soul is similar to the union of qualities in things, we have left the case of contrary sensations unexplained. Hence he thinks that either discrimination of contraries can only be effected by means of memory, not by present sensations, or that it is by the central organ (the heart) being affected in different parts simultaneously (just as it must be different parts of the same object that have contrary determinations) that we can at the same time distinguish different sensations. Hence, though the simultaneous *experience* (πάθος) of two opposite qualities is not possible, simultaneous discrimination (κρίσις) is.

This seems to me to be an untenable position. Though, in perception, there can be distinguished the two different aspects of discrimination and experience or reception of the sensations, yet they cannot exist apart from each other; at any rate the discrimination of the diversity cannot exist without the presentation of the differents, and simultaneous discrimination of the differents cannot exist without simultaneous modification of the same thing by the differents.

Besides, this theory seems to be exactly that which Aristotle, in anticipation of his final solution, is going to disprove below in the passage from 448 b 19—449 a 9: ἅμα μὲν, ἑτέρῳ δὲ τῆς ψυχῆς αἰσθάνεσθαι. This is impossible, he says, even though the different parts belong to one continuous whole—οὕτω δ' ἀτόμῳ ὡς παντὶ ὄντι συνεχεῖ (cf. *infra* 23 sqq. and notes). This would be a good description of the central organ functioning by means of different parts.

The way out of the difficulty is found by paying close attention to the conclusion established in *De An.* III. ch. 7.

There is no essential difference, Aristotle says, between the discrimination of differents and of contraries. Similarly we might add there is no essential difference between the way in which both classes of qualities are realised in things. Incompatible qualities must, if realised in one thing (by belonging to different parts of it), meet in a common point which is two or one according to the way of looking at it, just as much as a particle of matter which is both sweet and white has both a dual and a unitary aspect.

If this is Aristotle's final opinion, what is to be thought of the purport of the earlier part of this chapter? It might be suggested that in the *De Sensu* he is talking of αἰσθάνεσθαι in the sense of πάσχειν, in the *De Anima* as κρίνειν. But this can hardly be accurate; the final verdict in the *De Sensu* is the same as in the *De Anima*, while there is no indication that he is at the end thinking of αἴσθησις merely as κρίσις. As we have seen, there cannot be simultaneous κρίσις without simultaneous πάθος, while again sensation is always with him a δύναμις κριτική, always cognitive. Perhaps the meaning to be extracted from the discussion is as follows—Sense qualities as such cannot be perceived simultaneously. True, if the sensations they give rise to can combine, as they may do if they belong to the same sense (since the corresponding stimuli are in closer proximity than in other cases—μᾶλλον γὰρ ἅμα ἡ κίνησις 447 b 9 sq.), they can both be experienced. But in combination they cannot be discriminated, hence not perceived. But since, as we learn in the *De Anima*, to be discriminated they must be simultaneously apprehended, it is to their objective realisation in things, to their unity κατὰ συμβεβηκός, *i.e.* as accidents of the same substance, that we must look for the grounds of the possibility of their discrimination, while their discrimination is effected by a consciousness which has a unity, not like that of different spatial parts in a whole, but like that of the different qualities in one object.

If this be the meaning of our author, it forms a remarkable foreshadowing of the psychological doctrine that discrimination and objectification go together and, if objects can exist only in space, it is an argument for the necessity of the spatial form of things for the development of knowledge.

Aristotle says that this faculty which distinguishes the sense qualities belonging to the different genera is still a form of sense, for the qualities distinguished are sense qualities (αἰσθητὰ γάρ ἐστιν, *De An.* III. ch. 2, 426 b 15). Yet it cannot be ἰδία αἴσθησις, which merely discriminates qualities belonging to a single sense. It is not located in the organ of any special sense, nor in the flesh. Its organ he calls τὸ κύριον αἰσθητήριον, which is evidently to be identified with what he elsewhere calls τὸ κύριον αἰσθητήριον, *De Som.* ch. 2,

455 a 21 sqq., τὸ πρῶτον αἰσθητήριον *ibid.* 456 a 21, etc., and τὸ κοινὸν αἰσθητήριον *De Juvent.* ch. 1, 467 b 28, *ibid.* ch. 3, 469 a 12, namely the heart or some constituent found in it. This is the organ of the κοινὴ αἴσθησις, one function of which we have already discussed, namely the perception of the 'common sensibles,'—number, figure, magnitude, motion, and unity. If we look however to *De Som.* ch. 2, 455 a 13 sqq. we find that the faculty by which we distinguish the various genera of sensations, *e.g.* white and sweet, is also called a κοινὴ δύναμις ἀκολουθοῦσα πάσαις, and this it is, too, which enables us to be not only conscious but self-conscious (ᾗ καὶ ὅτι ὁρᾷ καὶ ἀκούει αἰσθάνεται). It resides in the κοινὸν αἰσθητήριον (τινὶ κοινῷ μορίῳ τῶν αἰσθητηρίων πάντων).

Hence we come to the conclusion that the faculty by which we discriminate and hence objectify sense qualities is also the same as that in virtue of which we are self-conscious, a striking anticipation of Kant's doctrine of the objectifying function of the 'transcendental unity of apperception.' Cf. Introd. sec. IX.

448 b 22. ἀτόμῳ χρόνῳ. Cf. note to ἀτόμῳ above 447 a 15 ; this has been the sense in which Aristotle has used 'individual time' throughout. Cf. *Physics* VIII. ch. 8, 263 b 27 : οὐχ οἷόν τε εἰς ἀτόμους χρόνους διαιρεῖσθαι τὸν χρόνον, cf. also VI. ch. 9, 239 b 8.

448 b 23. ἑτέρῳ δὲ. This seems not to be exactly the theory rejected in *De An.* III. ch. 2, 426 b 17 sqq.: οὔτε δὴ κεχωρισμένοις ἐνδέχεται κρίνειν ὅτι ἕτερον τὸ γλυκὺ τοῦ λευκοῦ, κ.τ.λ.

There it was shown in general terms that it is not by separate organs or faculties that the soul discriminates diverse sensations. Here it is proved that not even though the different organs were to form a continuous whole could it be said that through them the distinction of the sensations is effected.

In short, both arguments are directed against the contention that it is by means of spatially different parts that the simultaneous presentation and discrimination of two different sense qualities is rendered possible. In the *De Anima* these different parts seem to be regarded as the various end organs, but as it might have been objected that they need not be regarded as separate in that way, since, on Aristotle's own theory, the various sense organs all connected with the heart, and the real organ of discrimination might hence be the various parts of that member, Aristotle here refutes this second version of the theory.

448 b 24. οὐ τῷ ἀτόμῳ. This is omitted by MSS. L S U and also by Alexander, who reads, instead of the subsequent οὔτω δ᾽ ἀτόμῳ, καὶ οὔτως ἀτόμῳ ὡς παντὶ ὄντι συνεχεῖ. This he takes to refer to the ἅμα in l. 21 above and to be a second attempt to define the sense in which the organ is individual (Alex. p. 157 ll. 17 sqq. [W.], p. 331 l. 7 [Th.]). This reading and interpretation is supported by Thurot and also Bäumker (*Jahrb. für Class. Philol.* 1886, p. 319) who, of course, assign the οὐ τῷ ἀτόμῳ to dittographia. But, if the interpretation is to be supported and οὔτως ἀτόμῳ is to be referred to time, we must read either καὶ ἐν οὔτως with Thurot or κἂν οὔτως with Bäumker. However, it is impossible that ὡς παντὶ ὄντι συνεχεῖ can elucidate the meaning of ἅμα or be a relevant description of the atomic time mentioned above (cf. previous notes). That is a time which relatively to the two sensations is atomic, which is such that the two sensations are not subsequent to each other, but both experienced concurrently throughout the whole duration of the time. But, though the time is continuous, one sensation may quite well be subsequent to another, for the time uniting two events in immediate succession is continuous.

It is true that the time in which the sensations are presented must be continuous, *i.e.* must be capable of resolution into still briefer times : cf. the general discussion of continuity in the notes to ch. 6, 445 b 3 and 28 sqq.

But to point this out in no way shows how the sensations are ἅμα; on the contrary, it would lead one to believe they were not really ἅμα, *i.e.* ἐν τῷ αὐτῷ χρόνῳ (*Physics* IV. ch. 10, 218 a 25, *Categ.* ch. 13, 14 b 25) in the sense of being concurrently present in all parts of it, but that one was ὕστερον, the other πρότερον. Cf. *Physics*, *loc. cit.*—ἅμα εἶναι κατὰ χρόνον = μήτε πρότερον μήτε ὕστερον τὸ ἐν τῷ αὐτῷ εἶναι.

Hence, if it was said that the individuality of the time in which two sensations were presented consisted in its being composed of continuous parts and that they were 'together,' ἅμα, merely in the sense of occupying different parts of this continuous whole, this would contradict the definition of their simultaneity given above in l. 22, which Alexander explains as not being merely immediate succession in time.

In short, if it can be asserted that a time of continuous parts is atomic in a sense (*i.e.* in the sense that no division in it has been made), yet this is not the sense in which the time in which sensations are simultaneously perceived is atomic.

Hence if οὕτω ἀτόμῳ refers to time, it is a misleading irrelevancy. It must refer to the organ or faculty of perception. (For the sense in which τὸ συνεχές is a unity cf. *Metaph.* x. ch. I, 1052 a 19 sqq.) The ancient translation runs 'et non indivisibili, sic autem indivisibili ut omni existenti continuo.' Biehl's conjecture καὶ οὐ τῷ ἀτόμῳ ἢ οὕτω[ς?] ἀτόμῳ seems to give little visible improvement.

448 b 28. ταῦτα. All MSS. except E M and all editors except Biehl read ταὐτά. Accordingly, following that reading we should have to interpret 'there will be a plurality of organs specifically alike.' Not only the interpretations but the readings also which we are to accept in the subsequent passage will depend upon our decision here.

Firstly, it is clear that whatever reading we accept we must not have the temerity to translate γένει in this line 'species.' Hammond reading ταὐτά renders : 'it will then have parts specifically the same. For its repeated sensations belong to the same species.' This is certainly to cut the knot and leave the difficulty unsolved.

Supposing that ταὐτά be read, then we may, throughout the subsequent lines also, follow pretty closely the version of the class of MSS. which gives us that reading.

Bekker gives καὶ γὰρ ἃ αἰσθάνεται, ἐν τῷ αὐτῷ γένει ἐστίν, which we may render 'for the objects of a single sense belong to the same genus.' This does not seem to be a confirmation of the ταὐτά unless we remember that, though the actual sensation is identical with the sense quality as actually perceived and that, hence, as qualities are specifically diverse so are sensations, yet as a δύναμις the sense is specifically a unit. The perception of black and of white is δυνάμει specifically one. What has a generic unity ἐνεργείᾳ has specific unity potentially.

The senses considered as faculties are only specifically distinct. Now the sense faculty and the sense organ are from many points of view one and the same thing. They are, of course, relatively to each other σῶμα ὀργανικόν and ἕξις—the ἕξις of the particular organ ; but they are often referred to by the same term ; αἴσθησις is often equivalent to αἰσθητήριον (cf. above ch. 3, 440 a 20, and ὄψις is even used for ὄμμα : cf. ch. 2, 438 a 13 : τὸ μὲν οὖν τὴν ὄψιν εἶναι ὕδατος ἀληθὲς μέν), and so ἀκοή for the ear, ὄσφρησις for the organ of smell (cf. *De An.* III. ch. I, 425 a 4 : ἡ δ' ἀκοὴ ἀέρος, κ.τ.λ. and *De Sens,* ch. 2, 438 b 21–22 and note).

Hence we might argue that, corresponding to the specifically identical faculty which perceives objects specifically distinct, there is, if it requires a separate organ to apprehend every separate determination, a corresponding plurality of sense organs which yet are specifically identical, for, if the faculty is specifically one, so are the organs.

Hence we should have to interpret εἰ δὲ ὅτι ὡς δύο ὄμματα, κ.τ.λ. 1. 29 sqq. in some such way as this—'If it be said that this may very well be the case because (*e.g.*) the eyes are specifically alike, and so the soul may have a plurality of similar organs, it must be observed that the cases are not parallel.

'The two eyes have an identical function, not two images but one alone is present when we see; but the case you try to explain is that of the perception of diversity.' (This would require to be the sense to be arrived at, whatever reading we follow.)

'Once more, if the organs are specifically alike, so will the faculty of perceiving black, white, etc., be specifically identical, *i.e.* you will have different sense faculties only numerically distinct (αἰσθήσεις αἱ αὐταὶ πλείους ἔσονται 1. 33) which is like saying that there may be different sciences of the same subject.'

But this last argument is sufficient to throw suspicion on the whole proof. If it is the case that, as the authors of this interpretation would themselves admit, the perception of black and the perception of white are only as actualised specifically different, and δυνάμει, or as a faculty, they are specifically identical and only numerically to be distinguished as different possible acts of the same sense (cf. Alex. *De Sens.* p. 158, l. 15 [W.], p. 333, l. 6 [Th.]: τῶν γὰρ ἐν τῷ γένει ἡ αὐτὴ κατ᾽ εἶδος αἴσθησις. Alexander, however, shows some perplexing hesitation between ὁμογενῆ and ὁμοειδῆ), then it is clear that Aristotle would not have the least objection to saying that the same sense faculty may be reduplicated, provided one understands what this means. If it mean, as is the only view consistent with the reading ταὐτά, that it is one sense faculty which is particularised and made determinate in the perception of black, white, etc., then this is precisely his theory.

(Compare 447 b 27 sqq. above. There he cannot maintain the unqualified assertion that, corresponding to a specifically identical object, there is a single (specifically identical) sense. A single sense corresponds to and discriminates specifically diverse objects (cf. 447 b 29). It is the single sense functioning in a determinate manner which gives specific identity in the object.)

Hence it would be Aristotle's own theory that the different organs by which we perceived white and black, if there were any, must be specifically alike, just as the eyes are alike.

But his argument is this—'If you postulate a diversity of organs, you will have to make them specifically *unlike* each other. Where we have different organs, as is the case with diverse senses, the unity of the senses is only generic; hence here too, within one sense, if you are to have separate organs, they will only have a generic resemblance to each other. You object and say there are the two eyes, specifically alike, but yet serving the one sense—sight. I reply that these have a single function; the sensations given by each combine to form one product. So too the different sensations mediated by specifically identical (εἴδει δὲ l. 31) parts of the same organ may form a compound, *e.g.* black and white, and sounds of various pitch, which combine. But, when that is so, the different sensations are not discriminated. Your proposal was to account for the perception, *i.e.*, discrimination of the sensations, by the diversity of the organs by which they are apprehended. If, as shown, a mere numerical difference in the organ does not render that possible, you will have to try specific disparateness. The different organs must be specifically diverse.

'But, if so, contained within each sense there will be diverse faculties, distinct from each other as the various sciences are distinct and as the admittedly different senses are distinct. Distinct sciences have each an appropriate δύναμις and so have distinct senses. The perception, then, of (*e.g.*) different colours will, because each has, as shown, its appropriate δύναμις, be distinct in the way that the sciences are.'

This carries us down to 449 a 3, after which the argument takes a new turn.

448 b 28–29. τῷ αὐτῷ γένει. Cf. 447 b 29–30; where you have different organs you have only generic identity in the sense.

448 b 29. If we read οὐδὲν κωλύει in this way as governing ὅτι (see translation), we must supply λεκτέον before ὅτι ἴσως in order to avoid an ugly anacoluthon. This, however, is very common in Aristotle. Cf. ἢ ὅτι πρῶτον l. 25 above. The ὅτι ἴσως clause can hardly be an argument against the suggestion that we may have different organs specifically alike, as in the case of the eyes; it will rather be in support of it. Alexander, however, wishes to take ὅτι ἴσως as an objection to a different thesis (cf. note to ταῦτα above).

If it is intended as an argument in support, it can only be the plea of an intelligent supporter. He (the supporter) says—'here you have two eyes of identical construction functioning alike and co-operating in the act of perception.' Aristotle in the next sentence replies 'that is exactly the point, the objects they perceive are numerically one, not diverse as is required in the case of the organs which are to perceive both white and black simultaneously.'

448 b 31–33. Bekker reads ἐκεῖ δέ, εἰ μὲν ἐν τὸ ἐξ ἀμφοῖν, ἐκεῖνο τὸ αἰσθανόμενον ἔσται, εἰ δὲ χωρίς, οὐχ ὁμοίως ἕξει, following L S U P and Alexander.

Biehl's text is εἰ δέ, ᾗ μὲν ἐν τὸ ἐξ ἀμφοῖν, ἐν καὶ τὸ αἰσθανόμενον κ.τ.λ.; he bases his restoration on readings in E M Y. This would give us—'But if that is so, then, consequent to the unity of the product, the perceptive organ (faculty?) is single, while again if the sensations are separate the case is altered.' We may extract a meaning out of it somewhat like that which Alexander gets from the other reading—viz. that in the case of the eyes you have really a single psychic faculty functioning through the two organs and not two, as is claimed. This will give a sense satisfactory to our argument; but it is difficult to see how τὸ αἰσθανόμενον could be said to be numerically single when it is quite as naturally an epithet for the eye as for the faculty, and the eyes are manifestly double.

Hence I propose, while following Biehl and the older class of MSS., to read εἴδει δὲ εἰ instead of εἰ δὲ in 448 b 31, and interpret as in note to 448 b 28. The point is, that two perceptive organs specifically alike will account for the perception of a single object, but that to account for the perception of two things (simultaneously), the organs must be specifically *unlike*.

Hammond translates, following Biehl's text, "If, however, the continuation of both forms a unit, then *that which is perceived* will be a unit and, if they remain uncombined, then the result will likewise be uncombined.'

448 b 33. ἔτι αἰσθήσεις κ.τ.λ. For Alexander's interpretation cf. note to b 28 above.

449 a 3. It seems to be the universal practice to take ταύτης as referring to ἐνέργεια in l. 2. We thus get a syllogism—if αἴσθησις then ἐνέργεια, if ἐνέργεια then οἰκεία δύναμις; hence all αἰσθήσεις have their οἰκεία δύναμις. But perhaps there was no need to prove this. Whether we read ταὐτά or ταῦτα in 448 b 28, we might prefer αἴσθησις here to be taken in the sense which it has in 448 b

33—as a distinct sense (not as *sensation* as I have translated). Now a sense is by definition a δύναμις (cf. *De An.* III. ch. 9, 432 a 16) and more accurately a δύναμις in the sense of ἕξις (cf. *De Sens.* ch. 1, 436 b 5, and note to ch. 4, 441 b 25, and *De An.* II. ch. 5). A sense is like a distinct science, a determinate potentiality; the actual exercise of both alike depends upon this, which may be called the οἰκεία δύναμις of the ἐνέργεια in each case. It may be of these principles that Aristotle reminds us here. It has already been shown that, if the organs by which we perceive white and black are distinct, they, and therefore the faculties which reside in them, must be distinct. Hence these latter will be distinct in the sense that sciences are distinct. The two clauses—οὔτε...δυνάμεως, οὔτε...αἰσθησις—will then form only a single premiss in the argument which proves that a distinct sense is like a distinct science.

449 a 4. Unless μὴ be read before αἰσθάνεται we get a shocking piece of bad reasoning; though if B can be perceived, *a fortiori* A can be perceived, we cannot infer that if A then B (B = τῶν τῷ γένει ἑτέρων, A = τὰ ἐναντία). Besides the presence of μὴ does not incommode the argument, in fact improves it.

The best defence of this emendation (which though authorised by no text is seen to be necessary by Alexander unless τούτων = ἐκείνων, *i.e.* heterogeneous objects, ἄλλων = ὁμοειδῶν. So St Hilaire and Leonicus) is by Bäumker in the *Jahrb. für Class. Philol.* 1886, p. 320. He points out that though in classical Greek if μὴ is read we should expect οὐδὲ not καὶ after ὅτι in the next clause, yet we find instances of the contrary usage in Aristotle, *e.g. De Coelo,* I. ch. 11, 281 a 16: οἷον ὁ χίλια βαδίσαι στάδια μὴ δυνάμενος, δῆλον ὅτι καὶ χίλια καὶ ἕν.

The presence of the καὶ, being so contrary to common usage, probably led to the omission of the μὴ.

For the principle compare above 447 b 7 sqq. and 448 a 15 sqq. ἐν ἑνὶ καὶ ἀτόμῳ must refer to time (cf. 448 b 22-24 and notes). It is the simultaneousness of the perception which is under discussion, and which cannot be accounted for by the theory that the faculty or organ is diverse.

449 a 7. From ἤτοι, l. 7, to ἐκ τούτων ἕν, l. 9, the passage is almost hopelessly obscure.

τούτων, l. 7, must surely refer to γλυκέος and λευκοῦ. The phrase τὸ ἐκ τούτων continually refers to a compound. Cf. *De An.* II. ch. 1, 412 a 9, where οὐσία συνθέτη, consisting of ὕλη and εἶδος, is so designated, and *Metaph.* VII. ch. 3, 1029 a 3, etc. Thus if here τὸ ἐκ τούτων refers to the organ or faculty of perception, it can hardly imply that it is a substratum or ὑποκείμενον, as Alexander (*De Sensu*, p. 162, l. 23 [W.], p. 343, l. 6 [Th.]) and Rodier (II. p. 390) take it.

However, apart from this, all except Simon (Simon, *De Sensu*, p. 261) admit that (τὸ) ἐκ τούτων in l. 9 refers to a compound of qualities or sensations, and it is hardly likely that in three lines Aristotle would employ the same expression to refer to two different things. Moreover the meaning of τὸ ἐξ ἀμφοῖν in 448 b 32 above, as well as ἐξ ὧν 447 a 23, ἐκ...ἐνίων 447 a 32, etc., all point to this phrase referring to a fusion of sensations, and so St Hilaire takes it. On the other hand, Alexander, Thomas, Simon, and Rodier wish to take it as referring to the soul or the central organ, the heart. The only advantage resulting from this is that the connection of ἀλλ᾽ ἀνάγκη ἕν and ἐν γάρ τι τὸ αἰσθητικόν ἐστι μέρος is quite clear, but it leaves the connection between the latter clause and those which follow it absolutely unexplained.

Simon is more consistent than others in thinking that the reference may be to the central sense and its organ throughout.

If we take τὸ ἐκ τούτων as referring on both occasions to a product of sensations, then the argument will be clear except as to the connection between ἀλλ᾽ ἀνάγκη ἕν and ἐν γάρ τι τὸ αἰσθητικόν ἐστι μέρος. The only way I can see for explaining this is as follows : 'It is claimed that we perceive black and white simultaneously by means of a single organ with spatially diverse though continuous parts. But in such a case the two sensations must coalesce and form a unity, and hence, if it is by the same means that we perceive sweet and white, then they too must form a unity. But such a unitary product does not exist. Hence it is not by the spatial diversity of the organ that those qualities are perceived simultaneously.'

The question is still as to the means of perceiving the two simultaneously (which he is sure can take place), and the objection to the solution proposed is not that it postulates different organs, for he admits that such exist (ἄλλο δὲ γένος δι᾽ ἄλλου, l. 11), but that it is through a spatial diversity of the organ that they are supposed to be related in the same moment of time.

Thus, in the whole of this section from 448 b 19 onwards Aristotle has been working up to his own theory. He rejects the solution proposed in the form in which it is offered but, *more suo*, abstracts from it the legitimate part. There are different faculties, but it is not *quâ* located in different physical organs that they are able to allow their different contributions to be correlated in a single consciousness.

449 a 8. ἀλλ' ἀνάγκη. If Aristotle is still discussing the solution hazarded in 448 b 23-25, as he must be, this is proof positive that according to that theory the soul must be a unity of a kind, and so our interpretation of οὕτω δ' ἀτόμῳ in 448 b 24-25 is confirmed. If it were under dispute whether what perceives is something unitary or not, Aristotle could not bring in without proof the very statement which was denied—ἐν γάρ τι τὸ αἰσθητικόν ἐστι μέρος. Indeed if he knew this to be true and to be excluded by the other theory —ἄλλῳ μὲν γλυκέος ἄλλῳ δὲ λευκοῦ αἰσθάνεται ἡ ψυχὴ μέρει—he would need to start with a direct proof of it.

449 a 10. Biehl proposes to read δὲ instead of ἄρα, no doubt because, apparently, all that has been said is in opposition to what follows. But, as we have seen (note to 449 a 7), what precedes is directed not against the doctrine of a unitary principle (indeed that has been affirmed in l. 8), but against the interpretation of it given.

449 a 12. ᾗ μὲν ἀδιαίρετον κ.τ.λ. The meaning of this is elucidated in *De An.* III. ch. 2, 427 a 10 sqq. Cf. note to 448 b 19 above.

449 a 17. Alexander reads, l. 17, εἰ γὰρ μὴ χωριστὰ κ.τ.λ. The sense then is—'One and the same thing numerically can be white and sweet and have many other qualities, for, though the qualities do not exist in separation from each other, yet in mode of existence they are different from each other.'

Bekker and Biehl both reject γὰρ, though Rodier accepts it. The latter also translates τὸ εἶναι by 'essence.' Cf. next note.

449 a 18. τὸ εἶναι. Alexander seems to countenance Rodier's translation of 'essence' by giving as equivalents λόγος and τὸ τί ἦν εἶναι. But, though not so far from λόγος in meaning, τὸ εἶναι is hardly as a rule equivalent to 'essential nature' or 'real being,' which is the special force of τὸ τί ἦν εἶναι. It is rather 'aspect of existence'; we might almost say 'existence for consciousness.' τῷ εἶναι almost = 'notionally': cf. note to ch. 6, 446 b 30, and for a typical case *De An.* III. ch. 2, 425 b 27, where it is said that though the ἐνέργεια of the sense object and that of the sense faculty are one and identical, yet in aspect of existence, *i.e.* as related to an external object in the one case and the human organism in the other, they are different—τὸ δ' εἶναι οὐ τὸ αὐτὸ αὐταῖς.

We may take λόγῳ in l. 22 (with Bonitz, *Ind.* p. 221 a 60) as equivalent to τῷ εἶναι and translate 'but notionally not the same,' or we may take λόγος here as equivalent to 'ratio' and say 'but not by means of an identical relation [to them],' *i.e.* to the two sensations.

449 a 24. ἄπειρον. Aristotle cannot mean that the point from which a thing ceases to be visible is infinitely far away. Of course the point from which it ceases to be δυνάμει, *i.e.* potentially visible, is infinitely far away, *i.e.* is non-existent. This is a consequence of the doctrine, that every magnitude is sensible, discussed in the first part of chapter 6. But here we are discussing the converse proposition which answers the question raised in ch. 7, 448 b 17 and mentioned in ch. 6, 445 b 10. Simon (p. 256) is wrong in thinking that it is this issue which is raised in ch. 3, 440 a 29 ; it is the other statement, πᾶν μέγεθος ὁρατόν.

Alexander at first takes ἄπειρον as πολύ τε καὶ σχεδὸν ἄπειρον, but later on gives the correct interpretation : οὐ γὰρ ἔστι λαβεῖν τὸ μέγιστον διάστημα ἀφ' οὗ οὐκ αἰσθανόμεθα (*De Sens.* p. 168, 1. 27 [W.], p. 356, 1. 6 [Th.]).

The argument is worked out in terms of sight, but applies to all other senses which employ a medium. It is—'as the distance between object and seer increases, we arrive at last at a point beyond which the object is invisible, though short of it vision is still possible. This is a single mathematical point, and the object, as it diminishes, will, if indivisible to sight anywhere, be indivisible when this point is reached. But this point is the first in the series from which vision is possible, the last where it is impossible. Hence, when at this point, the object will be both visible and invisible ; which is impossible.'

449 a 28. τοῦτο. Alexander takes this to refer to the μεταξύ, the mean point at which vision begins and invisibility ceases. Thus all others too. But, if we interpret it so, it is difficult to construe ὄντος, l. 30. The indivisibility of the point seems to be implied strongly enough in the last clause—ἔστι δέ τι ἔσχατον κ.τ.λ., and, at any rate, whether expressed or not, it is a necessary part of the argument that an indivisible αἰσθητόν will be found at this point if anywhere.

449 b 2. κοινῇ. For this sense of κοινός cf. ch. 1, 436 a 7.

DE MEMORIA

CHAPTER I.

449 b 4. μνημονεύειν is simply the verb corresponding to μνήμη, and means to have something (consciously and at the time) in one's memory. It is paraphrased by ἐνεργεῖν τῇ μνήμῃ in 450 a 21 beneath. It is to be distinguished from ἀναμιμνήσκεσθαι which implies the active search for the memory of some particular item of one's past experience. Though we employ 'to remember' for the former, 'to recollect' for the latter, the English words are hardly so sharply contrasted as the Greek; in fact, in ordinary use they are hardly to be distinguished, as is natural considering that both contain the prefix corresponding to the Greek ἀνά. But even in Greek, and sometimes in Aristotle himself, the terms are not used with perfect precision. Cf. Freudenthal in *Rheinisches Museum*, 1869, p. 403.

449 b 8. μνημονικοί. This is one of the characteristics enumerated in Aristotle's hardly complimentary list of the peculiarly feminine qualities. Cf. *Hist. Animal.* IX. ch. 1, 608 b 13.

449 b 10. ληπτέον = we must make an assumption. Aristotle is going to show grounds for this assumption, but he could not say ὑποκείσθω, because that would imply that the grounds had been already shown. Cf. note to *De Sensu*, ch. 1, 436 a 5. This seems to be the distinction generally maintained between λαμβάνειν and ὑποτίθεσθαι.

449 b 12. δοξαστόν. δόξα, as a faculty, means generally the power of forming opinions and thinking, in the widest sense of the term. When defined more closely, however, it takes rank as the lowest of the rational faculties; it is practically equivalent to ὑπόληψις in its most restricted application and is opposed to ἐπιστήμη, which has for its object necessary truth. Cf. *De An.* III. ch. 3; *Anal. Post.* I. ch. 33; *Metaph.* VII. ch. 15, 1039 b 32 sqq.

449 b 14. There is a special treatise Περὶ τῆς καθ' ὕπνον μαντικῆς 462 b 12 sqq., on supposed prevision of the future by means of dreams. Aristotle accounted for the phenomena in question by means of natural agencies.

449 b 16. Here Aristotle agrees with Locke (*Essay*, Bk. IV. ch. II. § 14 and ch. XI.) with whom 'sensitive knowledge' occupies pretty much the same place as αἴσθησις with Aristotle.

Though only the present is known by perception, this does not mean that only perception knows the present. In l. 18 beneath, τὸ θεωρούμενον is given as an example of τὸ παρόν.

449 b 17. Biehl prefers ὅτι before πάρεστιν instead of ὅτε, the reading adopted by all other editors. The point to be made out is that *quâ* present an object of consciousness is not an object of memory. One might remember, while he was looking at a white thing, that he had seen it before ; but he cannot remember that it is now present. This is the only point to be made out here, viz. that memory is the apprehension of a thing not as present but as past. How this is possible is discussed in 450 a 27 sqq. That which is present to consciousness when we remember, is not the object remembered but its copy (εἰκών). When the present object of consciousness is recognised as a representation of something in the past, then we have memory.

449 b 20. ἄνευ τῶν ἐνεργειῶν. Themistius and Michael read ἔργων. Themistius explains thus—ἔργα δὲ λέγω οἷον τοδὶ τὸ ζῷον ἢ τοδὶ τὸ λευκὸν καὶ τὸ ἐν τῷδε τῷ βιβλίῳ τρίγωνον, *i.e.* as practically equivalent to πράγματα = the real things. Whatever the reading be, the sense must be the same ; ἐνεργειῶν must mean the actual operation of the real objects, or something similar ; ἄνευ τῶν ἐνεργειῶν cannot mean 'without actually having knowledge or perception,' which would imply that only the ἕξεις providing for knowledge or perception existed, for these may persist throughout unconsciousness, *e.g.* in sleep. There really is perception or knowledge of something present whenever we remember ; an ἐνέργεια is realised (cf. 450 b 30 : ὅταν ἐνεργῇ ἡ κίνησις αὐτοῦ κ.τ.λ.), but to be memory it depends upon whether or not this ἐνέργεια is referred to something else (ἄλλου l. 32) existing in the past.

What is actually present in the act of memory we shall find to be a φάντασμα ; a φάντασμα is a persisting sensation or sense content. Now, though it is true that this is in most cases the intermediary employed by memory, yet that intermediary might in certain cases be an actual perception, as *e.g.* when we see a thing for the second time and remember we have seen it before.

449 b 22. Biehl and Freudenthal (*Rheinisches Museum*, XXIV. p. 394) wish to delete τὰς τοῦ τριγώνου...ἴσαι, on the ground that if these words are left standing we shall have to translate 'he remembers that the angles of a triangle are equal to two right, in the one case because he learned or thought of it, in the other because he heard or saw it or had some sense knowledge of the fact.' But Freudenthal points out that we cannot have sensuous knowledge of any mathematical principle according to *Anal. Post.* I. ch. 31, especially 87 b 34 sqq.: οὐδ' ἐπίστασθαι δι' αἰσθήσεως ἔστιν. ἀλλὰ δῆλον ὅτι καὶ εἰ ἦν αἰσθάνεσθαι τὸ τρίγωνον κ.τ.λ.

Freudenthal quotes Themistius, who paraphrases 'he remembers that the angles of a triangle are equal to two right angles, and that Socrates is white, in the one case because he learned, in the other because he heard or saw it' (Themist. *Sp.* II. p. 233, ll. 12 sqq.). The writer of the paraphrase, he thinks, felt the same difficulty and accordingly inserted καὶ τὸν Σωκράτην ὅτι λευκός as an example of sensuous memory.

This, however, is not convincing; it is not a case of *knowing* in the full sense of having scientific knowledge of a fact but of *remembering* it. Perception is of the particular, but there is no reason why we should not perceive in a particular case and without proof that the angles of a triangle are equal to two right angles; cf. *Anal. Post. loc. cit. infra*: we can perceive that the moon is eclipsed without knowing the reason. However, there is an additional reason for rejecting τὰς...ἴσαι (which is such a common Aristotelian example that it might easily have crept into the text); it is the necessity of translating ὅτι before ἔμαθεν and ἤκουσεν by 'that,' not by 'because.' The point to be brought out is that memory refers to the past; we are not here explaining *why* memory takes place. Cf. next clause— δεῖ γὰρ...λέγειν, ὅτι πρότερον. The disputed words are probably a gloss that has crept in at the wrong place. Some such expression inserted after ἐθεώρησεν would be quite in harmony with the thought here.

449 b 27. ὑπόληψις is here used in its widest sense as equivalent to conceptual thought. It seems to include θεωρία: cf. l. 18 above and 450 b 25, 35 etc. The present objects of consciousness are objects either of αἴσθησις or ὑπόληψις, sense or thought, αἰσθήματα or νοήματα.

In its more restricted application ὑπόληψις is the poorest of the intellectual faculties. Cf. *De An.* III. ch. 3, 427 b 17, 25, 28, and *Anal. Post.* I. ch. 33, 88 b 37, and cf. Rodier, II. p. 411.

449 b 29. Freudenthal (*op. cit.* p. 395) rejects καὶ πρότερον because these words cannot refer to a statement which immediately precedes, while here it is simply to the previous paragraph that reference is made.

Themistius, the ancient translation, and L M S U also omit the two words.

449 b 30. αἴσθησις. As we have seen above, ὑπόληψις also deals with the present; but Aristotle is here talking generally and, in fact, a sensuous element is always involved in knowledge of the present, because the object of thought, as we shall see, is always accompanied by imagery which, again, depends upon sense.

449 b 33. τούτῳ. The heart (or according to Neuhäuser, cf. Introduction, sec. VI., the σύμφυτον πνεῦμα contained in it) is the organ of the κοινὴ αἴσθησις : cf. *De Juvent.* ch. 3, 469 a 11, cf. also beneath 450 a 11 sqq. and notes.

At ἐπεὶ begins a protasis, the apodosis corresponding to which is not reached till 450 a 15 : ὥστε τοῦ νοητικοῦ κ.τ.λ. Φαντασία is treated in *De An.* III. ch. 3. There it is defined as a (psychic) change due to sensation (κίνησις ὑπὸ τῆς αἰσθήσεως τῆς κατ᾽ ἐνέργειαν γιγνομένη 429 a 1). Again we find in ch. 8, 432 a 9 : τὰ γὰρ φαντάσματα ὥσπερ αἰσθήματά ἐστι, πλὴν ἄνευ ὕλης, *i.e.*, an image is identical in character with a perception except that in the former case the real concrete thing which contains ὕλη is absent; only the εἶδος of the sensible object is present. As Themistius (*Sp.* II. p. 237, l. 18) says, it is that which is left over (after perception), and remains even though the sense object is not present, which is called φαντασία. Besides the fact of the absence of the real object in φαντασία, the only other difference between it and sensation seems to be its greater liability to error (428 a 26 sqq.), and that it is weaker in intensity : cf. *Rhet.* I. ch. 11, 1370 a 28 : ἡ δὲ φαντασία ἐστὶν αἴσθησίς τις ἀσθενής. It is like Hume's 'idea' as opposed to his 'impression.'

On the other hand it does not seem to be perfectly necessary that the real object should cease to be present; *e.g.* in 428 b 2 the appearance of the sun as of a foot in diameter is given as a case of φαντασία, and again, from 428 b 28, it is clear that φαντασία and αἴσθησις can synchronize. But the φαντασία is probably to be distinguished as the κίνησις which has penetrated to the heart—the ἀρχή; cf. *De Insom.* ch. 3, 461 b 12, 461 a 6; cf. also ch. 2, 459 a 23 sqq.: at least special emphasis is laid on this aspect. Sensations or stimuli travel from the end organ to the central one and persist after the exciting object is removed, καὶ ἐν βάθει καὶ ἐπιπολῆς. It must be the former which is the φάντασμα proper, for we hear in 450 a 11 sq. below that it belongs to the κοινὴ αἴσθησις and the πρῶτον αἰσθητήριον (cf. note to 450 a 11).

This all goes to emphasize the sensuous character of imagination, but however they are to be related to each other, we must not go so far as Themistius, who practically makes φαντασία a genus, which is known as αἴσθησις if the object is present, as μνήμη if it is absent, and makes the φαντασία in both cases the presentation of a τύπος or imprint left by the external object in the sensorium—the heart. But, after all, τύπος is only a metaphor to Aristotle. The αἴσθημα (sensation) is not strictly a τύπος; it is rather the λόγος of the αἰσθητόν, and the φάντασμα present in memory is not *per se* a τύπος, but only in so far as it represents the original perception. Even then it is only οἷον ζωγράφημα. Themistius himself sees that, according to his theory, only the very vaguest sense could be given to τύπος (238, l. 10: χρὴ δὲ κοινότερον τοῦ τύπου ἐπὶ τῆς φαντασίας ἀκούειν).

449 b 34. νοεῖν οὐκ ἔστιν κ.τ.λ. Cf. *De An.* III. ch. 7, 431 a 16: διὸ οὐδέποτε νοεῖ ἄνευ φαντάσματος ἡ ψυχή and 431 b 2: τὰ μὲν οὖν εἴδη τὸ νοητικὸν ἐν τοῖς φαντάσμασι νοεῖ, also ch. 8, 432 a 8: ὅταν τε θεωρῇ, ἀνάγκη ἅμα φαντάσματι θεωρεῖν.

The reasons which Aristotle adduces for this contention seem to be twofold, (1) firstly that brought forward in chapter 8 of *De Anima* III., that nothing self-dependent or 'isolated' (κεχωρισμένον 432 a 4) exists beyond the extended things given by sense perception; knowledge can occupy itself only with the εἴδη, forms of or concepts realised in sense objects. Hence, when the actual object is not present, thought is possible only if the φάντασμα originated by perception is present to the mind. Secondly (2) there is the reason obscurely implied in ch. 7, which culminates in the statement in 431 b 10 that truth and falsehood, the distinctions applicable to theoretical consciousness (cf. 431 a 14: τῇ διανοητικῇ ψυχῇ) are generically the same as good and evil, the objects of pursuit and avoidance in the practical life (cf. also *Eth. Nic.* VI. ch. 2, 1139 a 26); cf. Rodier, II. p. 515; affirmation and negation are at bottom the same as pursuit and avoidance (the germ of Pragmatism). Now, it is by means of sense that animals are able to distinguish between the pleasant and the unpleasant (cf. 431 a 10). Hence the pursuit of truth, which is distinguished from the quest of the good merely by having an absolute as opposed to a relative end (431 b 12), will employ the same sensuous images as the latter. This doctrine seems to be implied in Aristotle's statements, and we must remember that it in no way conflicts with what he elsewhere teaches—that there are entities capable of existing in isolation from the things of sense. There are τὰ ἀκίνητα τοῦ οὐρανοῦ εἴδη—the intelligible natures of the heavenly bodies (cf. Alexander *ap*. Simp., *De An*. 284, 23; Rodier, II. p. 524) which seem to be referred to by τὰ μὴ ἐν χρόνῳ ὄντα beneath (450 a 9-10). Again νοῦς—Reason—is said to be χωριστός, and we need not understand this of the human reason, but as applying to the mind of God, who is held to exist beyond the confines of the world and to stand to it in the relation of τὸ πρῶτον κινοῦν—the ultimate source of change in it. His activity is νόησις, and, if he exists in isolation from things sensible, one would expect that the contents of his thought would be likewise transcendent, and would not exist merely as realised or realisable in the world of change and decay. (Whether, if that is so, the object of the divine consciousness is a differentiated scheme of distinct intelligible entities existing apart from the material world, or whether the activity of God, the νόησις νοήσεως, is merely the affirmation of a blank identity—the eternal assertion of 'I am I'—it would be difficult to decide.)

But such statements constitute no assertion of the real separability of certain *concepts*, the Platonic doctrine of transcendent εἴδη, which is so consistently attacked by Aristotle. Though he continually talks of κεχωρισμένα or ἀκίνητα καὶ χωριστά as being the objects of metaphysical science (*De An*. I. ch. 1, 403 b 15; *Metaph*. VI. ch. 1, 1026 a 8 sqq.), φαντασία may be necessary for the realisation of such science in the mind of man. (In the passage in *De An*. III. ch. 8, where Aristotle says, 'as it appears no objects but sensible magnitudes exist,' we need find no denial of the objective existence of χωριστά, but merely his reiterated doctrine, that for human reason, which is not ἀπαθής, there are no objects of thought not realised in a sensuous material.)

450 a 9. ἄνευ τοῦ συνεχοῦς. Quantity, τὸ ποσόν, which is either discrete (as in number) or continuous (as in space or time) is here alluded to in the latter form, in which indeed it has been illustrated just above. It is the continuity which forms the perceptual element in the concepts of mathematical objects. We read in *De An*. III. ch. 8, 432 a 5 that concepts, including those belonging to mathematics, exist in the perceptual forms of things (ἐν τοῖς εἴδεσι τοῖς αἰσθητοῖς τὰ νοητά ἐστι) which, therefore, when we think, form the total object of consciousness from which the mind disengages the higher concept or νόημα. νοῦς is εἶδος εἰδῶν, whereas perception (as actualised) is the εἶδος αἰσθητῶν. The perceptual setting, as opposed to the higher concept, will form the ὕλη νοητή of which Aristotle tells in *Metaph.* VII. ch. 11, 1037 a 4 and ch. 10, 1036 a 9 sqq. : ὕλη δ' ἡ μὲν αἰσθητή ἐστιν ἡ δὲ νοητή, αἰσθητὴ μὲν οἷον χαλκὸς καὶ ξύλον καὶ ὅση κινητὴ ὕλη, νοητὴ δὲ ἡ ἐν τοῖς αἰσθητοῖς ὑπάρχουσα μὴ ᾗ αἰσθητά, οἷον τὰ μαθηματικά. (Cf. the discussion of *De An.* III. ch. 4, 429 b 10–22 in Rodier, II. p. 442 sqq. The ὕλη αἰσθητή is the actual matter of the physical substance apprehended. It is not this which gets into the soul when we perceive, but the εἶδος of the thing; cf. *De An.* III. ch. 8, 431 b 29 : οὐ γὰρ ὁ λίθος ἐν τῇ ψυχῇ ἀλλὰ τὸ εἶδος.) But this perceptual form itself supplies a matter for the higher concept, *e.g.* in mathematics. The pure mathematical concept is not τὸ εὐθύ or τὸ κοῖλον, the straight line or the curved, but τὸ εὐθεῖ εἶναι and κοιλότης—straightness or curvature (cf. *loc. cit.* 429 b 18 and ch. 7, 431 b 12, also *Metaph.* VI. ch. 1, 1025 b 30 sqq., x. ch. 8, 1058 a 23, etc.). But these concepts cannot exist apart, though they are for mathematical purposes assumed to exist apart (τὰ ἐξ ἀφαιρέσεως)—τὰ μαθηματικὰ οὐ κεχωρισμένα ὡς κεχωρισμένα νοεῖ. The general expression for this matter, 'matière logique,' without which these concepts cannot exist, is τὸ συνεχές (cf. 429 b 19 : μετὰ συνεχοῦς γάρ, and Philop. *De An.* 531, 15, ὕλη γάρ ἐστιν, ὥς φησιν, τῶν σχημάτων τὸ συνεχές).

ἄνευ χρόνου. Aristotle here mentions a different class of objects from the mathematical entities referred to in the last clause. He seems in particular to mean the heavenly bodies (cf. note to 449 b 34), which he continually refers to as ἀίδια and ἄφθαρτα (cf. *Phys.* IV. ch. 12, 221 b 3), and as not being in time. They differ from other bodies in not having a ὕλη which admits of growth and decay, but one which admits of motion only. Cf. *Metaph.* VIII. ch. 4, 1044 b 7.

One may say with Freudenthal (*op. cit.* p. 396) and Hammond that Aristotle here refers also to 'eternal laws'; they must be those of existence generally, and not merely the laws governing the motions of the heavenly bodies, as is implied by Hammond, for we hear in *Phys.* IV. ch. 12, 222 a 5 : τὸ ἀσύμμετρον εἶναι τὴν διάμετρον ἀεί ἐστιν. He does not, however, talk of laws or principles as existing apart from the objects which obey them. They at least are not on the same level of objectivity as the objects.

To suppose him to do so would be to impute to him the Platonic theory of εἴδη χωριστά. The concepts involved in thinking of the things of sense are not οὐσίαι, *e.g.* neither the point (στιγμή, cf. *Metaph.* VIII. ch. 5) nor the infinite (τὸ ἄπειρον, cf. *Phys.* III. ch. 5, 204 a 23, and *Metaph.* XI. ch. 10, 1066 b 13 sqq.) are οὐσίαι. Again, τὸ ἀγαθόν and τὸ καλόν are not εἴδη χωριστά. Though in the case of some concepts their essence and their existence is identical (*De An.* III. ch. 4, 429 b 12, and Rodier, *ad loc.* pp. 442 sqq.) this does not mean that these are to be regarded as substances (*e.g.* that their essence involves their existence, as according to Spinoza's definition of substance), but that their existence is a purely conceptual one. The ὅσα ἄνευ ὕλης mentioned in *De An.* III. ch. 6, 430 b 30, which are the ultimate simple constituents of intellect or objects of νοῦς (ἀδιαίρετα, τὰ ἄνευ συμπλοκῆς, πρῶτα νοήματα, *De An.* III. ch. 8, 432 a 12) and which are to be identified in part with the categories (cf. Rodier, II. p. 474, and *Metaph.* VIII. ch. 6, 1045 a 33 sqq.) partly with vague conceptions like the Good, Being, and the One, or again with τὸ ἄπειρον, στιγμή, μονάς, etc., are not to be regarded as existing apart from sensible things. If Aristotle says that they have neither ὕλη νοητή nor ὕλη αἰσθητή (*Metaph.*, *loc. cit.*), that simply means that they are ultimate and simple and are not formed by a complex of constituents, even mental constituents. These concepts must in fact be the constituents out of which the complex ones are formed. In that sense they themselves must be ἄνευ ὕλης but they are not χωριστά nor οὐσίαι in the sense in which the individual is οὐσία.

The connection with the thought here and the main contention— that thought cannot function apart from φαντασία—is not quite plain. Why should the impossibility of a thing being thought apart from time require the presence of a φάντασμα when it is apprehended? Doubtless it is because of the continuous nature of time which accrues to it owing to its connection with change. Cf. *Phys.* IV. ch. 11, 219 a 12 : διὰ γὰρ τὸ τὸ μέγεθος εἶναι συνεχὲς καὶ ἡ κίνησίς ἐστι συνεχής, διὰ δὲ τὴν κίνησιν ὁ χρόνος· ὅση γὰρ ἡ κίνησις, τοσοῦτος καὶ ὁ χρόνος ἀεὶ δοκεῖ γεγονέναι. Time is the 'measure' or 'number' of change ; cf. ch. 12, 220 b 8 sqq. (though not number in the proper sense, for that implies discreteness): and change is the great characteristic of the sensible world. No doubt it is because the heavenly bodies are μεγέθη and participate in κίνησις, though merely κίνησις κατὰ τόπον, that they must be represented as in time—a characteristic of the sensible world, and that they too can be apprehended only by means of φαντασία (cf. note to 449 b 34).

450 a 11. ᾧ. By this, as we have seen, Aristotle refers indifferently to the faculty or the organ and there is no ground for Freudenthal's refusal to think that the organ is here referred to. μέγεθος is certainly here not the simple equivalent of τὸ ποσόν above ; it is, rather, a particular example of quantity. Aristotle in this clause merely particularises what he had said before more universally of ποσόν in general, and at the same time the mention of κίνησις and χρόνος carries us beyond the particular example of spatial quantity which was indicated by the triangle. μέγεθος, κίνησις, and χρόνος, are all united (cf. previous note) as species of τὸ συνεχές, and it is pointed out that, in consequence, it must be the same function (and hence faculty and organ) which apprehends them all. If we keep the following sentences in the order given in the text, the argument will then be, " Magnitude, motion and time are perceived by the same faculty. But they (being *continua*, cf. previous note) form the sensuous and hence imageable element in consciousness. Now imagery belongs to the *sensus communis*. Hence the apprehension of these determinations of quantity belongs to the organ of the common sense—the primary sensorium. But memory, even that which deals with concepts, implies imagery. Hence it is a function of the primary organ of sensation directly, though indirectly it concerns the faculty of thought."

The whole argument as it stands is not well arranged and hence Freudenthal proposes to remodel it, but it is not much more confused than many others in the *Parva Naturalia* and the want of order can be explained. There are two conclusions to prove, (1) the minor premiss of the final conclusion—that thought must employ imagery, enunciated first in 449 b 34 sq. ; (2) that, since that is so, even the memory which deals with the objects of thought must be a function of the organ to which imagery is due. Involved in all this there is also the briefer argument that memory in general, employing imagery, must be attributed to the primary organ of sensation.

It is the involution of these three difficult discussions which causes the apparent want of coherence. There is moreover one premiss which is merely implicit and never formulated—that which identifies the imageable element—τὸ φανταστόν—with τὸ συνεχές. Aristotle simply assumes their identity as obvious, and any arrangement of the passage would have to fall back upon this principle as a constituent in the proof. Freudenthal proposes (*op. cit.* p. 397) to pass from χρόνον, l. 11, to ὥστε, l. 12, and insert the clause καὶ τὸ φάντ. ...πάθος ἐστίν after φαντάσματός ἐστιν, l. 14. For this he has the support of Themistius. Accordingly he gives the following as the sketch of the argument—"Every memory is bound up with a perception of time, every concept accompanied by a φάντασμα. To perceive time is identical with the perception of magnitude and motion, and is provided for by the πρῶτον αἰσθητικόν. Memory also uses concepts, but not apart from imagery, and this belongs to the πρῶτον αἰσθητικόν. Hence, memory belongs to it also."

But this does not do justice to the real complexity of the argument or bring out the main point—that even conceptual memory is a function of the primary sensorium. To prove that memory which does not specially deal with νοητά is a sense function would not cost so much argument.

Freudenthal seems to have been led astray by his misunderstanding of the reference to χρόνος in ll. 9 and 11. He thinks that there Aristotle refers to memory as a sense of time, as in 449 b 31. But there is no particular reference to this here. Aristotle is forced to talk of χρόνος because he wishes to illustrate the objects of thought which cannot be apprehended without an image in the mind, not only by the concepts of mathematics, τὰ ἐξ ἀφαιρέσεως, *e.g.* τὸ τρίγωνον, the scientific interest in which does not affect the matter in which they are realised, but by the eternal substances, which, though appearing in time, are not conditioned by it.

450 a 15. The texts all have νοουμένου, which must be a mistake instead either of νοητικοῦ or of διανοουμένου (Bywater, *J. of Philol.*, xxviii. p. 243). Biehl relying on the vet. tr. "intellectivi" has νοητικοῦ.

450 a 16. καὶ ἑτέροις. Cf. *De An.* iii. ch. 3, 428 a 10, 11, where φαντασία is attributed to the ant and the bee but not to the worm. Themistius brings in the dove (περιστερά) also.

450 a 20. The reading of all mss. is θνητῶν, but Rassow, *Prog. d. Joachimsth. Gym.* 1858, suggests θηρίων, which Biehl accepts. Most of the commentators certainly take θνητῶν as referring to the lower animals. Themistius writes ἀλόγων. If Aristotle meant to refer to them, certainly θηρίων is the more suitable term.

But Simon (p. 287), who also leans to the view that by θνητῶν "bruta" are meant, suggests as an alternative an interpretation which gives its proper sense to θνητῶν.—If Memory belonged to the faculty of pure thought it would not belong to many animals (for few possess reason), and perhaps to none that have a perishable body (which requires their thinking to be mediated by imagination). Relying on the famous passage at the end of *De An.* III. ch. 5, where the impassivity of the eternal νοῦς is set forth, and it is declared that we have no memory of a previous state of existence, because our thought depends upon the perishable reason which alone can experience impressions, he contends that, in Aristotle's opinion, memory does not belong to the superior and divine reason but only to the human, being exercised by the latter only through the instrumentality of φαντασία.

Whatever be the exact interpretation of the passage in the *De Anima* referred to, it is clear that, according to the Aristotelian teaching, νοῦς, in the sense of a faculty of pure thought, cannot exercise memory. Its function is the ἀδιαιρέτων νόησις (*De An.* III. ch. 6, 430 a 26) which must be something totally different from the apprehension of time in which there is no part which is indivisible. Again, in its characteristic sense, it is not a faculty of synthesis (*ibidem*) such as human thought and memory must be. (When we remember we must affirm that the image is like the real object, *i.e.* there must be synthesis : cf. below.)

Simon, however, takes the next clause (ἐπεὶ οὐδὲ νῦν πᾶσι, κ.τ.λ.) to refer to the lower animals which have not even got φαντασία (cf. *De An.* II. ch. 3, 415 a 10 : ἀλλὰ τοῖς μὲν οὐδὲ φαντασία); but, if that is so, it is difficult to see what it has to do with the previous statement. Even though we read θηρίων or interpret θνητῶν as θηρίων, we should have to render—"If memory were an affair of the intellect not many, perhaps none, of the lower animals would possess it, and, as a fact, as things are (memory being not an affair of the intellect), not all the lower animals do possess it, seeing that they do not all have the sense of time." But ἐπεὶ can hardly carry this meaning, and, even if it did, the latter clause adds nothing to the argument. That some animals, being without φαντασία, do not remember, does not in the least show why, if memory were a matter of pure thought, none would remember.

Yet it must be in some such way that Rassow and Biehl, reading θηρίων, take the sentence; and Simon, taking the last clause as he does, rather inclines to give up his first interpretation and follow the other commentators.

Hammond (p. 198) translating Biehl renders "perhaps in none

of the brutes, seeing that they do not, as a matter of fact possess it, because they all lack the sense of time." This is an impossible rendering of οὐδὲ νῦν πᾶσι and διὰ τὸ μὴ πάντα...ἔχειν, and, besides, contradicts ll. 16–17 immediately above, where memory is said to be found in certain other animals—διὸ καὶ ἑτέροις τισὶν ὑπάρχει τῶν ζώων.

Rassow, defending his emendation, maintains that it could not be said that if memory depended on thought it would be absent in man, one of the θνητά. But that is not so : memory exists in man only because he possesses the faculty of φαντασία ; if he were a being whose sole activity was pure thought he would not remember. It should be clear that, if memory depends solely upon the νοῦς παθη-τικός (which involves φαντασία and αἴσθησις), a being whose reason is not similarly to be described as passive will not remember.

Hence the solution of the difficulty is to take ἐπεὶ οὐδὲ νῦν πᾶσι, κ.τ.λ. as referring to that being or those things whose sole activity is the exercise of νοῦς—θεωρία, i.e. θεός—God, or perhaps to the heavenly bodies. Hence, after πᾶσι we are not to understand τοῖς θνητοῖς but τοῖς ζώοις.

It is not at all unprecedented for ζῷον to refer to living beings generally, nor is it impossible for it in this wide acceptation to include θεός and the heavenly bodies. Cf. De An. II. ch. 3, 414 b 15 sqq. : τῶν ζώων...ἐνίοις δὲ...ὑπάρχει καὶ τὸ κατὰ τόπον κινη-τικόν, ἑτέροις δὲ καὶ τὸ διανοητικόν τε καὶ νοῦς, οἷον ἀνθρώποις καὶ εἰ τοι-οῦτον ἕτερόν ἐστιν ἢ τιμιώτερον. By the latter Simplicius (De An. 106, 27) tells us the stars are meant ; cf. also De Caelo, II. 12, 292 a, 20 sqq. and ch. 8, 290 a 32. The stars are in the last passage called ζῷα. Cf. De An. I. ch. 1, 402 b 7, where it is implied that θεός is a species or particular example of ζῷον. Cf. also Metaph. XII. ch. 7, 1072 b 28 : φαμὲν δὲ τὸν θεὸν εἶναι ζῷον ἀίδιον ἄριστον, also XIV. ch. 1, 1088 a 10. Since the activity of God is νόησις (1072 b 18), and since, being ἀίδιος and ἄφθαρτος, he is not in time, it would be a safe deduction that he has not the χρόνου αἴσθησιν which is indis-pensable to memory.

Hence, the sense of the passage is clear—"Memory is not a function of pure thought for, if it were, none of the living creatures that are mortal, i.e. have perishable bodies and think by means of the sensuous images which are bound up with bodily changes would have memory. (Cf. De An. I. ch. 1, 403 a 13 sqq. The psychical changes we experience are λόγοι ἔνυλοι 403 a 25.) In fact certain living beings, which are freed from the conditions of human life, do not possess it."

450 a 22–23. Rassow (*op. cit.*) proposes to read ἢ ἔμαθε πρότερον, αἰσθάνεται and make αἰσθάνεται govern ὅτι εἶδε κ.τ.λ. The chief ground for the change is that προσαισθάνεται seems to be a ἅπαξ λεγόμενον. But Biehl lets it stand, reading ἐνεργῇ τῇ μνήμῃ as equivalent to μνημονεύει and as governing ὅτι εἶδε.

450 a 27. ὅσα μὴ ἄνευ φαντασίας. The question is whether there are any concepts which can be divorced from all imagery. Cf. previous notes.

450 a 32. Freudenthal (*op. cit.* p. 401) proposes either to omit τὸ πάθος or to read it after τοιοῦτον, l. 30. Certainly the words seem out of place and Rassow, who proposes either to delete τὸ after τοιοῦτον or to read τι, interprets the sentence following an order which places τὸ πάθος, οὗ...εἶναι after νοῆσαι l. 30.

450 a 34. Aristotle uses the metaphor of the seal-ring in another connection in the *De Anima*, III. ch. 12, 435 a 2. The object as it were stamps an impression on the air which as it were transmits it onwards until it meets the sensory organ. Again in II. ch. 12, 424 a 19 the impression on the organ produced by the sense object is compared to the impression left by a seal-ring on a surface. But cf. above note to 449 b 33.

450 b 1. πάθος Themistius renders by νόσου. Cf. *De An.* III. ch. 3, 429 a 7.

450 b 2. δι' ἡλικίαν. This, in consonance with the common use of ἡλικία (cf. Bonitz, *Ind.*), seems to refer both to the aged and the young. In both the mind seems to be too "fluid" to retain impressions, cf. ῥέουσι, l. 7 beneath.

450 b 4. τὸ ψήχεσθαι. This may be another simile for the minds of the aged, and Aristotle may have in view the crumbling condition of an old stone surface. But in the light of its conjunction with σκληρότητα l. 5, perhaps it refers to the inner walls of a building that had originally a prepared surface in which a design was cut, but which gets worn off and leaves nothing but the hard layer beneath. This is suggested by a perusal of the famous passage in the *Theaetetus* (191 c sqq. especially 194 c sqq.) from which Aristotle seems to have drawn almost all the illustrations here employed. There the heart is compared to a waxen tablet (κήρινον ἐκμαγεῖον) on which impressions are stamped. The surface must be neither too soft nor too hard, for, in the former case, the mind, though easily receiving an impression, soon loses it (ὧν μὲν ὑγρόν, εὐμαθεῖς μέν, ἐπιλήσμονες δὲ γίγνονται), while, with the hard surface, the opposite is the case. For a mind of good capacity, the waxen surface must be not only of the proper consistency but deep (βαθύς τε καὶ πολὺς καὶ λεῖος καὶ μετρίως ὠργασμένος). People with such an organ are both εὐμαθεῖς and μνήμονες.

Now an ἐκμαγεῖον or prepared surface need not be composed of wax; it may consist of gypsum (cf. L. and S.), and probably the decorated parts of Greek houses and buildings (where marble was not employed) may have had a layer of plaster imposed on the stone, with bas-reliefs cut thereon.

450 b 6–7. Cf. also ch. 2, 453 b 5.

450 b 18. Freudenthal proposes to read ἢ τούτου αἴσθησις instead of τούτου αὐτοῦ ἡ αἴσθησις with Themistius (*Sp.* ii. p. 239, l. 25). The change is not important.

450 b 27. Biehl brackets θεώρημα, while Freudenthal (*op. cit.* p. 401) deletes both it and φάντασμα, on the ground that if we read αὐτό τι καθ' αὑτὸ εἶναι θεώρημα the next line ἢ μὲν οὖν καθ' ἑαυτὸ, θεώρημα ἢ φάντασμά ἐστιν forms a tautology and, if we read ἄλλου φάντασμα, is contradictory.

Biehl has the support of L S U, Themistius and the ancient translation, in omitting θεώρημα. If we read θεώρημα it will be better to follow E Y and read καὶ αὐτὸ καθ' ἑαυτὸ εἶναι θεώρημα καὶ ἄλλου φάντασμα—"is both an object of consciousness *per se* and the image of something else." Then the next sentence goes on to explain and correct this statement. "*Per se* it is an object of consciousness or an image; so far as it is the appearance of something else it is a copy and souvenir."

The contradiction, or rather the duality, in the use of φάντασμα here, which causes Freudenthal to expunge it from the former clause, is really one which goes right down into the heart of the concept of φαντασία and φαίνεσθαι as used by Aristotle. A φάντασμα is at once a sensuous image posited like a simple sensation or a fundamental concept before the mind, and at the same time it claims to represent something objective. In its first aspect, as a simple element in the content of consciousness, it has nothing to do with either truth or falsity; in its second capacity it falls within the domain of synthesis, in which truth and error reside. (Cf. note on φαντασία above 449 b 33.) Here Aristotle uses it first in the second of the two above senses, but immediately reminds us that properly and *per se* the

R. 17

φάντασμα has no reference to the object, that, so far as it has this, it is considered in a new light—as an εἰκών.

Hence, if Aristotle is in the second sentence really guarding his former statement, it would not be out of place to repeat that part of the former statement with which part of the second is identical. Hence, we may retain θεώρημα; it is no doubt used to signify the direct, immediate object of consciousness, something that is present as if to the senses (cf. Bonitz, *Ind.* p. 328). It would include a present perception and so cover the case, never separately treated by Aristotle, of the recognition that an object in present perception has been seen before.

On the other hand νόημα is substituted in 451 a 2, which rather makes it appear as though θεώρημα meant a concept specially. But probably this change is not significant.

450 b 29. Freudenthal proposes to omit καὶ after εἰκών, tr. "a memorial after the fashion of a copy." μνημόνευμα is a ἅπαξ λεγόμενον in Aristotle.

450 b 33. μὴ ἑωρακώς. It is not hereby implied that we can remember without a prior sensuous experience. That would contradict what has been already said (cf. 449 b 24 sqq. above). μὴ ἑωρακώς must mean—without having then had present to vision the veritable Coriscus.

450 b 34. ἐνταῦθα κ.τ.λ. All commentators from Michael Ephesius to Freudenthal notice that this paragraph is mere repetition. If more condensed and obscure it is not thereby less Aristotelian.

451 a 13-14. Cf. chapter 2, 451 b 15 and 32, ἔθει.

CHAPTER II.

451 a 21. ἐν τοῖς ἐπιχειρηματικοῖς λόγοις. Themistius (*Sp.* II. p. 241, l. 7) says ἐπιχειρηματικοῖς καὶ προβληματικοῖς, and, if we trust Diogenes Laertius, *R.V.* § 23–24, there was more than one work falling under the first title, viz. ὑπομνήματα ἐπιχειρηματικά γ΄ and ἐπιχειρημάτων α΄ β΄. Hence it is probably to them that we are here referred. Michael Ephesius thinks rather that the *Problems* are indicated, but in the extant *Problems* no such discussion is found.

An ἐπιχείρημα is defined in *Topics*, VII. ch. 11, 158 a 16 as συλλογισμὸς διαλεκτικός, and ἐπιχειρεῖν very often means to discuss controversially (cf. Bonitz, *Ind.* p. 282 b 59). Now Aristotle frequently, even in the same book, prefaces his proper scientific treatment of a subject with a 'dialectical' account. This seems to be necessary in his view in order to attain a preliminary clearing up of notions, and hence we may conjecture that he wrote several popular tentative tractates (the literal sense of ἐπιχειρέω, = to attempt, seems to linger about ἐπιχείρημα) on various matters, and that these, owing to their tentative character, have been dropped out of the canon. Certainly we cannot here translate with Hammond 'treatise *On Argumentation.*' A reference to recollection could occur only as an illustration in a logical work, and λόγοι ἐπιχειρηματικοί could not be discussions *on* dialectical argumentation but discussions *of* a dialectical nature.

451 a 23 sqq. We may set aside Simon's theory that by λῆψις is here meant not λῆψις μνήμης but the acquirement of fresh knowledge. There is no evidence that that is an Aristotelian usage, nor will the Greek bear the interpretation.

At the same time it is difficult to see what relation this statement bears to the following one. Having asserted that recollection is neither the reacquirement nor the first acquirement of memory, he goes on to point out that in μάθησις—the first acquirement of *knowledge,* there is no such thing as recovery or acquisition of *memory.*

The doctrine that recollection is to be thus described is, as Freudenthal, *Rheinisches Museum,* p. 404, points out, not a Platonic one; but, of course, the teaching that μάθησις is ἀνάμνησις is the famous tenet set forth in the *Meno* and other dialogues; cf. esp. *Meno,* 85 D: τὸ δὲ ἀναλαμβάνειν αὐτὸν ἐν αὑτῷ ἐπιστήμην οὐκ ἀνάμνησις; Πάνυ γε. *Phaedo,* 72 E sqq. Hence the tortuous argument here seems to be...'When you recollect, you do not reacquire or acquire memory. If you take ἀνάμνησις with the Platonists as equivalent to μάθησις it is certainly not so (ὅταν γὰρ l. 23...ἐγγίνεται l. 27), nor when taken in the ordinary sense, as the remembering again of something forgotten, is it strictly defined either as the acquisition or reacquisition of a memory' (ἔτι δ' ὅτε κ.τ.λ. l. 27 sq.).

Freudenthal (*loc. cit.* p. 403) points out that Plato really anticipated the Aristotelian distinction between ἀνάμνησις and μνήμη (cf. *Phaedo,* 77 C sqq.). Recollection is a knowing again of what has been forgotten. It is to be reminded of something by oneself or by another; cf. *Phaedo,* 73 B, ἀναμνησθῆναι = commonefieri : μέμνηται = meminit. Recollection implies ζήτησις *Meno,* 81 D. But the scientific discrimination of the two functions belongs to Aristotle.

(Plato also noticed the three ways in which ideas may be associated; cf. 451 b 22 sq. *infra,* contiguity, similarity, and contrast. Cf. *Phaedo,* 73 (1) A lyre or garment belonging to the beloved one puts the lover in mind of him and from seeing Simmias you may remember Cebes. (2) From seeing the picture of Simmias you may remember him. (3) Recollection may be derived from things unlike as well as from similar things.)

451 a 25. If we translate ἐξ ἀρχῆς as 'at the beginning,' then this argument becomes practically identical with the next, and Freudenthal will be right in saying that we have here the same thought as is repeated in ἔτι δ' κ.τ.λ. ll. 27 sqq.

But perhaps the sense is rather...'when we learn, we neither have a memory reinstated in us, nor derive it (as a memory) from some origin, *i.e.* some other experience. Once the present experience is produced you may remember it; *quâ* present experience it is not remembered. To start memory you need present experience, and hence you cannot derive the present experience from the memory.'

Aristotle is thus dealing here not with the temporal but the logical priority of present experience. It is in the next paragraph that he goes on to show that memory requires, in addition to the originating experience, a period of time to have elapsed before it can be called memory. In addition, this is now brought in when he is dealing with ἀνάμνησις in the customary sense, not as identical with μάθησις, and hence the point of view is different.

But without adopting this hypothesis we may detect a note of individuality in the present passage. Perhaps in ὅταν δὲ κ.τ.λ. (ll. 25–27) the emphasis is on the necessity of there being a ἕξις—a disposition to remember—as well as an experience (πάθος) which is to be remembered, while in the next paragraph the lapse of time necessary becomes more prominent.

451 a 26. ἕξις. As I take it, this means the permanent disposition which itself *is* memory; it is not to be identified with τὴν ἕξιν in l. 30 beneath, which is a disposition produced by learning regarded as a *source* of memory. It is, however, somewhat misleading to think of that as being a source of memory in the same way as a πάθος is. Quâ ἕξις nothing is an activity (ἐνέργεια) of consciousness and all memory must start from a present activity.

451 a 28. τὸ πρῶτον ἐγγέγονε, Biehl and Bekker; τὸ πρῶτον ἐγγεγόνει ἐν, L S U.

Freudenthal proposes to insert τι after ἐγγέγονε in order to provide it with a subject, τὸ πρῶτον being taken adverbially.

τῷ ἀτόμῳ καὶ ἐσχάτῳ. All commentators take this as referring to time, and that would be the most likely meaning of the Greek if we read ἐν τῷ ἀτόμῳ with L S U. But the dative which ἐγγίγνεσθαι governs should rather indicate the real ὑποκείμενον in which the πάθος originates, not the time. Hence perhaps we should interpret τῷ ἀτόμῳ κ.τ.λ. as referring to the αἰσθητήριον which is the primary seat of sensation and which, we learn in *De Sensu*, 7, is αὐτὸ καὶ ἐν ἀριθμῷ and is also elsewhere called τὸ ἔσχατον αἰσθητήριον, *De An.* III. ch. 2, 426 b 16 and 7, 431 a 19. This is also Neuhäuser's interpretation: cf. Introduction, sec. VI.

The argument then is, that the mere realisation of the impression in the primary organ of sensation—the heart or its σύμφυτον πνεῦμα— is not memory. There must be lapse of time before it can function as an εἰκών of the absent object.

If we take ἀτόμῳ καὶ ἐσχάτῳ as referring to time, it is difficult to interpret ἐσχάτῳ. We should have to translate 'in the same individual and proximate moment of time.' But the proximate is *not* the same moment, unless in the improper sense in which the same thing may be said to be proximate to itself.

Michael Ephesius thinks that the reference here is to the moment *after* complete perception and that this is here distinguished from the moment of perception mentioned in the last sentence. Freudenthal finds this too 'spitzfindig' and accordingly chooses to regard this passage as another version of the former one (cf. note to l. 25 above).

451 a 31.   κατὰ συμβεβηκὸς.   Cf. ch. 1, 450 a 15–16.

451 a 32.   πρὶν χρονισθῆναι.   Cf. ch. 1, 449 b 28.

451 b 2.   Unless we accent ἔστι with Freudenthal the sentence will not construe.

The interpretation of ἐξ ἀρχῆς here confirms our rendering of the same phrase in 451 a 25.   The ἀρχή is the starting point in time rather than the original experience from which the continued consciousness known as memory is derived.

451 b 3.   ἀλλ' ὅταν κ.τ.λ.   Here at last is the distinction between ἀνάμνησις (in the proper and customary, as distinct from the Platonic sense) and μνήμη.

Recollection is the reproduction of a previous experience (apart, of course, from renewed sense perception or repetition of the experience, whatever its nature, afresh), which has passed out of the mind, and a revival—ἀνανέωσις (Themistius)—*quâ* experience, not *quâ* memory. The memory, holding the present experience as the εἰκών of the past, can be produced either by the continued presence in consciousness of the previous experience or by its reinstatement through recollection. It is a consequence (συμβαίνει l. 6) that, when we reinstate an experience identical in character with the previous one, we should remember, *i.e.* that it is an εἰκών of the previous one.   But it is the act of reinstatement which is accurately to be described as ἀνάμνησις, not the referring of the reinstated experience to the past.

451 b 6–7.   Michael (132 a), Simon (p. 301) and Gesner, apparently (cf. Freud. *Rh. Mus.*), read τῷ δὲ μνημονεύειν συμβαίνει καὶ μνήμην ἀκολουθεῖν. This Freudenthal (p. 407) approves of, objecting to the absolute use of συμβαίνει in the other reading and trying to make out that we should, if we kept it, have to distinguish as different from each other, (1) ἀνάμνησις, (2) μνημονεύειν and (3) μνήμη. That is surely captious and, on the reading which he approves, we should have (with Gesner) to interpret μνημονεύειν as ἀναμιμνήσκεσθαι; but Freudenthal admits (p. 403) that, where Aristotle is distinguishing the two functions, he never employs a term, which refers to remembering merely, to designate the act of recollection, however much he may depart from this rule on other occasions.

Themistius says—ἕπεται δὲ τῇ ἀναμνήσει ἐξ ἀνάγκης ἡ μνήμη, understanding by ἕπεται apparently (and if there is any sense in his explanation) mere logical implication. He explains 'recollection implies memory because, to recollect, you must remember something connected with the thing which you are trying to recollect...the starting point in the ζήτησις which is recollection' (cf. *infra* 26 sqq.). Not only, however, is this a strange interpretation of συμβαίνειν and ἀκολουθεῖν, but, if recollection may start ἀπὸ τοῦ νῦν (l. 22 *infra*) it is not necessary for its starting point to be an object of memory.

451 b 7. ταῦτα refers vaguely and inclusively to ἀναμιμνήσκεσθαι and μνημονεύειν. The sense is...'you do not get recollection and memory every time an experience which has lapsed from the mind is repeated. It may be repeated without your remembering you had it before. In such cases the repetition of the experience is not recollection.' This is pretty nearly Simon's interpretation. St Hilaire, evidently basing upon Themistius's interpretation of the preceding sentence, thinks that here Aristotle is making explicit his distinction between the revived and the non-revived elements in consciousness in the act of recollection. (St Hilaire, p. 123): 'Ce ne sont pas du reste des choses antérieures qui se reproduisent complètement de nouveau dans l'esprit; mais il y a alors une partie des choses qui se reproduit et une partie qui ne se reproduit pas; car la même personne pourrait très bien deux fois découvrir et apprendre la même chose.' But this interpretation can only be come at by reading ἐγγίνεται l. 8 (impossible Greek) or by supplying it after ἐγγένηται; further ταῦτα would have to refer to ἐπιστήμην etc., l. 4, which is rather too far back and would suggest the use of ἐκεῖνα; thirdly the thought is still more elliptical and loosely arranged than on the interpretation I give. 'The previous experience is not wholly reinstated for, if it were, it would be a case of μάθησις not ἀνάμνησις.' This renders ἀλλ' ἔστιν...ἔστι δ' equivalent to 'partly ...partly' and makes us refer δὶς γὰρ μαθεῖν not to the clause immediately before it but to the previous one.

Hammond (p. 204) gives a totally new rendering, 'Neither do the phenomena of recollection, if their occurrence is the repetition of a previous recollection (*sic*), follow absolutely the same order, but sometimes they occur in one way, sometimes in another. It is possible for the same individual to learn and discover the same thing twice. Recollection then must differ from learning and discovery, and there is need of greater initial latitude (*sic*) here than is the case with learning.' He elucidates this in a note, 'In the case of learning and discovery there is a definite and exact process by which a given result may be twice arrived at.' (What Aristotelian doctrine is this?) '...In the case of recollection, on the other hand, there is not the same fixity of procedure. There are not only many forms of suggestion and association, but a given suggestion may not effect the same result in two instances.' This is to introduce a point mentioned in 452 a 27 below but not relevant here. It is in no way apparent that Aristotle ever meant to compare the acquisition and the revival of knowledge with regard either to the relative fixedness of the processes or the fixity of the starting point.

St Hilaire quite fails to see that τούτων (l. 11) refers to μαθεῖν καὶ εὑρεῖν, and so he completely distorts the sense.

451 b 11. καὶ ἐνούσης κ.τ.λ. On the whole this favours my interpretation of the previous passage rather than St Hilaire's. On his theory, relearning a thing implies complete reinstatement of everything in consciousness and it is difficult to see how there would be any ἀρχή at all in that case.

It is Aristotle's theory that in learning (either for the first or second time) as well as in recollection there is an ἀρχή from which we set out. We find no contradiction to this in 451 a 25 above; there he simply says that in the process of learning memory does not begin concurrently with the initial step. Here he merely distinguishes learning and recollection according to the *amount* of the ἀρχή involved; but we can gather his doctrine from other passages. We learn either by deduction or induction (*Anal. Post.* I. ch. 18, 81 a 38 sqq.) and, in either case, we must have some previous knowledge which is the starting point of our deduction or our induction. (Cf. *Anal. Post.* I. ch. 1, 71 sqq. and *Metaph.* I. ch. 9, 992 b 30 sqq.) In the one case we must know the premises of any particular conclusion and ultimately the constituents of the definitions of the terms (which enter into our premises); δεῖ γὰρ ἐξ ὧν ὁρισμὸς προειδέναι καὶ εἶναι γνώριμα (992 b 32). In the latter, the knowledge of particular cases which are given in perception (τὰ καθ' ἕκαστα, τὰ ἐγγύτερον τῆς αἰσθήσεως *Anal. Post.* I. ch. 2, 72 a 2, 3) and which are less intelligible naturally (τῶν ἧττον γνωρίμων φύσει *Metaph.* VII. ch. 4, 1029 b 4), is required before we can gather from them the universal law. But in learning by induction we do not have previous knowledge of the universal law, nor in deduction have we a prior acquaintance with the particular case. (It is only in so far as the particular is implicit in the universal that it is previously known. In its particularity and in the full sense of the word it is not known : ἁπλῶς δ' οὐκ ἐπίσταται 71 a 28.) If it had been explicitly thought of previously, then we should have a case of recollection not of μάθησις, which must be distinguished from ἀνάμνησις and is thus to be distinguished.

Another point of difference is that mentioned below in 452 a 5 sqq. Learning requires a teacher ; the process of recollection is self-originated.

There is also a sense in which the act of learning is not a process. Cf. *Phys.* VII. ch. 3, 247 b 10 sqq. and also *De An.* I. ch. 3, 407 a 32. This however comes to no more than the familiar doctrine that *per se* the intellectual life is not a σωματικὸν πάθος like memory and recollection. But in this sense it cannot apply without qualification to the functioning of the νοῦς παθητικός which is realised in finite individuals.

451 b 14. ἐξ ἀνάγκης. Hamilton (*Reid*, p. 894) points out that Locke too, in Essay II. ch. 33 § 5, distinguishes between those ideas which are naturally connected by a 'union and correspondence which is founded in their peculiar beings' and those that are associated 'through chance or custom.' By those necessarily connected Aristotle means notions which objectively imply one another, like centre and circumference. As Hamilton indicates, it was typical of members of the empirical English school (other than Locke) to ascribe all collocations of ideas to custom.

451 b 16–17. Freudenthal's reading (*op. cit.* p. 407)—συμβαίνει δ' ἐνίας μᾶλλον ἢ ἑτέρας πολλάκις κινουμένας—seems unnecessarily to anticipate the doctrine of 452 a 3 sqq. *infra.*

451 b 20. Freudenthal's conjecture of τινὰς instead of τινὰ makes the reading smoother, 'we experience a *number* of previous changes conducting to the stimulation of that one' etc.

451 b 22. τοῦ νῦν ἢ ἄλλου τινός. By this Aristotle cannot mean merely 'a time present or otherwise.' It is difficult to see how one could start a process of reflection otherwise than from the present time. The idea is that the object, the thought of which starts the train of recollection, can be given either in present perception or in memory.

ἀφ' ὁμοίου κ.τ.λ. This describes the character of the object or content of the notion which starts the process.

It is the first recorded formulation of the celebrated laws of association, though they are all to be found instanced in the *Phaedo.* Cf. above note to 451 a 23.

451 b 24. τῶν δ' ἅμα. This evidently is capable of being illustrated by the ἐναντίαι κινήσεις which, being affections of a single sense organ, must be ἅμα; cf. *De Sens.* ch. 7, 447 b 9 sq.: μᾶλλον γὰρ ἅμα ἡ κίνησις τῆς μιᾶς ταύτης (αἰσθήσεως) ἢ τοῖν δυοῖν. Here of course the κινήσεις seem to be regarded as existing in the central not in the end organ, but evidently the characteristic of being ἅμα, which distinguishes ἐναντίαι κινήσεις in the end organ, is regarded as attaching to them when they are transferred to the heart.

If this interpretation be correct 'Association by Contrast' is to be assigned to 'Contiguity.'

451 b 27. δ' οὕτως. δ' ὅμως Freudenthal, G. A. Bekker. The change is immaterial unless with Themistius, Leonicus, and Simon we take the οὕτως with ζητοῦντες and translate 'and we recollect, even though we do not search in this way.' But we see from 453 a 18 sqq. below, that Aristotle does not limit ἀνάμνησις to the volitional process which reinstates an idea. Recollection is there said in some cases *not* to be ἐπ' αὐτοῖς, *i.e.* subject to the will.

Cf. also Hamilton *op. cit.* p. 902, note.

451 b 30. μεμνήμεθα here must be used inaccurately for ἀναμιμνησκόμεθα: cf. 452 a 8, 11.

τὰ πόρρω. Hamilton, *op. cit.* p. 903, takes this as 'things remote and irrelevant to our inquiry' and (apparently) not as the object of μεμνήμεθα. This is surely very unnatural; the use of τὰ πόρρω and τὰ σύνεγγυς to denote something else than objects and processes which are connected in the train of recollection, just where the series has been described in terms of similar notions, would be a most flagrant instance of slipshod writing on the part of Aristotle. Hamilton translates, ' Nor is there any necessity to consider things remote [and irrelevant] how these arise in memory; but only the matters coadjacent (and pertinent to our inquiry). For it is manifest that the mode is still the same—that, to wit, of consecution,—[in which a thing recurs to us, when] neither pre-intentionally seeking it, nor voluntarily reminiscent. *For [here too], by custom, the several movements are concomitant of one another—this determinately following upon that.*' Hamilton, reading τρόπος πῶς (λέγω δὲ τὸ ἐφεξῆς) οὐ κ.τ.λ., thinks that reference is still being made to the case of voluntary and involuntary reminiscence, and that it is the manner of occurrence of these two which is said to be identical. But προζητήσας and ἀναμνησθείς cannot distinguish intentional as opposed to unintentional recollection. (What can 'pre-intentionally' mean?) It is the method of recalling τὰ πόρρω and τὰ σύνεγγυς which is the same. As the remoteness of two distantly connected ideas can be bridged over by inserting intermediate ones, it is the mode of connection of these latter we have to consider.

451 b 31–32. λέγω δὲ...ἀναμνησθείς. A gloss according to Freudenthal. But, if we let it stand, it simply points out the fact that he refers to the order of a series of psychic changes determined, not by any previous act of recollection, but by the way in which they are accustomed (τῷ γὰρ ἔθει l. 32) to be experienced together.

451 b 35. ἀρχὴν κινήσεως. This is simply the term for efficient cause used in *Phys.* II. ch. 7, 198 b 1, *Metaph.* I. ch. 3, 984 a 27, etc. Here we are dealing with that class of efficient causes or sources of change which are themselves motions or changes. The series of changes in conscious process is conceived by Aristotle quite in the same way as all other changes occurring in the world of generation and decay. The whole series is a κίνησις which is made up of parts which are themselves κινήσεις. Hence Themistius's illustration of the series of mental sequences by a chain in which, if one link be lifted, the next will also be moved (*Sp.* II. p. 243, l. 12) is inadequate. The links in the series are themselves nothing static but processes also.

So far as we have gone, the κινήσεις which are stimulated in the act of recollection seem to be dormant in the soul or its organ the heart prior to stimulation, and this is apparently the view maintained through the *De Memoria*. In *De An.* I. ch. 4, 408 b 15 sqq., however, a rather different attitude is taken up. In recollection the κίνησις is said to pass from the soul to the affections (also κινήσεις) or their traces (μονάς) existing in the sense organs; this is opposed to what occurs in sense perception, where the κίνησις proceeds in the reverse way. In neither case is the process *in* the soul.

By this however Aristotle probably means no more than to emphasize the fact that in the higher faculties the mind is an originating cause. Of course, in all cases the soul is an ἀρχή (cf. *De An.* I. ch. 1, 402 a 7) and to be regarded as an efficient as well as a final cause (*De Part. Animal.* I. ch. 1, 641 a 27). But, just as none of its modifications, even a primitive one like perception, is mere passivity (cf. *De An.* II. ch. 5) so we seem to find a progressively greater absence of passivity as we pass from lower to higher faculties; *e.g.* scientific knowledge—ἐπιστήμη—is not passive change of the type ἀλλοίωσις in the proper sense at all (417 b 6). A mechanical determination of psychic processes by each other may go on and be beyond the control of the individual in whom they occur (cf. 453 a 18 sqq. *infra*). This is held to show the corporeal nature of such changes, or rather their dependence upon corporeal conditions. Hence it is suggested by implication that a function which was exclusively psychical would not be determined in this mechanical way but would be completely under control (ἐπ᾽ αὐτοῖς : 453 a 22). Notwithstanding Aristotle's determination to make out all human faculties to be conditioned by the bodily organism, and thus establish a thorough-going parallelism of psychical and corporeal changes, notwithstanding the fact that he declares the human νοῦς to be παθητικός, there seems to be this tendency to free itself from bodily conditions which is always manifested by that which is most characteristically psychical. It is significant that in this passage where Aristotle talks of the process in recollection proceeding outward from the soul, he immediately goes on (as if impelled by association of ideas) to talk of the νοῦς which is impassive and imperishable, and practically identifies ψυχή with it. The decline of the mental faculties is just like the dimness of sight in an old man, due to the bodily organ becoming impaired. It is not the ψυχή which suffers change but its organ (ὥστε τὸ γῆρας οὐ τῷ τὴν ψυχήν τι πεπονθέναι, ἀλλ᾽ ἐν ᾧ, 408 b 22). Hence the ultimate core of the ψυχή seems to consist of this imperishable νοῦς, which, no doubt, relatively to the body will be like the divine νοῦς in its relation to the world, the prime source of movement—τὸ πρῶτον κινοῦν.

Aristotle, however, does not state this explicitly, and though, indeed, he tells us that the νοῦς enters the living being from outside and its activity has nothing in common with that of the body (*De Gener. Animal.* II. ch. 3, 736 b 28) yet the relation of this to the other mental faculties is most obscure in his philosophy, and really leads to difficulties much the same as those surrounding the relation of the Platonic ἰδέα to the things of time and sense.

452 a 2. τὰ πράγματα (the facts) may be either static elements, *e.g.* contiguous objects or different parts of a mathematical theorem, or events themselves. The series may be either temporal or not.

452 a 4. φαῦλα is the version of L S U. Themistius and Michael read φαύλως καὶ χαλεπῶς. For φαῦλος in the sense of inexact cf. Thuc. vi. 18. Cf. also *Metaph.* vii. ch. 4, 1029 b 10.

452 a 8. μέμνηται. Referring a reinstated process to the past is a characteristic of remembering as distinct from learning a second time : cf. 451 b 6. Hence Aristotle is justified in using memory here as the generic term to include recollection.

452 a 10. κινοῦντι πολλά. This surely refers to many different starts not to many different items in a single series.

452 a 11–12. τὸ γὰρ μεμνῆσθαι κ.τ.λ. The *act* of memory cannot be the merely potential existence of a process in the mind.

δυνάμει. δύναμιν L S U, Themistius, vet. tr. But we do not elsewhere hear of a special δύναμις κινοῦσα in the mind. It is an *actual* process which functions in recollection.

452 a 14. ἀπὸ τόπων. This, surely, as the illustration below bears out, refers to the τόποι—commonplaces of thought in general which Aristotle defines in their most universal sense in *Rhet.* i. ch. 2, 1358 a 12 : (οἱ τόποι) εἰσὶν οἱ κοινῇ περὶ δικαίων καὶ φυσικῶν καὶ περὶ πολιτικῶν καὶ περὶ πολλῶν διαφερόντων εἴδει, οἷον ὁ τοῦ μᾶλλον καὶ ἧττον τόπος : cf. also l. 32. The τόπος is a rule or general statement that will readily recur to one and hence it may be used as the ἀρχή of a train of ideas in recollection. *E.g.* it is a τόπος of the Aristotelian philosophy that air is damp, and apparently from *Meteor.* iii. ch. 4, 374 a 2 that it is λευκός ; that milk is white and the autumn damp are given by ordinary perception.

Unfortunately Aristotle in illustrating the use of τόποι in recollection by those drawn from his own philosophy gives a series of ideas which would hardly with plausibility be used in the purposive recall of an idea. Hence Hamilton (followed by St Hilaire) proposes to read ἀπ' ἀτόπων. But if the series is an absurd one still less likely is it to be employed in voluntary recollection, which is now being discussed. Themistius (*Sp.* ii. p. 247, ll. 8 sqq.) gives a variety of alternative explanations to τόπων. τόπους δὲ ἢ ἃς ἀρχὰς ἐνεῖναι δεῖν τῇ ψυχῇ λέγομεν, ἢ τοὺς κατὰ τὰ σύστοιχα καὶ ὅμοια καὶ ἀντικείμενα ὡς ἐν τῇ διαλεκτικῇ εἴρηται, ἢ τοὺς σωματικοὺς καὶ τὰς ἐν τῷδε τῷ μέρει θέσεις. Thomas interprets it as meaning the last merely. In that case, the reference would be to the art of memorising objects by attaching each to a special point in a spatial series—an art said to have been discovered by Simonides of Ceos and referred to by Cicero in *De Oratore*, ii. ch. 86.

So Hammond and Freudenthal, *loc. cit.* p. 409 (who indeed in consequence wishes to read τάχιστα instead of ἐνίοτε in l. 15). But it is strange that Aristotle after mentioning this method of memorising should give an example which has no reference to it.

452 a 18. τὸ καθόλου is read by L S U Y, Themistius and Michael. Both those commentators, however, render it by ὡς ἐπὶ τὸ πολύ, a meaning which, according to Freudenthal (*Archiv für Gesch. d. Philos.* II. 1887, p. 11) καθόλου can certainly have. They thus interpret τὸ καθόλου as though the τὸ were inessential. Siebeck however in *Philol.* 1881, pp. 350–2, and his *Untersuchungen zur Philosophie der Griechen*, p. 155, wishes to retain τὸ and to make it essential. He thinks that here Aristotle identifies the middle of a series of terms employed in reminiscence with the μέσον of logical inference which is a universal and furthest from sense. The connecting bond in recollection is a universal concept which binds together various particulars by means of their implication in it.

This comes to pretty much the same as Mr Bradley's doctrine that 'Association marries only Universals,' or more simply, that there is a bond of identity between the thing remembered and the thing that brings it to mind. This however has been already made clear enough in 451 b 21–26 above, and it is strange that Aristotle should confuse that implication of a predicate in the middle term of a syllogism, which accounts for the truth of the conclusion, with that relation between psychical states which causes the presentation of the one to entail the presentation of the other. In the latter case you are accounting for a process, in the former for a connection which is independent of process. Moreover the 'universal' which connects different ideas in reminiscence is hardly the universal of logic—that which is 'furthest from sense'; it is often of the most sensuous character. Once more, it would be unfair to represent it as a separate member in the train of connected ideas; it is rather the identical element pervading any two.

In the details of the subsequent passage Siebeck's interpretation is beset with at least no fewer difficulties than Freudenthal's. Cf. also next note *sub fin.*

452 a 21. ἐφ' ὧν ΑΒΓΔΕΖΗΘ κ.τ.λ.

Biehl's text, which I print, follows Freudenthal's reconstruction of the passage. I have translated it as it stands. But it can hardly be said that all difficulties have been removed even by this radical alteration of Bekker's text. The general drift seems to be that the middle term of a series of connected ideas is of unique importance because from it you can go in either direction to the other members. If you have a series of ideas A B C D E F G H and want to remember F or G and are not able to do so when you think of H, by thinking of E you may be able to recall them. Then from E you can get either to D or F, or from C you can pass to B, the term before it.

But this is not at all persuasive. Why should the final possibility of recall be the starting from A, which is an extreme in the series, if it is the employment of the middle term which Aristotle is illustrating? Besides, as Freudenthal himself points out, there is no single middle term in a series of eight.

Again, Freudenthal does not seem to give sufficient weight to the objection that this makes Aristotle talk of recollection as proceeding in a reverse order with equal facility.

Bekker's text is as follows (l. 21) : εἰ γὰρ μὴ ἐπὶ τοῦ E μέμνηται, ἐπὶ τοῦ E Θ ἐμνήσθη· ἐντεῦθεν γὰρ ἐπ' ἄμφω κινηθῆναι ἐνδέχεται, καὶ ἐπὶ τὸ Δ καὶ ἐπὶ τὸ E. εἰ δὲ μὴ τούτων τι ἐπιζητεῖ ἐπὶ τὸ Γ ἐλθὼν μνησθήσεται, εἰ τὸ H ἢ τὸ Z ἐπιζήτει. εἰ δὲ μή, ἐπὶ τὸ A (ll. 19–23, Bek.).

Now, perhaps Aristotle only means that, after all, it is the connecting link, the intermediate term, which accounts for and must universally account for the recollection. If one does not remember by thinking of another term in the series one does so by coming to *it*. It is the proximate and universal (καθόλου, l. 18) cause of the recall of the idea in question. Hence I propose to read and translate as follows, 452 a 21 sqq.:

$$\begin{pmatrix} A\ B\ \Gamma\ \Delta\ E\ \ Z\ H\ \Theta \\ A\ B\ C\ D\ E\ F\ G\ H \end{pmatrix}$$

εἰ γὰρ μὴ ἐπὶ τοῦ E ἐμνήσθη ἐπὶ τοῦ H τὸ (τοῦ?) Θ μέμνηται· ἐντεῦθεν γὰρ ἐπ' ἄμφω κινηθῆναι ἐνδέχεται, καὶ ἐπὶ τὸ H καὶ ἐπὶ τὸ Z. εἰ δὲ μὴ τούτων τι ἐζήτει, ἐπὶ τὸ Γ ἐλθὼν μνησθήσεται, εἰ τὸ Δ ἢ τὸ E ἐπιζητεῖ· εἰ δὲ μή, ἐπὶ τὸ A· καὶ οὕτως ἀεί.

'If one has not remembered at E, at G one does remember H. The reason why one does not remember at E is that from that point one can pass to both G and F. If one does not want to remember these he will remember by going to C if he is seeking for D or E; if he is not seeking for these he goes to A. This is universally the process.'

MS. Y reads τοῦ HΘ (l. 20, Bek.). The omission of the τοῦ before Θ would easily occur. For the other changes of letter no MS. authority is available, except that the vet. tr. reads Z in l. 23 (l. 22, Bek.), a change approved by both Siebeck and Freudenthal. The other alterations are mild in comparison with those made by Freudenthal. The point is that it is the term just before the one to be recalled that you must get. There is no intention of dealing with a fixed middle term of the whole series. When Aristotle says the middle term may be considered as the ἀρχή, he means that in a way it is really πρῶτον. It is πρῶτον in the sense of being the proximate cause. Now it is anything πρῶτον in this way that is universally (καθόλου) a cause.

Hence καθόλου may be read in l. 18 and its normal meaning 'universally' given to it, if my conjecture as to the meaning of the subsequent passage is adopted. It is the intermediate link between any two terms which is universally the cause of the transference from one to the other, just as it is the proximate cause which universally produces an effect, or as it is *quâ* triangle, the middle term, that we can universally predicate equality of the angles of any figure to two right angles. Cf. *Anal. Post.* I. ch. 4, 73 b 25 sqq.

But another interpretation has been suggested to me (by Mr W. D. Ross, of Oriel College). It is proposed to adopt the following text instead of that of Bekker:

452 a 21 sqq. εἰ γὰρ μὴ ἐπὶ τοῦ Α μέμνηται ἐπὶ τοῦ Ε ἐμνήσθη· ἐντεῦθεν γὰρ ἐπ᾽ ἄμφω κινηθῆναι ἐνδέχεται, καὶ ἐπὶ τὸ Δ καὶ ἐπὶ τὸ Ζ. εἰ δὲ μὴ τούτων τι ἐζήτει, ἐπὶ τὸ Ζ ἐλθὼν μνησθήσεται, εἰ τὸ Η ἢ τὸ Θ ἐπιζητεῖ· εἰ δὲ μή, ἐπὶ τὸ Δ.

The only changes here for which there is no MS. authority are A instead of E in l. 22 (l. 20, Bek.) and Z instead of Γ in l. 24 (l. 22, Bek.), while the other variations from Bekker and Biehl follow the best MSS.

The translation will then be as follows :

'If one does not remember at A he remembers at E, for from that point he can pass in both directions—both to D and to F. But if he is not searching for one of these (D or F), by going to F he will remember, if he is looking for G or H ; while if he is not (looking for G or H, but those in the other direction—C and B) he goes to D.'

In explanation of this interpretation it is maintained that A is not included in the series of terms of which τὸ μέσον πάντων is said to be the ἀρχή (hence they form an odd number and E becomes a real middle term). A is rather a term immediately outside the group in which the idea to be recalled is contained.

Aristotle is held to be illustrating the well-known process of recall in which, when we wish to revive an idea, we pass first of all to the group of former presentations within which we must already know it to lie. E, then, will symbolize the central idea or nucleus of this group from which it is possible to pass, in more than one direction, to the idea lying in the outskirts of the group.

This interpretation is ingenious and gets rid of minor difficulties, *e.g.* it does not require that Aristotle should be held to commit himself to the statement that we can recall ideas by proceeding backwards among terms experienced in a linear series like the letters of the alphabet. Though Aristotle symbolizes his terms by the letters of the alphabet he is thinking not of a series following the direction of the time process but of a set of notions formed by those notions being frequently thought of together and grouped round one striking topic.

452 a 28. Freudenthal, in conformity with his interpretation of the above passage, proposes to read E instead of Γ (C). The associative process may go in either direction. But the meaning is quite satisfactory and does not involve the special difficulties of this contention if we keep the ms. version. Aristotle has just before said that the intermediate term is universally the ground of recollection. But it is objected that from a given term sometimes you pass to a certain other one and sometimes not. That will be true, he says, of the remoter terms in the series, for sometimes from C we pass all the way along to F, sometimes to the next member D only. Again, the particular series CDEF may become obliterated and the association branch off in some other direction that has become more familiar. Hence, though starting from C, we may not arrive at F.

452 a 28-29. ἐὰν οὖν δι' ἃ πάλαι οὐ κινηθῇ. All editors except Biehl, following L S U, read ἐὰν οὖν μὴ διὰ παλαιοῦ κινῆται and Freudenthal wishes to follow the same text with the omission of μή. All difficulties, however, vanish when we take πάλαι as 'lately,' a sense which it often bears in Aristotle (cf. Bonitz, *Ind.* p. 559 a 19: 'τὰ πάλαι λεχθέντα, οἱ πάλαι λόγοι refertur ad ea quae antea in eodem libro exposita sunt') and in other writers.

One may not have lately experienced the succession CDEF, and hence when C occurs one goes off on some more familiar route.

452 a 30. πολλάκις ἅ: L S U and all editors before Biehl read ἃ πολλάκις, especially since the explanation is based upon the frequency of the repetition; cf. 452 b 1 below: τὸ δὲ πολλάκις φύσιν ποιεῖ. But the idea of frequency or continued action is contained in the imperfect tense ἐννοοῦμεν.

452 b 1. ἐνεργείᾳ. Mr Cook Wilson (*Journal of Philol.* XI. p. 120) conjectures συνηθείᾳ; but this makes the sentence simply a repetition of ll. 29-30 above. Though Themistius reads οὕτω καὶ ἔθει, that is no guide. It is just the practice of that commentator to reduce significant statements to idle repetitions.

Every one of those who read ἐνεργείᾳ will have it that the reference is to the activity of mind and, as it is the function of intellect which is most appropriately styled an ἐνέργεια, the term may perhaps be used absolutely as referring to that without further qualification. But the meaning will not be, as some think, that the order of connection of things in nature must be reproduced in the mental process of recollecting. That would only be the case if the order of recall was always identical with the order of notions in science, which is admittedly a reproduction of the objective order. (Cf. *De Interp.* ch. 9, 19 a 33: ὁμοίως οἱ λόγοι ἀληθεῖς ὥσπερ τὰ πράγματα and *Metaph.* IX. ch. 10, 1051 b 3.) It is only the order of experience, though at times that might coincide with the scientific order, which is reproduced in association, and it is doubtful if it could be said that that takes place φύσει. The meaning would then rather be that, just as in the order of nature things succeed in a definite sequence, so it is in the functioning of thought. It is the occurrence of a particular order which is common to both.

Perhaps, however, the meaning is much wider than this. One of the MSS. (M) inserts ἢ δυνάμει after φύσει and this, which seems to be a gloss, may, however, give us a clue to an interpretation— 'Things when actually produced in a definite order do so by virtue of a natural disposition (or δύναμις) to do so. Now frequency of repetition produces this φύσις, and hence you explain the way in which we actually associate such and such ideas, since the ἔθος produced by frequent repetition is a kind of φύσις.' This φύσις might well have been called a ἕξις, as the tendency to virtuous action produced by practice is called in the *Ethics*. This ἕξις is, it must be noticed, a δύναμις, though determinate, and from φύσις you can never dissociate the idea of potentiality. Thus it can quite well be opposed to ἐνέργεια. In fact φύσις as the world of Nature is, apart from actual sensation, merely the potentiality of a sensible object, a ὑποκείμενον. Cf. *Metaph.* III. ch. 5, 1010 b 31 sqq.: τὸ μὲν οὖν μήτε τὰ αἰσθητὰ εἶναι μήτε τὰ αἰσθήματα ἴσως ἀληθές..., τὸ δὲ τὰ ὑποκείμενα μὴ εἶναι, ἃ ποιεῖ τὴν αἴσθησιν, καὶ ἄνευ αἰσθήσεως ἀδύνατον. Something must exist to cause sensation, but it is a ὑποκείμενον. Cf. also *De An.* II. ch. 5, 417 a 12 and III. ch. 2, 426 a 15 sqq. The one sense of φύσις is not totally dissevered from any of the others. It is not a homonymous term. Here in this line φύσιν is used in a way which would suggest 'natural tendency' or 'constitution' as a translation and it is used in the same connection as ἐν τοῖς φύσει and παρὰ φύσιν (452 b 2) which imply a reference to the world of Nature. Cf. Introduction, sec. IV.

452 b 2. παρὰ φύσιν. Cf. *Phys.* II. ch. 8, 198 b 35 sqq. and III. 215 a 2, etc. τὸ αὐτόματον or τύχη is the source of what we should call exceptions to the laws of Nature. Those deviations from the normal which we should ascribe to the operation of special subsidiary and counteracting laws Aristotle did not regard quite in the same light. As the action of Nature is not merely according to law, but purposive, Aristotle seems to consider these deviations from the general rule as being opposed to this purpose which aims for the best and as thwarting it. Hence the expression παρὰ φύσιν. Cf. Zeller, *Arist.* I. pp. 465 sqq. (τὸ αὐτόματον and τύχη may be distinguished, the former being specially the tendency to produce the unexpected found in *natural* phenomena). Cf. Bonitz, *ad Metaph.* XI. ch. 8, 1065 a 30.

452 b 5. ἀφέλκηται which Christ suggests, would make the reading smoother. But Aristotle continually works with an exceedingly indefinite subject, especially when discussing mental phenomena (cf. Rodier, *ad De An.* III. ch. 5, 430 a 25); it is, indeed, possible for the subject to be changed between κινηθῆναι and ἀφέλκῃ.

452 b 6. δέῃ ὄνομα : ἐπίῃ Christ : E Y have ἐπείῃ μόνον.

452 b 8. γνωρίζειν δεῖ τὸν χρόνον. This is not a special characteristic of recollection, but is common to it and memory: ch. 1, 449 b 32 *et passim*. From here up to 453 a 5 Aristotle deals with the perception of time, a common function of both activities, and thereafter he goes on once more to contrast the two.

452 b 9. τι. This is evidently the common sense or its organ, the ἔν τι τῆς ψυχῆς mentioned in *De Sensu*, 449 a 10. To perceive time is a function of the common sense: cf. above, ch. 1, 450 a 11 and notes.

452 b 10. τὰ μεγέθη. Compare the way in which the perception of time is illustrated by the perception of a spatial magnitude in *De Sensu*, ch. 7, 448 b 3 sqq.

452 b 11. ἀποτείνειν κ.τ.λ. This would be a device for effecting thought by contact. Plato suggests in the *Timaeus* that thought is effected by contact (cf. *De An.* I. ch. 3, 406 b 26 sqq. and Rodier, *ad loc.*). But thought would thus be itself a μέγεθος. Cf. *Timaeus*, 34 C sqq. and especially 37 A. Aristotle, however, does not disdain to speak of the activity of intellect as a contact with its object—which is itself. Cf. *Metaph.* XII. ch. 7, 1072 b 21: θιγγάνων καὶ νοῶν (ὁ νοῦς).

Plato, though making thought to be effected by contact, does not suggest that it issues from the body and reaches out to the things thought of, but as we see in *De Sensu*, ch. 2, he, along with Empedocles, holds this to be true of sight.

452 b 14–16. Bekker reads τίνι οὖν διοίσει, ὅταν τὰ μείζω νοῇ; ἢ ὅτι ἐκεῖνα νοεῖ, ἢ τὰ ἐλάττω; πάντα γὰρ τὰ ἐντὸς ἐλάττω, ὥσπερ ἀνάλογον καὶ τὰ ἐκτός. This is pretty nearly the traditional version of the commentators and it seems to have given rise to the interpretation descending from Themistius, which is to the effect that Aristotle is comparing the relation of external magnitudes and objective time to subjective processes by some relation between a whole and its parts. The inner processes in the subject are ἐλάττω, but so are the parts contained in a whole. Themistius takes the ἐντός as referring to the parts which are contained *in* the whole, not, apparently, as referring to ἐν αὐτῇ (sc. τῇ διανοίᾳ), l. 13. Nevertheless, τὰ ἐντὸς—the parts contained in the whole—do correspond to the subjective processes but, when they are described as ἐλάττω, that primarily characterises their relation to the whole (τὰ μείζω) and only secondarily the relation of inner process to the external reality.

The argument then is (Themistius, *Sp.* II. p. 250) that, if you know the whole, the knowledge of the part is annexed to it, but that knowledge first attaches to the parts (τὰ ἐντὸς) and then, because they are analogous to each other, and to the whole, proceeds to the whole. The relation between whole and parts is like that in the *Timaeus* between the demiurge, or rather the animal of perfect figure which is to contain all others (*Timaeus*, 33 A), and the created gods which are within it and yet like to it.

It looks as though Themistius, having consulted the *Timaeus* in connection with the passage above, has been led on by some similarities of expression in the two works (τὰ ἐντός, ὁμοιότης and the notion of figures containing one another) to introduce as a parallel something perfectly irrelevant. As Freudenthal points out, though a whole contains its parts, the parts do not contain the whole and it is impossible merely from the relation of part and whole to understand how a part can represent a whole. Among the commentators Simon and Thomas dismiss all this construction and take τὰ ἐντὸς as referring simply to the inner psychic affections which correspond to the external objects and periods of objective time.

It might seem at the first glance that τὰ ὅμοια σχήματα which reside within the soul or its organ are what corresponds to the external spatial magnitudes, the κινήσεις what answers to the periods of real time; but this distinction can hardly be maintained. All internal affections must be κινήσεις and those by which time is apprehended must themselves be spatial, *i.e.* capable of being represented by figures (cf. *De Insom.* ch. 3, 461 a 8–11). The relation of inner to outer is represented by similar triangles (cf. 18–19 below). Though Themistius employs such triangles (the one including the other) in his elucidation of the passage, the one does not, according to him, represent the psychic states, the other the external realities, but one is held to symbolize time, and its smaller parts the subjective processes apprehending time, the other the objective thing, with its parts representing the concepts by which we know the objective, and what is asserted is not merely a proportion between the inner elements of each triangle and the whole, but between the two triangles as a whole and consequently between the inner elements of each triangle. Cf. Themistius, *Sp.* 11. p. 250, l. 23: ὡς τὸ ἔλαττον πρᾶγμα πρὸς τὸ μεῖζον ἔχει, καὶ ὁ ἐλάττων χρόνος πρὸς τὸν μείζονα ὁμοίως ἔξει, καὶ ἐναλλάξ, ὡς τὸ πρᾶγμα <πρὸς> ἅπαντα τὸν χρόνον ἔχει καὶ τὰ μέρη πρὸς τὰ μέρη. (Spengel conjectures πρὸς before ἅπαντα.) But Themistius has completely missed the point, which is—how can the internal represent the external? He is continually using νόημα and πρᾶγμα as interchangeable (cf. l. 21, *loc. cit.*); but the question is—*how* is it possible to use the νόημα (in the sense of psychic process) instead of being in actual contact with the πρᾶγμα? How are they related to one another?

Freudenthal, in *Rheinisches Museum*, XXIV. p. 415, conjectures practically the identical reading which Biehl reproduces and which makes quite plain to what τὰ ἐντὸς and τὰ ἐκτός refer. We must, however, depart from Biehl to some extent and delete before ἀνά-λογον in l. 16 the ὥσπερ which obscures the sense and may have easily crept in from the subsequent line. We read καὶ with Freudenthal.

452 b 17.   St Hilaire and Hammond take εἴδεσιν to mean figures (mathematical); 'just as a figure may contain a proportionate one within it, so with distances.' But εἶδος is never used as identical with σχῆμα—figure, though σχῆμα may be regarded as an instance of εἶδος in the most general sense; and besides, since the sides of geometrical figures are ἀποστήματα, in comparing the relations of ἀποστήματα to those which exist between proportionate figures, Aristotle would only be comparing a thing with itself.

Bender translates εἴδεσιν by 'Bildern,' and this may be founded on an illustration which Simon gives when he compares the psychic states to statuettes of equal size reproducing on the small scale the lineaments and features of two different men. Simon, however, seems to agree with Thomas that ἐν αὐτῷ (ll. 17–18) refers not to the εἶδος as Bender seems to take it (—'in der Sache'—but that would rather be ἐν αὐτῷ or ἐν αὐτοῖς) but to the perceiving subject— 'in ipso cognoscente,' and he thinks that Aristotle is comparing the function of the internal quantum in representing external quantity to the function of the internal εἶδος in representing that which exists in the objective universe.   In both cases the internal is analogous to the external.   This account of the εἶδος in the soul is rather different from the usual one.   Aristotle generally says that the εἶδος of the object gets into the soul.   For example, sense is a faculty for receiving the εἶδος—the form without the matter; cf. *De An.* II. ch. 12, 424 a 18, and so of νοῦς in III. ch. 4, 429 a 15, but again in 429 a 27 the soul is said to be the τόπος εἰδῶν.   Now, if the εἶδος of the sensible object only exists actually (ἐνεργείᾳ) when it is perceived or thought of, the εἶδος in the soul will be identical both numerically and specifically with that in the object so far as the latter exists ἐνεργείᾳ, and this seems to be from one point of view the Aristotelian theory: cf. *De An.* III. ch. 2, 426 a 15 sqq., and *Metaph.* III. ch. 5, 1010 b 30; but here we seem to have the more common-sense position that the εἶδος exists realised in the external object independently of the percipient mind and that what exists in the mind is at least numerically different from the objectively existing one.   Here indeed Aristotle would seem to go so far as to suggest that the εἶδος in the mind is only *analogous* to that existing in the external world.

In this passage, then, Aristotle's purpose is to illustrate the representation of an external ἀπόστημα by an internal σχῆμα, by the function which the εἶδος of an external object communicated to the sense organs has in giving us knowledge of that object.   He refers to the latter operation as to something already agreed upon. Cf. *De Interp.* ch. 1, 16 a 6 : παθήματα τῆς ψυχῆς, καὶ ὧν ταῦτα ὁμοιώματα, πράγματα κ.τ.λ.

452 b 18. In the following lines, while I adhere to one of the emendations which Biehl adopts from Freudenthal (ΓΔ for ΑΔ in l. 19), I disagree with the latter in his interpretation of the passage. My interpretation enables us to read ΑΓ with Bekker and all other editors and MSS. instead of ΑΖ in l. 21, and I instead of M in l. 22, a lection supported by MSS. E M Y.

The figure I give in illustration of the text (for which, along with this interpretation, I am indebted to Mr W. D. Ross of Oriel College) differs from that suggested by Freudenthal as much as from the one found in Themistius ; it will be found to be simpler than either and open to fewer objections. My contention is that Aristotle's sole point is to show how external ἀποστήματα and κινήσεις may be reproduced *in parvo* in the psychical organs. His explanation is that the internal σχήματα and κινήσεις are analogous to the external ones, just as the sides of a small triangle are in the same proportions as those of one any number of times larger, obtained by producing the sides to any distance and drawing the base parallel to the base of the small one.

He accordingly draws the triangle ΑΓΔ with ΒΕ near the apex and parallel to ΓΔ. (That this is the first figure to be drawn is evident from the fact that the letters round it succeed each other in the order of the alphabet.)

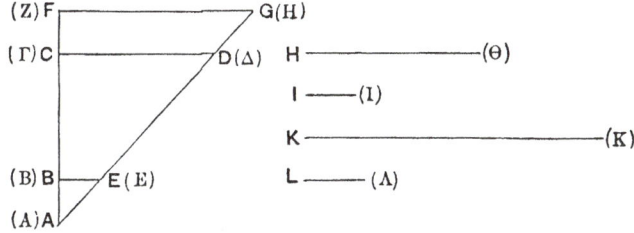

The internal σχῆμα or κίνησις then represents the external just as the sides AB, BE represent ΑΓ, ΓΔ by being proportional to them.

But the question arises, why should the internal σχῆμα or κίνησις symbolized by AB, BE represent the external ΑΓ, ΓΔ rather than ΑΖ, ΖΗ (obtained by producing ΑΓ and ΑΔ and drawing ΖΗ parallel to ΓΔ), which are equally proportional to AB, BE ?

Will not an internal σχῆμα which represents a length of six feet at a certain distance represent one of twelve feet at double the distance? Aristotle replies that this is so, but that in the two cases we are conscious of a different proportion between the external and the internal. We have some standard by which we measure *real* size. We are conscious of the *real* distance from the eye outwards of the various objects, and hence (to state the case in modern terms) we know that an affection of the retina, which may mean a size of two inches in a near object, may mean two miles in a distant one. This is what Aristotle means when he says that AΓ is to AB in the proportion of Θ to I, but AZ is to AB in the ratio of K to Λ.

This interpretation requires us to regard Θ, I, K and Λ as the names of single lines, not as referring to points at the ends of lines as Freudenthal and Themistius would have it. This usage is common in Euclid. On the other hand it is impossible that τῶν ΘI or τὰς KΛ could refer each to single lines as Freudenthal maintains; nor is there anything in the passages he quotes (*Phys.* VIII. ch. 10, 266 a 16, *Meteorol.* III. ch. 5, 6, 7, 8, 9, 11) to show that Aristotle could, by Θ or M (I) in l. 22, be referring to a single line by means of a point at one end of it, if the point at the other end is denoted by another letter. The difficulty is increased by the fact that his interpretation requires the full designation of the former line to be [M] Θ, of the latter [K] M. There is nothing to show that M was in Aristotle's original scheme; it seems to have crept into some of the MSS. from the figure of Themistius where it is found along with several other superfluous letters. For further criticisms of the figure of Themistius, cf. Freudenthal in *Rheinisches Museum, loc. cit.*

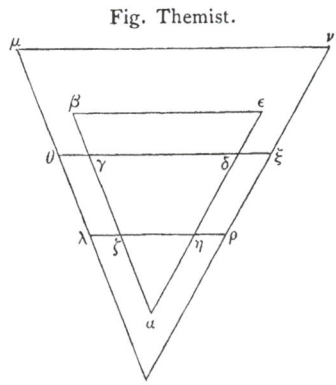

Fig. Themist.

Freudenthal's text is as follows: 452 b 18 sqq. :—ὥσπερ οὖν εἰ τὴν AB BE κινεῖται, ποιεῖ τὴν ΓΔ· ἀνά-λογον γὰρ ἡ AΓ καὶ ἡ ΓΔ. τί οὖν μᾶλλον τὴν ΓΔ ἢ τὴν ZH ποιεῖ; ἢ ὡς ἡ ΔZ πρὸς τὴν AB ἔχει, οὕτως ἡ Θ πρὸς τὴν M ἔχει. (The rest is identical with the version followed here.) He constructs two diagrams.

1. αζη and μθι are two similar triangles one inscribed in the other and both are intersected by a

line κβελ drawn parallel to θι or ζη so that μκ : κθ :: αβ : βζ.   γδ is
also drawn parallel to ζη.

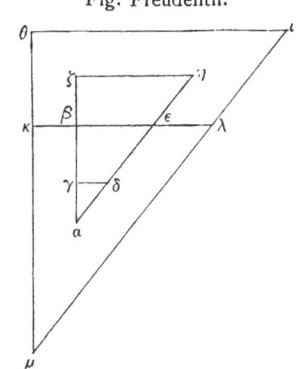

Fig. Freudenth.

Then the following result will hold :

$$\frac{a\gamma}{\gamma\delta} = \frac{a\beta}{\beta\epsilon} = \frac{a\zeta}{\zeta\eta}.$$

Also $\dfrac{a\zeta}{a\beta} = \dfrac{\theta}{\mu}$ i.e. $\dfrac{\theta\mu}{\kappa\mu}.$

Finally $\dfrac{\zeta\eta}{\beta\epsilon} = \dfrac{\theta\iota}{\kappa\lambda} = \dfrac{\zeta a}{\beta a}.$

According to Freudenthal, αβ, βε
represent inner affections; αγ, γδ concepts ; αζ, ζη are objective magnitudes,
while μκ, κλ represent our idea of time,
μθ, θι actual objective time.

This scheme is not wholly unlike that of Themistius whose outer
triangle represents time and its subjective apprehension, while the
inner one symbolizes objects and the ideas by which they are
thought.

But, as the whole point of the argument is, that the internal
σχήματα and κινήσεις, though much smaller, are still analogous to the
external magnitudes and periods of time, it is strange to find the
internal κίνησις, which is the means of apprehending time, symbolized
by lines in the external triangle.   If there is any point at all in
drawing inserted triangles to represent the relation in question, the
inner one should certainly represent the subjective and 'smaller'
process.   A series of similar triangles, the one enclosing the other,
would be a much better means of bringing out Aristotle's contention.
It would thus be shown that differences in magnitude are non-
essential ; the proportions in the sides of the smallest interior triangle
are still analogous to those of the largest exterior one.   There is no
need for Aristotle to represent objective time by different lines and
symbols from those which represent external spaces (cf. *De Sensu*,
ch. 7, quoted above), nor need the internal κίνησις be distinguished
by different letters from the internal σχῆμα.   In fact, the internal
state corresponding to both spatial and temporal magnitudes must be
a κίνησις (and perhaps it is this that Aristotle means when he says in
De An. III. ch. 1, 425 a 17–18, that we know both figure and
magnitude by means of κίνησις).   But this κίνησις can be represented
by a figure, *i.e.* it is spatially determined, it is a kind of φορά, and it

is as such that it can represent the objective magnitudes whether of time or space. What the difference is between the κίνησις which represents a magnitude which is itself a κίνησις (as in time) and that which represents a space, Aristotle does not say; he seems merely to be bent on describing everything internal in terms of κίνησις.

Again, it is difficult to believe that here Aristotle is distinguishing inner affections ('innern Affectionen,' Freudenthal in *Rheinisches Museum*, p. 417) from concepts (Begriffe). In the previous sentence (ll. 16-18) he had (by implication) distinguished the apprehension of εἴδη from that of ἀποστήματα, holding that in both cases there is something analogous in the soul which corresponds to the objective εἶδος or ἀπόστημα. Now the distinction between εἶδος and ἀπόστημα —magnitude or spatial figure generally—is quite different from that between inner affection (φάντασμα?) and concept. Further, εἶδος is not a psychological term; it could not be used to mean concept as opposed to image. Though the εἶδος of a thing means the concept or knowable character of a thing, it is used only in the epistemo-logical reference not in the psychological. The appropriate term to designate the concept as a psychical entity is νόημα not εἶδος. Com-pare the usage all through this treatise as in *De An.*, especially 432 a 12, 430 a 28. Further, even though one did take εἶδος in the sense of νόημα and held that the lines αγ, γδ represent νοήματα or εἴδη, yet, as they are not of the nature of spatial quantity, what is here said about their analogy to the objects they represent will be the merest metaphor. A concept represents the external reality by having the same λόγος, or in fact being the λόγος of the external thing (cf. *De An.* II. ch. 12, 424 a 24); but that λόγος is not a spatial proportion, neither in the external object (for that would be the Democritean theory) nor, consequently, in the soul. On the other hand the φάντασμα is spatial in character; as we saw in ch. 1, 450 a 9, not to be able to think without φαντάσματα is just the same as not being able to think ἄνευ τοῦ συνεχοῦς. (This συνέχεια, as we saw, forms the ὕλη νοητή of the concept.) Hence the analogy between the φάντασμα (or αἴσθημα which is equally a spatial κίνησις) and the objective magnitude whether temporal or not, can be ade-quately symbolized by spatial figures, *e.g.* by the identical ratios which may be found in similar triangles of diverse magnitudes, whereas the analogy between the νόημα proper and its external object must be something very different.

Hence, even though we were to keep Freudenthal's figure, we need not appropriate special lines to the symbolization of particular classes of psychical states. The point seems to be merely that within a triangle of the same apex the shorter lines may be proportional to those obtained by producing the sides.

2. Freudenthal gives another illustration with three triangles, the smaller progressively inscribed in the larger, but the alteration is not material.

The only reason for following Themistius's explanation of the passage—the alleged correspondence of the 'triangulum rei' and 'triangulum temporis'—would be the difficulty of accounting for οὖν at the beginning of the next paragraph (l. 26) by any other. 'Hence, (since the process corresponding to the time and that corresponding to the thing may themselves correspond), we may explain memory. When they occur together we remember, etc.' But the alleged correspondence of time-apprehending and object-apprehending processes does not account for the fact of remembering. It is their *coincidence* that does so. It is also difficult to see what sense there is in making out a correspondence between an object and the time in which it is apprehended or between the subjective processes produced by each. Both may be illustrated by the same lines and figures as above, but that need not imply an analogy other than generic between the two classes of processes. The οὖν does not imply that the act of memory is explained by the previous passage ; all that has been accounted for is the possibility of an internal process representing external reality, whether that be spatial magnitude or temporal process. Memory, as such, is accounted for by the coincidence merely of the two subjective processes.

(In l. 22 γάρ instead of οὖν would give a smoother sense, but the change is not necessary.)

453 a 1–2. Bekker reads οἷον ὅτι τρίτην ἡμέραν ὁδήποτε ἐποίησεν, ὅτε δὲ καὶ μέτρῳ. This gives no material difference. But Freudenthal, (*op. cit.* p. 419) pointing out that τρίτην ἡμέραν makes one think of an exact interval of time, and hence can hardly be employed as an instance of indeterminate time, wishes to read οἷον ὅτι τρίτην ἡμέραν, ὅτι μέντοι ποτὲ ἐποίησεν· ὅτι δὲ καὶ μέτρῳ. ὅτι μέντοι is read by L S Michael and vet. tr.

The change is surely not essential. I take ὅτι τρίτῃ ἡμέρᾳ ὁδήποτε ἐποίησεν to be an example of remembering μέτρῳ. Aristotle says that sometimes one does not remember the exact interval, as *e.g.* that it was an interval of three days, but at other times one does.

Freudenthal's objection against ὁδήποτε is not convincing. The indefiniteness of the subject acting need not entail any indefiniteness in the act performed.

453 a 7–8. Evidently to have recollection proper one must remember μέτρῳ.

453 a 10. γνωριζομένων. The reading of L S U γνωρίμων is perhaps a little smoother.

453 a 12. οἷον συλλογισμός τις. This would point either to Siebeck's theory or to the one I have given as to the meaning of 452 a 18 sqq. Beginning with your present thought, as it were with a minor premiss, you develop it further by a series of middle terms which finally lead to the idea you are in search of, just as your middle terms in a deduction finally bring you the ultimate predicate which is to be attached to the subject.

Here Aristotle lays emphasis on the purposive character of ἀνάμνησις. He treats it as a ζήτησις depending on will. It is evidently as such only that it is the exclusive possession of man. But ἀνάμνησις is not in all cases purposive: cf. 451 b 26, and l. 28 below.

453 a 14. βούλευσις is also a species of ζήτησις: cf. *Eth. Nic.* VI. ch. 10, 1142 a 32, and again we have in 1142 b 1: ὁ δὲ βουλευόμενος ζητεῖ καὶ λογίζεται. Cf. also III. ch. 5, 1112 b 20 sqq. It is a search for means to an end and for means which are in our power. There is another kind of ζήτησις—theoretic, such as in mathematics is a kind of ἀνάλυσις. Aristotle calls it in *Metaph.* IX. ch. 9, 1051 a 22 sqq., διαίρεσις (at least he says διαιροῦντες γὰρ εὑρίσκουσιν. This is of course not the Platonic διαίρεσις). The process involved is thus explained by Mr Burnet in *The Ethics of Aristotle*, p. xxxv. 'Figures are resolved by making actual the divisions into other figures which are there potentially. If they were already actually divided the proof would be plain; as it is, we must make a construction which is always in the long run some form of division. For instance, why are the angles of a triangle equal to two right angles? It is because the angles about one point are equal to two right angles. If the line parallel to the side were already drawn, the truth would be plain at first sight.'

This process is obviously just ἀπόδειξις—demonstration, or συλλογισμός—the finding of the middle term. Scientific analysis and demonstration are just the same thing, as is borne out by the name of the treatises on demonstration—τὰ ἀναλυτικά. Recollection is then like a syllogism in being an analysis, though a psychological one, corresponding to the logical analysis involved in scientific reasoning.

453 a 16–17. σωματικὸν τὸ πάθος. σωματικόν τι πάθος is read by L S U, the commentators and all editors other than Biehl.

ἐν τοιούτῳ. Cf. *De An.* I. ch. 4, 408 b 17 and above, note to 451 b 35, ἀρχὴν κινήσεως.

453 a 19. ἐπέχοντες. For this Christ is responsible. If we read ἐπέχοντας with the mss. and Bekker we must place a comma after ἀναμνησθῆναι and, taking the ἐπέχοντας along with ἐπιχειροῦντας, translate it 'and though they restrain their thoughts.' The vet. tr. however, though taking it along with ἐπιχειροῦντας, has 'adhibentes intellegentiam.'

453 a 20. After οὐδὲν ἧττον I understand with Simon παρενοχλεῖν. It is this which it is the purpose of the proof to maintain. So Thomas also. Themistius explains that the *search* still goes on. This is not far wrong though it is difficult to see how what is against one's will can be a ζήτησις (cf. Themistius, *Sp.* II. p. 253, l. 29). Hammond and Bender wish to have it that people remember when they are not trying and in fact trying not to. This does not suit the Greek so well and is hardly the point. Aristotle does not attempt to show the bodily nature of recollection by its occurring involuntarily (though that it does so is also implied, cf. ll. 27 sq.). In fact he has lately understood by ἀνάμνησις the voluntary recall of an idea. He wishes rather to show its corporeal connection by pointing out that it may stimulate bodily disturbances beyond the control of the will. This is the meaning of τοῦ μὴ ἐπ' αὐτοῖς εἶναι τὸ ἀναμιμνήσκεσθαι (ll. 22 sq.) and the subsequent illustration.

453 a 25. σωματικόν τι. The heart, according to everyone but Neuhäuser: cf. Introduction, sec. VI. In *De An.* I. ch. 4, 408 b 18 Aristotle talks of the κινήσεις stimulated in recollection as being in the sense organs (ἐν τοῖς αἰσθητηρίοις), but that is probably only a vaguely worded statement.

We have seen above in ch. 1, that the organ of κοινὴ αἴσθησις and φαντασία is the heart, or is situated in it. Cf. also *De Juvent.* ch. 3, 469 a 12. These κινήσεις or πάθη are φαντάσματα.

453 a 28. ἐπανέλθη L S U. Michael, Themistius, and almost all editors read ἐπέλθη, which does not give the sense of *returning* which is involved in ἐπανέλθη and seems to be required.

453 a 34. εἰσὶ δὲ κ.τ.λ. Another proof of the bodily nature of memory and recollection. Dwarfs are people with the upper parts of their bodies more developed than the lower extremities just like young children.

453 b 5–6. διὰ τὴν κίνησιν. Cf. ch. 1, 450 b 7 sqq.

APPENDIX I.

THE ARISTOTELIAN THEORY OF LIGHT.

It is difficult to reconcile Aristotle's doctrine that light is a ἕξις (cf. pp. 211–14 above) with his other statements which imply that, if not a motion, it at least has direction in space.

We must, indeed, disregard those passages (e.g. *Meteorol.* I. ch. 8, 345 b 10 and II. ch. 9, 369 b 13–14) where his use of language which has such an implication is due to the fact that some Empedoclean doctrine is under discussion ; and again in *Anal. Post.* II. ch. 11, 94 b 29 sqq., where he talks of the passage of light through the enclosing walls of a lantern, he expressly safeguards himself by saying εἴπερ φῶς γίνεται τῷ διιέναι. Once more, statements in the *Problems* (e.g. 904 b 17 : τὸ μὲν φῶς κατ' εὐθεῖαν φέρεται) may be set aside as not being of necessity genuinely Aristotelian.

Nevertheless, in *Meteorol.* III. ch. 4, 374 b 4, Aristotle speaks of rays proceeding from the sun, and the whole of his account of the phenomena of eclipse and illumination rests on the assumption that light has direction ; in *De An.* II. ch. 8, 419 b 29 sqq. he explains the diffusion of daylight by the reflection of the sun's light from the spots directly illuminated.

It is noteworthy, however, that when he talks of the formation of images in mirrors and tries to show that rainbows, haloes, etc. are due to reflection (*e.g.* in *Meteorol.* III. ch. 2, 371 b 17 sqq.) he always speaks of the reflection of *sight*, not of the reflection of light. Moreover it is evident that he was as far as his predecessors from understanding that the visibility of an object which is not self-luminous is a phenomenon of reflection.

It is precisely when he comes to explain the perception of such an object that his theory, like that of prior philosophers, breaks down. The perception of anything which is a source of light (τι πυρῶδες) is relatively a simple matter. The luminous body, by producing a ἕξις in the medium intervening between it and the eye, is enabled to act upon the organ of vision and so cause perception of itself. But the non-luminous object must also act upon the eye, if it is to be seen, and yet, not being of the nature of fire, it cannot produce a ἕξις in the medium. The fact that it is illuminated, *i.e.* endowed with the ἕξις produced in the transparent medium (which penetrates it to a greater or less extent) by the presence of a source of light, may be a prior cause of its visibility (τὸ γὰρ φῶς ποιεῖ τὸ ὁρᾶν), but does not explain how it acts upon the eye. Light can be the proximate cause of vision only in the case of a self-luminous body. We may think it strange that Aristotle, whose general doctrine of perception involved the action of all visible objects upon the eye, and who in *De Sensu*, ch. 2, 438 b 5, is content to call this a κίνησις, did not leap to the conclusion that illumination is itself due to a κίνησις which is identical with this. As things stand, his theory of the perception of bodies which are not self-luminous is left incomplete and is not reconciled with the rest of his teaching. It can only be described as an advance upon the Empedoclean doctrine, which made the act of vision a phenomenon of illumination— the illumination of an object *by the eye*, and thus took as obvious the fact most in need of explanation, namely the perception of an illuminated object.

APPENDIX II.

THE ARISTOTELIAN THEORY OF TIME-PERCEPTION

A TENTATIVE rendering of the difficult passage 452 b 8–25 (Bek. 7–22) has been suggested to me by Mr J. A. Smith and Mr W. D. Ross. The same figure is retained in illustration of the text and the explanation is of the same general type as that which I have adopted in pp. 279 sqq. But the reading in ll. 14–16 (Bek. 13–15) is altered to—τίνι οὖν διοίσει, ὅταν τὰ μείζω νοῇ, ὅτι ἐκεῖνα νοεῖ ἢ τὰ ἐλάττω; πάντα γὰρ τὰ ἐντὸς ἐλάττω, ὥσπερ ἀνάλογον καὶ τὰ ἐκτός. 'When one thinks of the greater (and more distant) objects, what is the difference between thinking of them and of the smaller (and nearer)? For all the internal (subjective) are smaller (than the external) as it were in proportion to the external (objective).'

The internal AB, BE is smaller than AΓ, ΓΔ, but preserves the same proportion as AΓ, ΓΔ, and also as AZ, ZH. What then is the difference between interpreting AB, BE as meaning AΓ, ΓΔ and interpreting it as meaning AZ, ZH? The difference lies in the power (assumed by Aristotle l. 9 above—ἔστω δέ τι ᾧ κρίνει τὸν πλείω καὶ ἐλάττω) of knowing the distance in space *or time* of the object for which our mental object stands, and knowing, therefore, by what to multiply AB and BE—whether by $\frac{\Theta}{I}$ or $\frac{K}{\Lambda}$. This tells us (to take the case of μεγέθη) whether the image in us stands for a cat at ten yards' distance or a tiger much farther away. Similarly it enables us to say whether the κίνησις in us represents an event which took ten minutes a week ago or twenty minutes a fortnight ago. When the image is multiplied by us in the same ratio as that in which its distance from us is multiplied, we think of (or recollect) the right object at the right distance of space or time. When different ratios are used we get a false thought or a false recollection.

According to this interpretation AB is the ἀπόστημα of the *image* from us, AΓ and AZ the ἀποστήματα (in space or time) of the objects from us. BE represents our subjective image or κίνησις, ΓΔ and ZH the objects (spatial or temporal) which we think of. If you wish to think of ZH rather than ΓΔ you must think of the ἀποστήματα as being different too, and multiply AB by $\dfrac{K}{\Lambda}$ not by $\dfrac{\Theta}{I}$.

The chief objection to this interpretation is that it implies that Aristotle thought of the image in the mind as existing *at a distance* from us, as though there were within us an inner spectator (the real self) whose relation to mental images merely reproduced on a small scale the relation between a percipient being and the spatial objects external to his organism. In fact we have the scholastic and Cartesian theory of the relation of the soul to the motions in the 'animal spirits.' But surely such a doctrine is definitely non-Aristotelian. Further if AΓ and AZ can be interpreted as being designed to represent distances in time of past events, AB will also (when compared with these) represent an ἀπόστημα in time. But how can a present image or κίνησις (BE) be said to be distant from us in time? It will thus be seen that there are difficulties in working out the consequences of this tempting and ingenious theory. I myself cannot believe that Aristotle meant his symbols to be anything more than a general illustration of the relation which internal κινήσεις bear to external κινήσεις and μεγέθη. The fact that motion always implies extension made it possible for the former class to symbolize both the latter.

APPENDIX III.

LIST OF PRINCIPAL AUTHORITIES REFERRED TO

Texts :

Aristotelis *Parva Naturalia*, ed. Biehl, Leipzig, 1898 (Teubner).
Bekker's *Aristotle*, Berlin, 1831.

Translations :

Barthélemy St Hilaire : *Psychologie d'Aristote*—Opuscules—Paris, 1847.
Bender : *Parva Naturalia*, Stuttgart.
Hamilton : Note D** in Reid's *Works* (Commentary on and translation of part of the *De Memoria*).
Hammond : *Aristotle's Psychology*, 1902.
Ziaja : *De Sensu* 436 a 1—439 b 18, Breslau, 1887 (Prog.).

Commentaries :

Alexander : *De Sensu*, ed. Wendland, Berlin, 1901 ; ed. Thurot, Paris, 1875.
Maynetius : *De Sensu*, Florence, 1555.
Michael Ephesius : *De Memoria* (Aldine).
Simon Simonius : *De Sensu et De Memoria*, Geneva, 1556.
Themistius : *Paraphrases Aristotelis*, ed. Spengel, Leipzig (Teubner).
Thomas Aquinas : *De Sensu et De Memoria*, Parma ed., vol. xx.

Works bearing on the Subject :

Bäumker : *Des Aristoteles Lehre von den äussern und innern Sinnesvermögen*, Paderborn, 1877.
Bonitz : *Index Aristotelicus ; Aristotelis Metaphysica*, Bonn, 1848.
Burnet : *Early Greek Philosophy*, 1892 ; *The Ethics of Aristotle*, 1900.
Bywater—in *Journal of Philology*, xviii.

Cook Wilson—in *Journal of Philology*, XI.

Freudenthal—in *Rheinisches Museum*, 1869 ; *Archiv für Geschichte der Philosophie*, 1889.

Hayduck : *Prog. Kön. Gym. zu Meldorf*, 1876–77.

Neuhäuser : *Aristoteles Lehre von dem sinnlichen Erkenntnisvermögen und seinen Organen*, Leipzig, 1878.

Rassow : *Prog. d. Joachimsth. Gym.*, 1858.

Rodier : *Traité de l'Âme*, Paris, 1900 (2 vols.).

Siebeck—in *Philologus*, 1881 ; *Untersuchungen zur Philosophie der Griechen*.

Torstrik : *De Anima*, Berlin, 1862.

Trendelenburg : *De Anima*, Berlin, 1877.

Wallace : *Aristotle's Psychology*, 1882.

Zeller : *Presocratic Philosophy* (English Translation, 1881), *Plato and the Older Academy* (E. Tr., 1876), *Aristotle and the Earlier Peripatetics* (E. Tr., 1897).

INDEX I (*Greek*).

ἀδιαίρετος 448 b 17; 449 a 12, 23, 29, 31
ἀδυνατεῖν 452 a 8
ἀέντων (Emped.) 437 b 31
ἀήρ. ὁ ἀὴρ ὑγρὸν τὴν φύσιν ἐστίν 443 b 6; 443 a 7. οὐκ ἔστιν ἀὴρ ἐν τῷ ὕδατι 443 a 5, 6
αἰθομένοιο πυρός (Emped.) 437 b 29
αἰσθάνεσθαι. οὐ κατὰ τὸ μανθάνειν ἀλλὰ κατὰ τὸ θεωρεῖν ἐστι τὸ αἰσθάνεσθαι 441 b 26. καὶ εἰ ἅπαν ἀκούει καὶ ἀκήκοε καὶ ὅλως αἰσθάνεται καὶ ᾔσθηται 446 b 3. ἑκάστου μᾶλλον ἔστιν αἰσθάνεσθαι ἁπλοῦ ὄντος ἢ κεκραμένου 447 a 19, 27. πῶς ἐνδέχεται ἅμα πλειόνων αἰσθάνεσθαι 448 b 19 sqq.; 449 a 21. αἰσθάνεσθαι ὀξέως 444 b 15. ὅτε αὐτὸς αὑτοῦ τις αἰσθάνεται 448 a 28. χρόνος ἐν ᾧ αἰσθάνεται 448 b 2
αἴσθησις. κοινὴ τῆς ψυχῆς καὶ τοῦ σώματος 436 a 9, b 7. περιτταὶ αἱ αἰσθήσεις 445 a 5. εἰ μή τις παρὰ τὰς πέντε αἰσθήσεις ἑτέρα 444 b 21. αἱ αἰσθήσεις ἀπτικαί dist. αἱ δι᾽ ἄλλου αἰσθητικαί 445 b 7, 8; 436 a 20. τῷ κινεῖσθαι τὸ μεταξὺ τῆς αἰσθήσεως ὑπὸ τοῦ αἰσθητοῦ γίνεσθαι τὴν αἴσθησιν 440 a 20, 21; cf. 438 b 5. ἡ κοινὴ αἴσθησις 450 a 12; cf. 442 b 4 sqq. ἡ αἴσθησις τοῦ παρόντος ἐστίν 449 b 14, 30. πάθη, ἕξεις αἰσθήσεως 436 b 5, 6. ἡ τῆς αἰσθήσεως ὑπεροχὴ 446 a 11
αἰσθητήριον. ἐν οἷς αἰσθητηρίοις ἐγγίγνεσθαι πέφυκεν ἡ αἴσθησις, ἔνιοι ζητοῦσι κατὰ τὰ στοιχεῖα τῶν σωμάτων 437 a 21; 438 b 20. ὅπως μὴ αἰσθητήρια δύο ποιῇ (ἡ φύσις) 444 b 5
αἰσθητικός. ἄγει (τὸ αἰσθητὸν) τὸ αἰσθητικὸν εἰς ἐνέργειαν 441 b 24. οὐκ ἐπὶ τοῦ ἐσχάτου ὄμματος ἡ ψυχὴ ἢ τῆς ψυχῆς τὸ αἰσθητικόν ἐστιν 438 b 10. θετέον καὶ ἐπὶ τῆς ψυχῆς τὸ αὐτὸ καὶ ἓν εἶναι ἀριθμῷ τὸ αἰσθητικὸν πάντων 449 a 19, 8. τὸ πρῶτον αἰσθητικόν 450 a 13, 16; 451 a 18. πολὺ βάρος ἔχειν ἐπὶ τῷ αἰσθητικῷ 453 b 2

αἰσθητός. τῶν αἰσθητῶν τῶν καθ᾽ ἕκαστον αἰσθητήριον, ...τί τὸ ἔργον αὐτῶν dist. τί ἐστι ἕκαστον αὐτῶν 439 a 7, 18. ἔστιν ἕκαστον διχῶς λεγόμενον, τὸ μὲν ἐνεργείᾳ τὸ δὲ δυνάμει 439 a 14, 15. τὸ αἰσθητὸν ἐνεργεῖν ποιεῖ τὴν αἴσθησιν 438 b 24; 445 b 7. οὔτε σώματα (τὰ αἰσθητά), ἀλλὰ πάθος καὶ κίνησίς τις, οὐδ᾽ ἄνευ σώματος 446 b 28. τὸ αἰσθητὸν πᾶν ἐστὶ μέγεθος 449 a 22; cf. 448 b 14 sqq.; 440 a 30; 445 b 10. τὰ αἰσθητὰ ἢ αἱ κινήσεις αἱ ἀπὸ τῶν αἰσθητῶν 446 a 23. τὰ παθήματα τὰ αἰσθητά 445 b 4; cf. 439 a 8. τὰ κοινὰ opp. τὰ ἴδια (αἰσθητά) 442 b 4 sqq.; 437 a 8. πᾶν τὸ αἰσθητὸν ἔχει ἐναντίωσιν 445 b 26; 442 b 19. τὰ μικρὰ πάμπαν λανθάνει· δυνάμει γὰρ ὁρατά, ἐνεργείᾳ δ᾽ οὔ 446 a 5 sqq. πάντα τὰ αἰσθητὰ ἁπτὰ ποιεῖ Δημόκριτος καὶ οἱ πλεῖστοι τῶν φυσιολόγων 442 b 1. αἰσθητός, dist. νοητός 445 b 17
αἴτιος 437 a 13
ἀκαραῖος 446 a 10
ἀκοή 437 a 10, 12. πρὸς τῇ ἀκοῇ 446 b 7
ἀκούειν 446 b 3, 18
ἄκουσις κατ᾽ ἐνέργειαν αἴσθησίς ἐστιν 439 a 17
ἀκουστός 437 a 13. τὸ ἀκουστόν 445 a 11
ἄκρατος 447 a 20
ἀκριβής 441 a 3; 442 b 16
ἀκριβῶς 444 b 10
ἄκρος 448 a 12
ἀκτίς. ἀκτίνεσσιν (Emped.) 437 b 33
ἀλλοιοῦν 447 a 1, 2
ἀλλοίωσις 446 a 31 sqq.
ἀλλοιωτικός 441 b 24
ἁλμυρός 441 b 4. τὸ ἁλμυρόν 442 a 19
ἀλουργός 440 a 1; 442 a 26
ἅλς. ἅλες γῆς τι εἶδός εἰσιν 441 b 5. ἅλες ὀσμώδεις εἰσίν 443 a 14
ἅμα. δυεῖν ἅμα αἰσθάνεσθαι 447 a 14 sqq. ἅμα κινεῖσθαι 448 b 22, 26
ἀμβλύνειν 443 b 16
ἄμικτος 445 a 23
ἀμνήμων 453 b 1, 5; 450 b 7

ἀμοργούς (Emped.) 437 b 30
ἀμφινάοντος ὕδατος (Emped.) 438 a 2
ἀνάγειν 442 b 11, 13
ἀνάγκη. ἐξ ἀνάγκης dist. ἔθει 451 b 13
ἀναθυμίασις 443 a 23 sqq. ἡ πνευματώδης ἀναθυμίασις 445 a 29. ἡ τῆς τροφῆς ἀναθυμίασις 444 a 14
(τὰ) ἄναιμα 438 a 25
ἀναίσθητος 440 a 23; 441 a 6; 448 a 27, b 4, 19
ἀνακαλύπτειν 444 b 27
ἀνάκλασις 437 b 12; 438 a 10
ἀναλαμβάνειν μνήμην 451 a 24
ἀνάληψις μνήμης 451 a 23
ἀνάλογον. ἀνάλογον εἶναι τὰς ὀσμὰς τοῖς χυμοῖς 443 b 13. ἀνάλογον τὰ ἐκτὸς τοῖς ἐντός 452 b 16 sqq.
ἀναμιμνήσκεσθαι 451 a 20 sqq.; dist. μνημονεύειν 451 b 2; 453 a 10; dist. πάλιν μανθάνειν 451 b 10
ἀνάμνησις; cf. ἀναμιμνήσκεσθαι
ἀναμνηστικός dist. μνημονικός 449 b 8; 453 a 6
ἀναπνεῖν; cf. ἀναπνοή
ἀναπνοή. γίγνεται (τὸ ὀσμᾶσθαι) διὰ τῆς ἀναπνοῆς 444 a 21 sqq.
ἀναφέρειν 444 a 24
ἄνθος 443 b 31; 444 a 36
ἀνθρακώδης 437 b 19
ἄνθραξ 444 b 33
ἄνθρωπος. πλεῖστον ἐγκέφαλον καὶ ὑγρότατον ἔχει τῶν ζῴων 444 a 33. μόνον χαίρει ταῖς τῶν ἀνθῶν ὀσμαῖς 444 a 36. ἔχει δόξαν καὶ φρόνησιν 450 a 17; cf. 453 a 11
ἄνισος 445 b 29; 447 b 1
ἀντικείμενος 448 a 10
ἀντικινεῖν 453 a 29, 31
Ἀντιφέρων ὁ Ὠρείτης 451 a 10
ἀόρατος 439 b 22; 440 a 30
ἀόριστος 439 a 29, b 4
ἄοσμος 443 a 11
ἅπαξ 451 b 15
ἀπατᾶσθαι 442 b 9
ἄπειρος opp. ὡρισμένος 440 b 26. vel πεπερασμένος 445 b 29, 3; cf. 449 a 24; 442 b 28, 29
ἀπέχειν 444 b 11; 448 a 15
ἄπηκτος 438 a 22
ἁπλοῦς 445 a 21; 447 a 20
ἁπλῶς dist. μεμιγμένως 442 a 3
ἀποδιδόναι 438 b 19
ἀποπλύνειν 443 b 8
ἀπορεῖν 438 a 11; 444 b 16; 445 b 3; 446 a 22; 450 a 27
ἀπορία 437 a 29; 446 b 29; 447 a 13; 448 b 20
ἀπόρροια 438 a 4; 440 a 17, 21; 443 b 2
ἀποσβεννύναι 437 b 15; 438 b 16
ἀπόσβεσις 437 b 17

ἀποστέγειν (Emped.) 438 a 2
ἀπόστημα 440 a 30; 449 a 24, 27; 452 b 18
ἀποτείνειν 438 a 27; 452 b 11
ἀποτέμνειν 438 b 16
ἀπόχρη 444 b 5
ἅπτειν. ἅψας (Emped.) 437 b 30
ἅπτεσθαι 442 a 5; 450 b 12
ἁπτικός. τὸ ἁπτικὸν (αἰσθητήριον) 439 a 1. αἱ ἁπτικαὶ αἰσθήσεις 445 a 7
ἁπτός. τὸ ἁπτόν 441 b 31; 445 a 13. τὸ ἁπτὸν γένος 445 a 10
ἀριθμός. ἀριθμὸς περιττός 445 a 6. κατ' ἀριθμούς sive ἐν ἀριθμοῖς 442 a 16, 18; 439 b 30, 33; 440 a 4, 6, b 21. εὐλόγιστοι ἀριθμοί 439 b 34. ἐν τῷ ἀριθμῷ 446 b 25; 447 b 26; 449 a 16 sqq.
(οἱ) ἀρχαῖοι 440 a 16
ἀρχή 451 b 35; 452 a 7, 19, 27; ἐξ ἀρχῆς 451 a 25, b 2
ἀσύμμετρος 439 b 32
ἀσφαλτώδης 444 b 35
ἄτακτος 440 a 5
ἀτμίς. ἡ τῶν ἀνθράκων ἀτμίς 444 b 33; dist. ἀναθυμίασις 443 a 28 sqq.
ἄτομος. ἐν τῷ αὐτῷ καὶ ἀτόμῳ χρόνῳ 447 a 15; cf. 448 b 22; 449 a 4. τῷ ἀτόμῳ (opp. ἑτέρῳ τῆς ψυχῆς) αἰσθάνεσθαι 448 b 24; cf. 451 a 23. τὰ ἄτομα μεγέθη 445 b 19
ἄτοπος 448 a 10; 442 b 1
αὐγή 439 b 3
αὐξάνειν 442 a 5
αὔξησις 442 a 1; 450 b 8; 453 b 6
αὐστηρός 442 a 20; 443 b 11
αὐτόσε 452 b 5
ἀφαιρεῖν 441 b 32; 441 a 13; 444 b 24, 25; 448 b 7; med. 447 a 25
ἀφανίζειν 443 b 16, 17; 447 a 22
ἀφέλκειν 452 b 5
ἁφή 436 b 14; 439 a 1; 441 a 3, 4; 442 b 8
ἀχλύς 440 a 12
ἄχυμος 441 a 6; 443 a 12

βαδίζειν 448 b 9; 445 a 30
βάθος. τὰ ἐν βάθει 440 a 15
βάρος 445 b 5; 442 a 7; 453 b 1
βαρύς opp. ὀξύς 447 b 4
βαφή coni. πλύσις 445 a 15
βηλός. κατὰ βηλόν (Emped.) 437 b 33
βιάζεσθαι 444 a 2
βλέπειν 437 b 27
βλέφαρον 444 b 26
βούλεσθαι. ἡ τοῦ ὕδατος φύσις βούλεται ἄχυμος εἶναι 441 a 4; cf. 447 b 12
βουλεύεσθαι 453 a 16

INDEX I (GREEK)　　　　　295

βουλευτικός. τὸ βουλευτικόν 453 a 15
βραδύς. μνημονικώτεροι οἱ βραδεῖς 449 b
9

γένεσις 446 b 5. ἐν τοῖς περὶ γενέσεως
442 a 4
γένος 443 b 27, 32 ; 448 a 16-20, b 29 ;
449 a 20; 445 a 10; 441 a 19
γέρων 450 b 7 ; 453 b 5
γεύεσθαι 447 a 7
γεῦσις 436 b 15; 439 a 3; 441 a 3,
b 23; 442 b 15, 17
γευστικός. τὸ γευστικόν 439 a 1
γευστός 442 a 2, b 26
γεώδης 441 b 20
γῆ. γῆς ἴδιον τὸ ξηρόν 441 b 13.
χυμοί ... ὑπάρχοντες καὶ ἐν τῇ γῇ
441 b 1. οἱ ἅλες γῆς τι εἰδός εἰσιν
441 b 5. ἡ καπνώδης ἀναθυμίασίς ἐστι
κοινὴ γῆς τε καὶ ἀέρος 443 a 26, 30.
τὸ ἀπτικὸν γῆς ἐστίν 439 a 1
γῆρας 436 a 15
γίγνεσθαι 446 b 5, 6
γλισχρότης 441 a 28
γλίχεσθαι 437 a 23
γλυκύς. ἐκ γλυκέος καὶ πικροῦ (μίξεως)
οἱ χυμοί 442 a 14. τὸ γλυκύ 442 a 3
sqq.; 448 a 17, 18; 449 a 6
γνωρίζειν 449 b 15; 453 a 5, 10
γράφειν 450 a 4, b 23; 451 a 1
γραφεύς 440 a 9
γραφή 450 b 17, 33

δεκτικός. δεκτικὸν φωτός 439 b 11.
δεκτικὸν τῆς χρόας 439 b 8. τόπος
δεκτικὸς τῆς τρόφης 445 a 26
δημιουργεῖν 442 a 5; 443 b 17
Δημόκριτος 438 a 5; 442 a 31, b 12
διαγιγνώσκειν 443 a 27
διαγράφειν 450 a 2
διαθρῶσκον (Emped.) 437 b 32; 438 a 3
διαιρεῖν. εἰς ἄπειρα (σῶμα) διαιρεῖν
445 b 3. εἰς τὰ ἐλάχιστα 440 b 5
sqq. ἡ ποδιαία...διαιρεθεῖσα 446 a 8.
διήρηται τὰ εἴδη 444 a 7 ; cf. 439 b
20
διαιρετός 449 b 13
διακρίνειν 442 b 16
διαλύειν 446 a 9
διάνοια. ἐπέχοντες τὴν διάνοιαν 453 a
19. ἔστι γὰρ ἐν αὐτῇ τὰ ὅμοια
σχήματα καὶ κινήσεις (τοῖς ἐκτός)
452 b 11
διασκιδνᾶσιν (Emped.) 437 b 31
διάστημα 446 a 3
διαφανής. τὸ διαφανὲς κοινὸν τοῦ ἀέρος
καὶ ὕδατος 438 a 14 ; 442 b 32 ; cf.
439 a 23 sqq. τὸ διαφανὲς χρώματος
ποιεῖ μετέχειν 439 b 9. διαφανές ἐστι
τὸ ἐντὸς τοῦ ὄμματος 438 b 11 sqq.

τοῦ ἐν τοῖς σώμασι διαφανοῦς τὸ ἔσχατον 439 a 30 sqq.
διαψεύδεσθαι 452 b 28
δίεσις 446 a 2
διηθεῖν 441 b 5, 20
διορίζειν 436 a 1, b 14 ; 439 a 6 ; 442 a
3 ; 443 b 21 ; 445 b 2
διστάζειν 451 a 6
δόξα 450 a 17
δοξαστόν 449 b 12
δριμὺς χυμός 442 a 20. δριμεῖα ὀσμή
443 b 10
δύναμις 437 a 6 ; coni. φύσις 439 a 25.
ἡ τοῦ θείου δύναμις 444 b 35. μίγνυν-
τες εἰς τὰ πόματα τὰς τοιαύτας δυνάμεις 444 a 2. δύναμις opp. ἐνέργεια
445 b 32 sqq.; 447 b 16 sqq.; 449 a 2.
ἡ γεῦσις ἡ κατὰ δύναμιν 441 b 23.
δυνάμει προϋπάρχον 441 b 25. ἐνεῖναι
δυνάμει 452 a 12
δυσανάπνευστος 443 b 13
δυσκατάποτος 443 b 13
δυσχεραίνειν 444 b 31
δυσώδης 444 b 31; 445 a 3
δυσωδία 445 a 2

ἐγκέφαλος 438 b 27, 31; 444 a 11,
33
ἐγρήγορσις 436 a 14
ἔγχυμος 442 b 31; 443 a 2, 17
ἐδώδη 445 a 4
ἐθέλειν 445 a 23; cf. βούλεσθαι
ἐθίζειν 451 b 17
ἔθος. ὥσπερ φύσις τὸ ἔθος 452 a 30.
ἔθει dist. ἐξ ἀνάγκης 451 b 15. δι᾽
ἔθος dist. φύσει 452 b 3
εἶδος = forma 452 b 17; dist. γένος 449 a
21, 5 ; 448 b 28, 31. εἴδη = species;
442 a 22, 23; 445 b 23 ; 439 b 20;
444 a 7. εἴδη = varietates 443 b 19.
εἴδει διαφέρειν 448 a 19. εἴδει ἕν,
447 b 16, 28. εἴδει ἕτερον 449 a 21
εἴδωλον 438 a 13
εἰκών 450 b 24, 26, 33 ; 451 a 15, 17
εἶναι. τὸ εἶναι = notio 449 a 18, 20;
cf. τῷ ἐνεῖναι vel εἶναι 446 b 30,
pp. 211, 212
εἰπεῖν. ὡς εἰπεῖν 444 a 35, 21; 441 a
19
εἴργειν. ἐεργμένον (Emped.) 437 b
34
εἷς. ἓν ἀριθμῷ dist. ἓν εἴδει 446 b 25 ;
447 b 16, 26, 28; 449 a 16 sqq.
εἰσαγγέλλειν 437 a 2
εἰσάπαξ 447 b 21
εἴωθα 453 a 3
ἐκκαίειν 443 a 20
ἐκκρούειν 447 a 16
ἐκλάμπειν 437 a 26
ἐκρεῖν 438 a 18

ἐκτέμνειν 438 b 14
ἔλαιον 441 a 26
ἕλκειν 441 a 15
ἐλπίς τοῦ μέλλοντός ἐστιν 449 b 30
ἐλπιστικός 449 b 13
ἐμμένειν 453 b 3
Ἐμπεδοκλῆς 437 b 12, 25; 441 a 6, 11;
    446 a 28
ἐμφαίνεσθαι 438 a 9, 12
ἔμφασις 438 a 6
ἐναντίος 441 b 10 sqq.; 442 b 22. τὰ
    ἐναντία b 25. αἱ τῶν ἐναντίων κινήσεις
    448 a 3
ἐναντιότης 441 b 16
ἐναντίωσις 442 b 20; 445 b 26
ἐναποπλύνειν 441 b 17
ἐναργής 440 a 10, b 31
ἐνεός coni. κωφός 437 a 17
ἐνέργεια; cf. δύναμις. ἐνεργείᾳ opp.
    φύσει 452 b 1. ἄνευ τῶν ἐνεργειῶν
    449 b 20
ἐνεργεῖν 446 a 24. ἐνεργεῖν τῇ μνήμῃ
    452 b 26, 30; cf. 449 b 24
ἐννοεῖν σφόδρα τι 447 a 18
ἐνοχλεῖν 453 a 26
ἐνσημαίνεσθαι 450 a 33
ἐξαπατᾶν 449 b 11
ἐξιέναι. ἐξιόντος τοῦ φωτός 437 a 26;
    cf. 438 a 26 sqq.
ἐξικμάζειν 441 a 16; 442 a 31; 443 a
    15
ἕξις. ἕξεις (τῆς αἰσθήσεως) 436 b 6.
    φαντάσματος ἕξις 451 a 17; 450 a 32;
    451 b 5. τὴν ἕξιν τὴν περὶ τὸν ἐγκέ-
    φαλον 444 a 10. ἕξις ἢ πάθος 449 b
    27; 451 a 30. ἡ ἕξις καὶ τὸ πάθος
    451 a 26. τὸ πάθος, οὗ φαμὲν τὴν
    ἕξιν μνήμην εἶναι 450 a 32
ἐξίστασθαι 451 a 11
ἔοικε νομίζοντι 437 b 25. ἔοικε ἀρχῇ
    καὶ τὸ μέσον 452 a 18
ἐπαλείφειν 440 a 10
ἐπαναμιμνήσκειν 451 a 14
ἐπέκεινα opp. ἐπὶ ταδί 449 a 29
ἐπεκτείνειν 441 a 27
ἐπέρχεσθαι 450 b 31; 438 a 10; cf.
    453 a 28. ἐπελήλυθεν ἡ ὄψις 446 a 1
ἐπέχειν τὴν διάνοιαν 453 a 19
ἐπί. τὸ μὴ ἐπ' αὐτοῖς εἶναι τὸ ἀναμιμνή-
    σκεσθαι 453 a 22
ἐπιζητεῖν 452 a 18, 22, 25
ἐπικαλύπτειν 437 a 28
ἐπιπολάζειν. ἐπιπολάζει ὁ ἀήρ 443 a 5
ἐπιπόλασις (χρωμάτων) 440 b 17
ἐπιπολαστικός 442 a 13
ἐπιπολῆς 440 a 15 sqq.
ἐπίσκεψις 436 a 3
ἐπίστασθαι 451 a 31
ἐπιστήμη 449 a 1; 451 a 29, 30
ἐπιφάνεια 431 a 33

ἐπιφέρειν 447 a 16; med. 443 a 24, 27
ἐπιχεῖν (Strattis) 443 b 34
ἐπιχειρεῖν 453 a 20
(οἱ) ἐπιχειρηματικοὶ λόγοι 451 a 21
ἔργον. ἐπ' αὐτῶν τῶν ἔργων δῆλον
    438 a 18. ἔργον dist. πάρεργον 444 a
    28, 17
ἔσχατος 449 a 26, 32. τὸ ἄτομον καὶ
    ἔσχατον 451 a 28. τὰ ἔσχατα 445 b
    24, 25; 447 b 2; cf. ἐναντίος
εὖ. τοῦ εὖ ἕνεκα 437 a 1
εὐήθης 438 a 30
εὐθυπορεῖν 453 a 28, b 4
εὐλόγιστος 439 b 34
εὔλογος 445 a 18. εὐλόγως 438 b 6;
    441 b 8; 445 a 19
εὐμαθής 449 b 9
εὐμνημόνευτος 452 a 3
εὐπίλητος 438 a 16
εὐπορεῖν 437 a 22
Εὐριπίδης 443 b 33
εὐσύνοπτος 441 a 12
εὐφύλακτος 438 a 15
εὔψυκτος 444 a 13
εὐώδης 444 a 19
ἕψειν 441 a 19; (Strattis) 443 b 34

ζητεῖν 451 b 26; 452 a 24
ζήτησις. οἷον ζήτησίς τις (ἡ ἀνάμνησις)
    453 a 14, 17
ζωή 436 a 16
ζῷον. ζῷον ᾗ ζῷον 439 b 12. πάντα
    τὰ ζῷα 445 a 26. τὰ ἄλλα ζῷα
    444 a 5–445 a 4; 450 a 16 sqq.
    τὰ γνωριζόμενα ζῷα 453 a 11

ἡδονή 442 a 17; 444 a 2; 436 a 10
ἡδύς. τὸ ἡδὺ καὶ τὸ λυπηρόν 443 b 23
    sqq.; 444 a 20. τὰ ἥδιστα χρώματα
    440 a 1
ἥδυσμα 442 a 11
ἡλικία. δι' ἡλικίαν 450 b 2. μέχρι
    πόρρω τῆς ἡλικίας 453 b 8
ἥλιος 440 a 11. τὸ ἀπὸ τοῦ ἡλίου φῶς
    446 a 29. εἰς τὸν ἥλιον 441 a 14
ἠρεμεῖν 437 a 31

θάλαττα 439 b 5, 443 a 13
θαλάττιος 444 b 13
θάνατος 436 a 15
θεῖον. τὸ θεῖον καὶ τὰ ἀσφαλτώδη 444 b
    35
θερμαίνειν 441 a 30
θερμός 441 b 33. θερμὴ τὴν φύσιν (ἡ τῆς
    ὀσμῆς δύναμις) 444 a 27. τὸ θερμόν
    441 b 13; 442 a 5
θέσις. ἡ παρ' ἄλληλα θέσις 440 b 8,
    17
θεωρεῖν 450 b 20, 25; coni. ἐννοεῖν 449 b
    17

θεώρημα 450 b 27, 28
θηρεύειν 451 b 21; 453 a 24
θιγγάνειν 447 a 9
θλίβειν 437 a 25
θολός (ὁ τῆς σηπίας) 437 b 8
θρεπτικός. τὸ θρεπτικόν 436 b 19;
    443 b 24; 445 a 9, 34. τὸ θρεπτικὸν
    εἶδος τῆς ὀσμῆς 444 b 10
θώραξ 444 a 29

(ἡ) ἰατρική 436 b 1
(ὁ) ἰατρός opp. ὁ περὶ φύσεως 436 a 21
ἴσος 445 b 29; 446 b 12; 447 a 27

καθαρός 440 a 6
καθίστασθαι 453 a 30
καθόλου 452 a 18
κάλλιστα 452 a 1
καπνός. εἰ πάντα τὰ ὄντα καπνὸς
    γίγνοιτο (Herac.) 443 a 26
(ἡ) καπνώδης ἀναθυμίασις 443 a 23 sqq.
κατακαίειν 442 a 30
καταλείπειν 442 a 7
καταχρῆσθαι 444 a 27
καττίτερος 443 a 21
κενός = vanus 437 b 17
κεραννύναι 447 a 20
κινεῖν 437 a 26; 440 a 26; 441 b 21.
    τὸ κινοῦν καὶ δημιουργοῦν 443 b 17.
    τὸ κινούμενον 446 a 31. τὸ πρῶτον
    κινῆσαν 446 b 23. κίνησιν κινηθήσεται
    441 b 15; cf. κίνησις
κίνησις dist. ἀλλοίωσις 446 b 31 sqq.
    ἡ μείζων κίνησις 447 a 16 sqq. ἡ διὰ
    τούτου (sc. τοῦ μεταξὺ) κίνησις 438 b 5.
    πάθος καὶ κίνησις 446 a 28. κίνησις
    καὶ χρῆσις 447 b 22. ἔστιν ἐν αὐτῇ
    (sc. τῇ διανοίᾳ)...κινήσεις 452 b 14; cf.
    451 b 12–453 b 6. ἐν κινήσει πολλῇ
    εἶναι 450 b 1
κνίψ 444 b 13
κοινός; cf. ἴδιος. τὰ κοινὰ αἰσθητά 437 a
    9; 442 b 9 sqq.
κόρη 438 a 16, b 17
Κόρισκος 450 b 34
κούρη (Emped.) 438 a 1
κοῦφος 442 a 6
κουφότης 444 a 25
κρῆναι 441 b 7
κρίνειν coni. γιγνώσκειν 445 b 16; coni.
    γνωρίζειν et νοεῖν 452 b 8 sqq. ἡ
    κρίνουσα αἴσθησις 447 b 28, 30
κριτικός 442 b 19
κρόταφος 438 b 14
κυανοῦς 442 a 26
κύκλωψ (Emped.) 438 a 1
κώδων 446 b 24
κωφός 437 a 18

λαμβάνειν 451 a 25. ἐντεῦθεν ληπτέον

437 a 33; 445 b 32; 449 b 10;
    cf. 441 b 28; 440 a 23
λάμπειν 437 a 34
λαμπέσκειν (Emped.) 447 b 33
λαμπτήρ 438 b 16; (Emped.) 437 b 30
λέγειν. λεκτέον 439 b 21; 440 b 30;
    ἐν τῇ ψυχῇ λέγειν 449 b 25; cf.
    447 b 27
λεῖος. τὰ λεῖα 437 a 34, b 7
λείπειν. λείπεται 441 a 22; 442 a 25
λεπτός. λεπτῇσιν ὀθόνῃσι (Emped.)
    438 a 1
λευκός. τὸ λευκόν 439 b 19; 442 a 13;
    447 b 26 sqq.
λῆψις dist. ἀνάληψις 451 a 23
λιβανωτός 446 b 24
λιπαρός. λιπαρὸς ὁ τοῦ γλυκέος ἐστὶ
    χυμός 442 a 18, 25
λόγος = oratio 437 a 13; 453 a 32.
    = disquisitio 445 b 21; 451 a 21.
    = argumentum 445 b 20. δῆλον διὰ
    τοῦ λόγου καὶ τοῦ λόγου χωρὶς 436 b
    9. = notio, λόγῳ ταὐτὸ 449 a 22.
    = ratio (mathematica) 439 b 29, 31;
    440 a 14, 16; 440 b 20; 448 a 10, 12
λοχάζετο (Emped.) 438 a 1
λύειν τὸν λόγον 445 b 20
λύσις 445 b 22
λύχνος 438 b 15; (Emped.) 437 b 28

μάθημα 452 a 4
μαθηματικός. σώματα μαθηματικά 445 b
    16
μανθάνειν. κατὰ τὸ μανθάνειν dist. κατὰ
    τὸ θεωρεῖν 441 b 25. μαθεῖν ἢ παθεῖν
    451 a 24. τὸ πάλιν μανθάνειν 452 a
    6; 451 b 9, 11
μαντική 449 b 14
μαρτυρεῖν 445 b 19
μέγεθος. ἔνια μεγέθη λανθάνει 446 a 17.
    πᾶν μέγεθος αἰσθητόν 445 b 10; cf.
    440 a 23, 29; 448 b 15–17. τὸ
    αἰσθητὸν πᾶν ἐστι μέγεθος 449 a 22
    sqq. μέγεθος καὶ χρόνου καὶ πράγ-
    ματος 448 b 4
(οἱ) μελαγχολικοί 453 a 21
μέλας. τὸ μέλαν 442 a 28; cf. λευκός
μελέτη 451 a 13
μέλιττα 444 b 12
(τὸ) μέλλον 449 b 11
μερίζειν 446 b 16
μέσος. τὸ τοῦ ὀφθαλμοῦ μέσον 437 b 1.
    μέση (ἡ ὄσφρησις) 445 a 7. τὸ μέσον
    πάντων 452 a 19
(τὰ) μεταλλευόμενα 443 a 18
μετασχηματίζειν 446 b 10
μετασχημάτισις 446 b 8
μετιέναι τὴν τέχνην 436 b 1
μετόπωρον 452 a 18
μῆνιγξ 438 b 2; (Emped.) 437 b 34

μῖγμα 447 b 12
μιγνύναι 440 b 5 sqq.; 444 a 1. τὰ
μεμιγμένα 440 b 19 sqq.; 447 b 12 sqq.;
cf. μίξις
μικρός 440 b 2 sqq.; 446 a 5
μικρότης 448 b 5
μίξις. χρωμάτων μίξις 440 a 31 sqq.;
442 a 13 sqq. τὰ περὶ μίξεως 440 b 4
μνήμη. περὶ μνήμης 449 b 4 sqq.; def.
449 b 26 sqq.; 451 a 14 sqq. ἐνεργεῖν
τῇ μνήμῃ 450 a 21; 452 b 27
μνημονεύειν; cf. μνήμη. τὸ μνημονεύειν
καθ᾽ αὑτό dist. κατὰ συμβεβηκός 451
b 31, 32; dist. τὸ ἀναμιμνήσκεσθαι
451 b 2 sqq.; 453 a 7 sqq.
μνημόνευμα 450 b 29; 451 a 3
μνημονευτός 449 b 10. τὰ μνημονευτὰ
καθ᾽ αὑτὰ καὶ κατὰ συμβεβηκός 450 a
26
μνημονικός. οἱ μνημονικοί dist. οἱ ἀναμνηστικοί 449 b 7; 453 a 6
(τὸ) μυριοστημόριον λανθάνει 445 b 33
μύρμηξ 444 b 12
μύρον (Strattis) 444 a 1

νανώδης 453 b 1, 7
νέος. οἱ σφόδρα νέοι 450 b 6; 453 b 5
νεότης 436 a 15
(ἡ) νήτη 447 a 21
νοεῖν 442 b 29; 451 b 21; 452 a 21.
τὰ ἐκτὸς νοεῖν 445 b 17; 452 b 10 sqq.
νοεῖν οὐκ ἔστιν ἄνευ φαντάσματος
449 b 34 sqq.
νόημα 450 b 31; 451 a 1
νοητικός. τὸ νοητικὸν μόριον 450 a 15, 18
νοητός. τὰ νοητά dist. τὰ πρακτά
437 a 3; dist. τὰ αἰσθητά 445 b 17;
450 a 14
(τὰ) νοσηματικὰ ῥεύματα 444 a 15
νοσώδης 444 a 19
νοῦς 445 b 17; cf. νοεῖν

ξανθός 442 a 24
ξηρός. τὸ ξηρόν 441 b 11 sqq.; 442 b
30 sqq.; 444 a 18
ξηρότης 443 a 2, 14, b 5
ξύλον 443 a 17

ὄγκος. ἐν τοῖς ὄγκοις 442 b 7
ὁδήποτε 453 a 2
ὀθόνη (Emped.) 438 a 1
οἰκεῖος 442 b 27; 444 b 11
ὅλος 448 b 5 sqq. ἐν τῷ ὅλῳ 446 a 20
ὄμμα 438 a 7 sqq. τὸ ἐντὸς τοῦ ὄμματος
438 b 6, 21. ἐπὶ τοῦ ἐσχάτου ὄμματος 438 b 9. τὸ λευκὸν τοῦ ὄμματος
438 a 21. οἱ πόροι τοῦ ὄμματος 438 a
15. πρὸ ὀμμάτων τίθεσθαι 450 a 5
ὅμοιος. ἀφ᾽ ὁμοίου (θηρεύειν, ἀναμιμνήσκεσθαι) 451 b 22

ὄνομα. τὰ ὀνόματα 437 a 15; 453 a 31.
ὄνομα μνημονεῦσαι 452 b 6
ὀξύς opp. ἀμβλύς 442 b 6; opp. βαρύς
447 b 4. ὀξὺς χυμός 441 b 7; 442 a
11, 21. ὀξέως αἰσθάνεσθαι 444 b 14
ὡπλίσσατο (Emped.) 437 b 28
ὁρᾶν 437 a 30 sqq.; 440 a 17. ἡ κίνησις
ἡ ποιοῦσα τὸ ὁρᾶν 438 b 5; cf. 447 a 12.
ὁρᾶν rel. ad ὁρᾶσθαι 446 b 12. ἅμα
τὸ αὐτὸ ὁρᾶν καὶ ὀσμᾶσθαι καὶ ἀκούειν
446 b 27; 448 a 25. εὐθὺς ὁρᾶν 444 b
29. οἴεσθαι τὸ ὁρᾶν εἶναι τὴν ἔμφασιν
438 a 6
ὅρασις 439 a 17
ὁρατικός. τὸ ὁρατικὸν τοῦ ὄμματος 438 b
21
ὁρατός. τὸ ὁρατόν 445 a 11
ὀργή 453 a 29
ὀρίζειν 439 b 7; 440 b 25; 450 a 3, 4
ὀσμᾶσθαι 443 a 34; 444 b 18; 445 a 12;
446 b 27
ὀσμή 438 b 26 sqq.; sed cf. 443 a 23 sqq.;
444 a 10–445 b 2. ὀσμὴ καὶ χυμός
440 b 29 sqq.; 442 b 29 sqq.; 443 b
9, 16; 447 a 8. τὸ θρεπτικὸν εἶδος
τῆς ὀσμῆς 444 b 12. αἱ τῶν ἀνθῶν
ὀσμαί 443 b 30. ἡ τῆς ὀσμῆς δύναμις
444 a 27. ἡ ὀσμὴ καὶ ὁ ψόφος 446 a
25
ὀσμώδης 443 a 15, 20
(τὰ) ὀστρακόδερμα 443 a 4
ὀσφραίνεσθαι 443 a 5; 445 a 5; 446 b
17 sqq.; cf. ὀσμᾶσθαι
ὀσφραντικός. τὸ ὀσφραντικόν 438 b 23
ὀσφραντός. τὸ ὀσφραντόν 443 a 1 sqq.
τὸ ὀσφραντὸν καὶ τὸ ἀκουστὸν κ.τ.λ.
445 a 9 sqq. τοῦ ὀσφραντοῦ τὸ αἰσθητήριον 445 a 28; cf. 444 a 31; 438 b
28. τὸ ὀσφραντὸν τὸ ἴδιον τῶν ἀνθρώπων 444 a 4 sqq.
ὄσφρησις; cf. ὀσφραίνεσθαι et ὀσμή
ὅτι pleonastice positum. ὡς...ὅτι 443 a
26
ὀφθαλμός; cf. ὄμμα. τοῦ ὀφθαλμοῦ τὸ
καλούμενον μέλαν καὶ μέσον 437 b 1
ὄψις 437 a 24 sqq.; cf. 437 a 4. τὸ
ἐξιόντι τινὶ τὴν ὄψιν ὁρᾶν 438 a 27;
452 b 12. ἀφικνεῖσθαι τὸ φῶς πρὸς
τὴν ὄψιν 446 a 30

πάγος 437 b 23
παθήματα 445 b 4
πάθος dist. ἕξις 436 b 5; 449 b 28; dist.
στέρησις 441 b 27; coni. ἕξις 451 a
26, 30. πάθος τῆς κοινῆς αἰσθήσεως
450 a 12; cf. 450 a 1, 28, 33, b 5;
437 a 25. τὸ πάθος τῆς θεωρίας ταύτης
450 b 34; cf. 453 a 17 sqq.; 440 b 30.
διὰ πάθος 450 b 1. διὰ τὸ πάθος
445 a 1. πάθη = τὰ παθήματα τὰ

αἰσθητά 445 b 13; 446 a 17; 449 a
17; 445 a 10
πανσπερμία 441 a 7, 20
παρακαλεῖν πρὸς τὴν τροφήν 443 b 32
παρασκευάζειν 441 b 21
παρεικάζειν 445 a 14
παρενοχλεῖν 453 a 18
πάρεργον 444 a 29
πάροδος 444 a 30
παρόμοιος 452 b 6
παρουσία 439 a 22
πᾶς. τὸ διὰ πασῶν 447 a 22. πάντῃ
πάντως 440 b 3
πάσχειν ὑπὸ τοῦ ἐναντίου 441 b 10, 15
πάχος ἔχειν 441 a 32
παχύνειν 441 a 30
περαίνειν 445 b 25. πεπερασμένα εἴδη,
μεγέθη 445 b 30; 446 a 20
πέρας (τοῦ σώματος) 439 a 32 sqq.
(τὸ) περιέχον 439 b 6; 446 a 9
περικάρπιον 441 a 14, 16, b 1
περιττός 445 a 7; 448 a 15
περίττωμα 445 a 21
περιφερής 442 b 23
πῇ 452 b 5
πηγνύναι 447 a 3, 4
πῆξις 443 b 15, 18
πικρός 442 a 7, 15, 19, 29
πίναξ 450 b 23
πληροῦν 443 b 25
πλήττειν 438 b 13
πλυντικός 443 a 1
πλύσις 445 a 16
πνεῦμα = ἀήρ 443 b 4; = κινούμενος ἀήρ
437 b 31; 444 b 23
πνευματώδης 445 a 29
ποδιαῖος. ἡ ποδιαία 446 a 7
ποιεῖν τὴν ΓΔ 452 b 19, 20. οἱ τὰ ἄτομα
ποιοῦντες μεγέθη 445 b 19; cf. 437 a
24
ποιόν τι τὸ ὑγρὸν παρασκευάζειν 441 b
21
πολύγωνος 442 b 22
πόμα 444 a 1
πορεύεσθαι (τὸ ὕδωρ) 441 b 3
(τὰ) πορευτικὰ τῶν ζῴων 436 b 20
(οἱ) πόροι τοῦ ὄμματος 438 b 14
πόρρω 446 b 14; 452 b 11. τὰ πόρρω
μεμνῆσθαι 451 b 30
πόρρωθεν 440 b 18
(ἡ) πορφύρα 444 b 13
ποσόν 445 b 11. ὡρισμένος κατὰ τὸ
ποσόν 450 a 3 sqq.
πότιμος 442 a 31
πρᾶγμα. ἐπὶ τῶν πραγμάτων opp. ἐπὶ
τῆς ψυχῆς 449 a 14; cf. 450 a 28;
452 a 2, 11, b 26. πρᾶγμα καὶ χρόνος
448 b 2, 4; 452 b 26, 32
πρᾶξις = ἐνέργεια 436 a 5
πράσινος 442 a 26

προαισθάνεσθαι 436 b 22
πρόοδος (Emped.) 437 b 28
προσαισθάνεσθαι 450 a 23
προσγίγνεσθαι 446 a 16
προσφέρειν. ἡ προσφερομένη τροφή
441 b 31, 33; 442 a 2
προϋπάρχειν 441 b 25
(οἱ) Πυθαγόρειοι 439 a 33; 445 a 18
πῦρ. ἡ τοῦ πυρὸς φύσις 441 b 12 sqq.;
437 a 24 sqq.; 438 b 22 sqq.
πυροῦν. τὰ πεπυρωμένα σώματα 437 b
24
πυρροῦν 441 a 14
πυρώδης 439 a 21
πῶμα 444 b 24

ῥεῖν 450 b 3, 7
ῥεῦμα 444 a 15
ῥυπτικός 443 a 2

σαπρός 443 b 12
σβεννύναι 437 b 18
σηπία 437 b 8
σκέπη 438 a 26
σκεπτέον 448 b 20; 449 b 3
σκέψις 442 b 27
σκληρόδερμος 438 a 25
σκληρόφθαλμος 444 b 28
σκοπεῖν 451 b 30
σκότος 439 a 22, b 18. ἐν σκότει 437 a
27, 34, b 6, 7
σκώπτειν 443 b 34
σολοικίζειν 452 b 7
στερεῖν 436 a 20; 439 b 17
στέρησις coni. φθορά 436 b 7; opp. παρουσία 439 a 22; opp. πάθος 441 b 28
στοιχεῖον 437 a 22; 443 a 11. τὰ περὶ
στοιχείων 441 b 14
Στράττις 443 b 34
στρυφνός 442 a 20; 443 b 11
συγκεῖσθαι 445 b 15
συζυγία 436 a 14
συλλογίζεσθαι 453 a 13
συλλογισμός 453 a 12, 16
συμβαίνειν 451 b 6; 437 b 3. ἐπὶ τῶν
συμβαινόντων (δῆλον) 438 b 13; cf.
439 b 32
συμβάλλεσθαι 443 b 32; 445 a 31
σύμβολον 437 a 15
σύμμετρος 444 a 36
συμμιγνύναι 442 a 9
συμφύεσθαι 438 a 28, 29, 30
συμφωνία 439 b 33 sqq.; 447 b 4;
448 a 22
συνάγειν 437 a 23
συναίτιος 441 a 33
συνέχεια 445 b 32
συνεχής 446 b 16; 448 b 25. τὸ συνεχές
445 b 29, 30; 450 a 9
συνήθεια 444 a 2

συνήθης 452 a 29
συνίστασθαι 438 b 31 ; 443 a 31
συνορᾶν 442 b 4
σύστοιχος 447 b 32 ; 448 a 18
συστοίχως 448 a 16
σφόδρα 447 a 17 ; 450 b 6 ; 453 a 33
σφραγίζεσθαι 450 a 34
σφραγίς 450 b 3
σχῆμα 442 b 21, 22
σῶμα 446 b 28 ; 445 b 12.   τὰ σώματα
437 a 7.   σῶμα ὡρισμένον 439 b 12
σωματικός 453 a 16, 25
σωματοῦσθαι 445 a 25
σωματώδης 445 a 24
σωτηρία 436 b 7

ταναός.   ταναώτερον πῦρ (Emped.) 437 b
32 ; 438 a 3
τάξιν ἔχειν 452 a 4
τάττειν 443 b 22 ; 444 a 5.   τεταγμένος
opp. ἄτακτος 440 a 5
ταχύς.   οἱ λίαν ταχεῖς 450 b 9
τέμνειν.   εἰς ἄπειρα τέμνεσθαι 445 b 29
(τὰ) τετράποδα 444 a 23
τέφρα 441 b 5 ; 442 a 30
τιθέναι.   ἄν τις τιθῇ τὸ φαιὸν μέλαν τι
εἶναι 442 a 23 ; cf. 443 a 7.   θετέον
449 a 18
(ὁ) Τίμαιος 437 b 13, 16
τραχύς 442 b 6
τρέφειν dist. αὔξησιν ποιεῖν 442 a 1 sqq.
τρέφεσθαι ταῖς ὀσμαῖς 443 a 19
τρίγωνον 449 b 22 ; 450 a 3
τροφή 441 b 29 sqq. ; 443 b 26 sqq. ;
445 a 20
τρόφιμος.   τὸ τρόφιμον ξηρόν 441 b 27.
τὸ τρόφιμον ὑγρόν 442 a 29.   λίαν
τρόφιμον (τὸ γλυκύ) 442 a 12 ; cf. τροφή
τυγχάνειν.   τὸ τυχὸν (φῶς) τῷ τυχόντι
οὐ συμφύεται 438 b 1
τύπος 450 a 33 ; 450 b 6, 17

ὑγίεια 436 a 18.   πρὸς βοήθειαν ὑγιείας
444 a 16 ; 445 a 32
ὑγιεινός 444 a 26
ὑγρός opp. σκληρός 450 b 10.   σβέννυσθαι
τῷ ὑγρῷ 437 b 18.   τὸ ὑγρὸν πάσχει
ὑπὸ τοῦ ἐναντίου 441 b 10 sqq. ; 442 b
30 sqq. ; 443 a 20.   ἐν ὑγρῷ εἶναι
447 a 8
ὑγρότης 444 b 2
ὑδατώδης 443 a 18, 22
ὕδωρ 438 a 17 ; 439 a 21 ; 441 a 4, 29,
b 3, 19 ; 442 b 31 ; 443 a 7, 33,
b 5, 14
ὕλη πανσπερμίας 441 a 20, 7
ὑπάρχειν.   τιθέσθαι ὡς ὑπάρχοντα 451 a
23
ὑπεροχή opp. ἔλλειψις 439 b 31 ; 440 b
22. =pars exigua 446 a 13

ὑποκεῖσθαι.   ὑποκείσθω 436 a 5 ; 447 a 19.
τὸ ὑποκείμενον dist. τὸ ἐπιπολῆς 440 a
27
ὑπολαμβάνειν.   ὑποληπτέον 438 b 21
ὑπόληψις 449 b 27

φαίνεσθαι.   φαίνεται τὸ τοῦ ὀφθαλμοῦ
μέλαν 437 b 2 ; cf. 439 b 2.   οὐ φαίνεται ὅσον (τὸ τοῦ ἡλίου μέγεθος)
448 b 15, 16
φαιός 442 a 23
φακῆ 443 b 34
φαντασία.   ἡ φαντασία τῆς χρόας 439 b
7.   περὶ φαντασίας 449 b 33 ; 450 a 25
φάντασμα.   νοεῖν οὐκ ἔστιν ἄνευ φαντάσματος 450 a 1 sqq.   θεώρημα ἢ
φάντασμα 450 b 29, 32.   θεώρημα
καὶ ἄλλου φάντασμα 450 b 28.   φαντάσματος ἕξις 451 a 17
φανταστός 450 a 26
φαῦλος.   τὰ φαῦλα coni. τὰ φθαρτικά
436 b 23.   τὰ φαῦλα opp. ὅσα τάξιν
ἔχει 452 a 4
φέρειν.   φερομένου τινὸς κίνησις 447 a
1 ; cf. 446 b 2
φθαρτικός 436 b 23 ; 444 b 32
φθείρειν 444 b 32 sqq.
φθόγγος 445 b 23 ; 446 a 2
φθορά coni. στέρησις 436 b 7
φιλόσοφος.   τῶν ἰατρῶν οἱ φιλοσοφωτέρως
τὴν τέχνην μετιόντες 436 a 21
φλόξ 437 b 20
φόβοι 453 a 29
φοινικοῦς 440 a 2, 13 ; 442 a 25
φορά 446 b 8 ; dist. ἀλλοίωσις 446 b 32
φρόνησις 437 a 1, 12 ; coni. δόξα 450 a
18.   ἡ τῶν νοητῶν φρόνησις dist. ἡ
τῶν πρακτῶν 437 a 3
φρόνιμος 437 a 16
φροντίζειν 445 a 2
φυλακή coni. σωτηρία 436 b 6
(τὰ) φυλόμενα 441 b 9 ; 445 a 3
φυσικός.   ὁ φυσικός 436 b 18
φυσιολογία.   ἡ περὶ τῶν φυτῶν φυσ.
442 b 28
(οἱ) φυσιολόγοι 442 a 32
φύσις.   τὰ περὶ φύσεως 436 b 2.   ἡ
φύσις 441 b 19 ; 444 b 4.   φύσει
dist. παρὰ φύσιν 452 a 31, b 2.   φύσις
coni. δύναμις 439 a 25.   φύσιν ποιεῖν
452 b 1.   ὥσπερ φύσις ἤδη τὸ ἔθος
452 a 29.   ἡ τοῦ ὕδατος φύσις 441 b
4 ; cf. 439 a 35 ; 441 b 12 ; 443 b
6 ; 444 a 11, 24 ; 450 a 6 ; 453 b 9
φυτόν 442 b 28
φῶς 437 a 34, b 14, 20 ; 438 a 31 sqq.
περὶ φωτός 439 a 20 sqq. ; 439 b
18 sqq. ; 446 a 28–447 a 12

χαίρειν ταῖς τῶν ἀνθῶν ὀσμαῖς 444 a 35

χαλκός 443 a 19
χειμερίην διὰ νύκτα (Emped.) 437 b 29
χρῆσις 447 b 21
χρόα sive χροία (cf. χρῶμα) 439 b 28;
  440 a 9, 17, b 17, 20, 28
χρονίζεσθαι 451 a 32
χρόνος 450 a 22. χρόνου αἴσθησις 450 b
  18; 450 a 11; 451 a 19; 452 b 8 sqq.
  ἡ τοῦ χρόνου κίνησις 452 b 27 sqq.
  μετὰ χρόνου 449 b 31, 28. διαφέρειν
  κατὰ τὸν χρόνον 453 a 8. τὰ μὴ ἐν
  χρόνῳ ὄντα 450 a 10 sqq. χρόνος
  ἀναίσθητος (οὐκ ἔστιν) 440 a 23;
  448 b 19. οἱ μεταξὺ χρόνοι (λανθάνουσιν) 448 a 26 sqq. χρόνος ἐν ᾧ
  κινεῖται τὸ κινούμενον 446 a 32
χρυσός 443 a 19
χρῶμα; cf. χρόα. περὶ χρώματος 439 a
  13 sqq. τὸ ἐνεργείᾳ χρῶμα 439 a 15.
  χρώματος μετέχειν 439 b 10; 437 a 8.
  τὰ χρώματα 439 b 20 sqq.; 442 a
  13 sqq. τὰ ἥδιστα τῶν χρωμάτων
  440 a 1. ἡ γένεσις τῶν χρωμάτων
  440 a 7 sqq. τὰ παρ' ἄλληλα τιθέμενα
  χρώματα 440 a 22, b 23. τὸ ἐπιπολῆς
  ...τὸ ὑποκείμενον χρῶμα 440 a 15, 26.
  τὰ εἴδη τῶν χρωμάτων 440 b 25; 445 b
  23 sqq.; 446 a 21
χρωματίζεσθαι 439 b 1, 2
χυμός 440 b 29 sqq. τὸ τῶν χυμῶν
  γένος 440 b 32; 441 b 9. τὰ γένη
  τῶν χυμῶν 441 a 6. οἱ χυμοί 441 a
  32; 442 a 14 sqq. τὰ εἴδη τῶν χυμῶν
  440 b 26; 445 b 23. οἱ τὴν ἡδονὴν
  ποιοῦντες χυμοί 442 a 17. ἀνάλογον
  εἶναι τὰς ὀσμὰς τοῖς χυμοῖς 443 b 9

χυτός coni. ὑγρός 445 a 16
χωρίζειν 446 a 8
χωρίς 446 a 6, b 22, 23
χωριστός 439 a 25; 446 a 12, 14;
  449 a 17

ψαθυρός 441 a 28
ψήχεσθαι 450 b 4
ψόφος 446 a 25 sqq.; 446 b 33. αἱ τοῦ
  ψόφου διαφοραί 437 a 10. τὸ τῶν
  ψόφων αἰσθητικόν 438 b 22
ψύξις 443 b 18
ψυχή. ἡ ψυχὴ αἰσθάνεται 450 b 31.
  λέγειν ἐν τῇ ψυχῇ 449 b 25. μένειν
  ἐν τῇ ψυχῇ 450 b 11. γίγνεσθαι ἐν
  τῇ ψυχῇ 450 a 30. τὰ τῆς ψυχῆς
  μόρια 436 a 1; 449 b 6; 450 a 18,
  24; 451 a 18; 453 a 17, b 11. τῆς
  ψυχῆς τὸ αἰσθητικόν 438 b 10. ἔν τι
  τῆς ψυχῆς, ᾧ ἅπαντα αἰσθάνεται 449 a
  10, 19; cf. 448 b 24 sqq. τὰ περὶ
  ψυχῆς 436 a 5, b 12, 16; 439 a 9;
  449 b 34. τὰ κοινὰ τῆς ψυχῆς ὄντα
  καὶ τοῦ σώματος 436 a 8, b 3. περὶ
  ψυχῆς καθ' αὑτὴν καὶ περὶ τῶν δυνάμεων αὐτῆς 436 a 1

ὠγύγιον πῦρ (Emped.) 437 b 34
ὡς. ἔστι μὲν ὡς τὸ αὐτὸ ἀκούει...ἔστι δ'
  ὡς οὔ 446 b 17-19. ἐκ τοῦ αὐτοῦ ὡς
  τροφῆς 441 a 22. ὡς εἰπεῖν 441 a 19;
  444 a 21. ὡς κατὰ μέγεθος 444 a 19;
  ὡς τὰ πολλά 451 b 28. ὡς ἐπὶ τὸ
  πολύ 449 b 8

INDEX II (*English*).

Alcmaeon, 134
Alexander of Aphrodisias, 121–286 *passim*
Anaxagoras, 163, 166
Apperception, 30–33
Association, 38–40, 266 sqq.
Atomists, 30, 150, 175
Atoms, 197 sqq.

Bäumker, 11, 15, 130, 235, 240
Bender, 138, 169, 209, 212, 278
Bonitz, 144, 150, 183, 187, 207, 221, 243, 273, 275
Bradley (F. H.), 270
Burnet (Professor), 128, 133, 137, 163, 182, 284
Bywater, 132, 253

Christ, 275, 285
Chromatic tones, 23, 154 sqq.
Cicero, 269
Colour, 20–23, 149–159
Cratylus, 132
Crustaceans, 139

Democritus—see Greek Index

Ear, 9, 144 sqq.
Elements, 10, 133
Empedocles—see Greek Index
Eye, 12, 142 sqq.

Faculty-Psychology, 123
Flavour, 24, 160–178
Freudenthal, 227, 244–288 *passim*

Gesner, 262
Grant (Sir A.), 186

Hamilton (Sir W.), 174, 265, 266, 269
Hammond, 137–288 *passim*
Hayduck, 144, 146, 187
Heart, 15 sqq., 147, 248
Heraclitus, 73, 182
Hume, 247
Hypotheses, 124

Insects, 139, 191

Joachim (H. H.), 158

Kant, 151, 234

Leonicus, 240, 266
Lewes, 11
Light, 20–23, 134 sqq., 150 sqq., 205 sqq., 287–288
Locke, 265

Meno, 260
Metrodorus, 166
Michael Ephesius, 258 sqq. *passim*
Mill (J. S.), 124

Nature, 168, 275
Neuhäuser, 15–20, 33, 39, 142 sqq., 171, 179, 247, 261, 285

Odour, 25–27, 179–194

Pearson (Professor Karl), 196
Phaedo, 260
Philebus, 156
Philoponus, 205
Physiology (Aristotle's), 9–20
Plato, 37, 126, 135, 137, 138, 249, 260
Poste, 124
Potentiality, 8

Quantitative character of Perception, 27–30, 194 sqq.; of Imagery, 36–38, 249 sqq.

Rassow, 206, 253, 255
Rodier, 32, 131, 161, 170, 208, 230, 241, 242, 251, 276
Ross (W. D.), 272, 279, 289

St Hilaire, 138–286 *passim*
Siebeck, 270 sqq.
Simon Simonius, 121–286 *passim*
Simonides of Ceos, 269

Simplicius, 255
Smith (J. A.), 289
Sound, 24, 206 sqq.
Spinoza, 251
Susemihl, 156, 159, 164, 168, 173, 188

Theaetetus, 37, 256
Themistius, 214–286 *passim*
Theophrastus, 133, 137, 138, 163, 174, 175, 177, 181
Thomas Aquinas, 138–286 *passim*
Thurot, 156, 164, 179, 235

Timaeus, 135, 138, 141, 173, 276
Torstrik, 179
Touch, 11, 143 sqq.
Trendelenburg, 163

Wallace (E.), 190
Wendland, 170
Wilson (Professor J. Cook), 180, 187, 189, 274

Zeller, 126, 130, 147, 163, 180, 205, 275
Ziaja, 135, 138, 144